Essential Obstetrics and Gynaecology

To my family

For Churchill Livingstone
Publisher: Peter Richardson
Editorial Co-ordination: Editorial Resources Unit
Design: Design Resources Unit
Sales Promotion Executive: Louise Johnstone

Essential Obstetrics and Gynaecology

E. Malcolm Symonds

MD FRCOG
Foundation Professor of Obstetrics and Gynaecology
University of Nottingham

Illustrated by Geoffrey Lyth BA

SECOND EDITION

CHURCHILL LIVINGSTONE
EDINBURGH LONDON MADRID MELBOURNE NEW YORK AND TOKYO 1992

CHURCHILL LIVINGSTONE
Medical Division of Longman Group UK Limited

Distributed in the United States of America by Churchill
Livingstone Inc., 650 Avenue of the Americas, New York,
N.Y. 10011, and by associated companies, branches and
representatives throughout the world.

First edition 1987
Second edition 1992
   Reprinted 1993 (twice)

ISBN 0-443-04337 X

British Library Cataloguing in Publication Data
A catalogue record for this book is available from the British
Library.

Library of Congress Cataloging in Publication Data
A catalog record for this book is available from the Library or Congress.

The
publisher's
policy is to use
**paper manufactured
from sustainable forests**

Produced by Longman Singapore Publishers (Pte) Ltd
Printed in Singapore

Preface to the second edition

There is always a considerable lag in the publication of textbooks so that by the time a second edition is needed, the original source material dates back the best part of a decade.

Whilst some subjects do not greatly change, others undergo major alteration in both scientific and social perspectives and this edition attempts to address those changes. The purpose of this textbook still adheres to the principle that undergraduate medical students have a limited time in the discipline and need a distillation of essential principles, rather than a comprehensive account of all aspects of Obstetrics and Gynaecology. In this second edition I have included a chapter on multiple pregnancy and expanded other sections such as the immunology of pregnancy and the importance of infections such as HIV in obstetrics and gynaecology.

There is always an uneasy truce between too many facts and inadequate documentation, and once again in this edition I have tried to steer a middle course. I hope it does not outrage too many specialists. It is, after all, written out of sympathy for the overburdened medical student.

I must acknowledge my gratitude to Dr Ian Symonds who has provided me with new sources of material and to Dr P. Twining and Mrs J. Swallow for supplying the new images for the section on ultrasound imaging. A series of new summary boxes has been included to promote recollection of important factual data, and in some chapters I have attempted to reinforce this process by including brief reports of actual case material.

Nottingham 1992   E.M.S

Preface to the first edition

This combined textbook of obstetrics and gynaecology presents the *essential* information required by medical students in their clinical course. At most medical schools obstetrics and gynaecology is given only 8 weeks of the clinical curriculum since there is a long-held belief that it is a postgraduate subject. Nothing, of course, could be further from the truth. Although obstetrics has become more hospital-based, gynaecology has become increasingly important in general practice, with all the problems related to fertility regulation and the increasing awareness by women of the many functional disorders of the menstrual cycle. However, the fact remains that 8 weeks is the usual allocation for undergraduate clinical training in obstetrics and gynaecology.

Therefore, this textbook has been written to provide the core of knowledge which medical students need to supplement their clinical experience and help them to master the essentials of obstetrics and gynaecology in that short 8-week period. It has been planned to bridge the gap between the vast postgraduate tomes and the very brief lists of facts in the 'pocket' books, providing students with one combined course book. I hope that it will also be of interest as an introduction to the subject for other health professionals.

As I have written each chapter, I have constantly reminded myself of a review written by an experienced paediatrician of an undergraduate textbook in which he counted 200 named syndromes. He had seen only four of these syndromes in a busy lifetime of clinical practice! I have tried to focus throughout on the common conditions encountered in clinical practice and not the small print required in an encyclopaedia text. Particular emphasis has been placed on certain chapters that form the physiological basis of obstetrical and gynaecological practice. For example, the chapters on physiological changes in pregnancy and on conception and nidation are essential platforms on which to build a knowledge of abnormal states of fertility and reproduction and therefore receive greater emphasis than many other sections.

Of course, some of the sections such as those related to the mechanisms of normal and abnormal labour remain essentially unchanged since these mechanisms were described by William Smellie and yet are still fundamental to an understanding of the management of parturition and its complications.

I owe a considerable debt to many people in compiling this textbook — first and foremost to Mr Geoffrey Lyth, who has thoughtfully designed and drawn the numerous diagrams and tables which have been planned to complement and enhance the text, and act as a series of 'aides-memoire'. The line drawings have been kept as simple as possible with a limited use of colour to emphasize particular points that are central to the narrative.

I also owe a great deal to my staff over the years who have helped in the formulation of the text. In particular, Mr G. M. Filshie and Mr R. R. Sanders played an important role in the evolution of the notes that formed the basis of many sections of this text. Dr Margaret Oates in the Department of Psychiatry, University of Nottingham, wrote the chapter on mental disorders in pregnancy. Dr Alexandra Tobert made a major contribution to the chapter on sexual disorders. I am particularly grateful for their contributions. Mr Martin Powell, Professor Brian Worthington and Mrs Josephine Swallow all provided invaluable assistance with the chapter on imaging. The book has been read and helpfully criticized by Dr Keith Louden, Dr Martin Walker and Mr Michael Martin. Dr Malcolm Lewis provided helpful information on serology and microbiology, and Dr Richard Madeley on perinatal and maternal mortality.

The text has been typed by Miss Catherine Greasley, Mrs Ann-Marie Kay, Mrs Gillian Bradshaw and Mrs Kathleen Nicholson, but the real problems of organizing and completing the text have rested in the capable hands of Mrs Sue Alvey.

Finally, I owe a great debt to Mrs Sue Symonds for patiently reading and correcting the text, and to my son, Matthew, for correcting the spelling errors!

Nottingham, 1987   E.M.S.

Contents

1. History and examination in obstetrics

INTRODUCTION

There are many features that are common to history–taking in any section of medical practice. However, there are also special areas that are central to the history in obstetrics and gynaecology, and knowledge of these factors is essential to good practice in these disciplines.

The term 'obstetrics' relates to the study and management of normal and abnormal pregnancy. The term 'gynaecology' describes the study of diseases of the female genital tract. There is a continuum between both subjects so that the division is sometimes arbitrary. Complications of early pregnancy, such as abortion, are often considered under the title of gynaecology, but more properly lie within the definition of obstetrics.

OBSTETRIC HISTORY

The relevant history in obstetrics can be considered under the present pregnancy, previous obstetric history, and previous medical and family history.

Present pregnancy

The commonest presenting symptom of pregnancy is the cessation of periods, i.e. secondary amenorrhoea, in a woman having regular menstruation. Therefore, it is important to ascertain the date of the first day of the last menstrual period. It must be remembered that this information is often inaccurate, simply because many women do not record the days on which they menstruate and, unless the date of the period is associated with some particular event, precise dates are not remembered.

The length of the menstrual cycle is also impor-

tant. Ovulation usually occurs on the 14th day before menstruation but the time interval between menstruation and ovulation – the proliferative phase of the menstrual cycle – may vary substantially. The length of the cycle always describes the time interval between the first day of the period and the first day of the subsequent period. This may vary from 21 to 42 days in normal women but menstruation usually occurs every 28 days.

It is important to ascertain the method of contraception employed prior to conception. The date of onset of the periods – the **menarche** – is recorded, although it is not particularly relevant to the obstetric history.

The **estimated date of confinement** can be calculated if one knows the date of the first day of the last menstrual period and the usual length of the menstrual cycle (Fig. 1.1). The average duration is

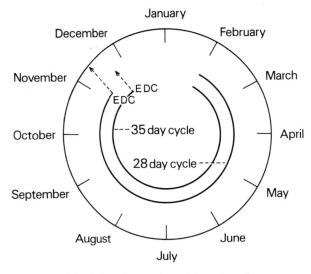

Fig. 1.1 Calculation of the estimated date of confinement (EDC)

269 days from the date of conception. In a 28-day cycle, the estimated date of confinement can be calculated by subtracting 3 months from the date of the first day of the last menstrual period and adding on 10 days. About 40% of women will deliver within 5 days of the estimated date of confinement and about two-thirds within 10 days.

If the normal menstrual cycle is less than 28 days or greater than 28 days, an appropriate number of days should be subtracted from or added to the estimated date of confinement. For example, if the normal cycle is 35 days, 7 days should be added to the estimated date of confinement. A history of taking oral contraceptive steroids may result in a delay in ovulation, particularly in the first cycle after discontinuation of the pill.

Obstetric history

- Period of amenorrhoea
- Previous obstetric history
- Condition of previous infants at birth
- Previous medical history
- Family history

Symptoms of pregnancy

In addition to the symptom of amenorrhoea, various other symptoms are common in early pregnancy.

Nausea and vomiting commonly occur within 2 weeks of missing the first period. Although described as morning sickness, vomiting may occur at any time of the day, particularly during the first 3 months of pregnancy. Thereafter, this symptom tends to disappear although it may sometimes persist throughout pregnancy.

Frequency of micturition occurs in early pregnancy and cannot be explained on the basis of pressure from the pregnant uterus as it tends to diminish after 12 weeks gestation.

Plasma osmolality falls soon after conception and the ability to excrete a water load is altered in early pregnancy. There is an increased diuretic response after water loading when the woman is sitting upright and this response declines by the third trimester. However, it may be sufficient to cause urinary frequency in early pregnancy.

Excessive lassitude is a common symptom of pregnancy and may be apparent even before the first period is missed. Again, it tends to disappear

after 12 weeks gestation but is often the most noticeable symptom experienced by many women.

Breast tenderness and *'heaviness'*, *symptoms* which are really an extension of those experienced by many women in the premenstrual phase of the cycle, are common, and are particularly apparent in the month after the first period is missed.

Fetal movements or *'quickening'* are not usually noticed until 20 weeks gestation in the woman having her first pregnancy and 18 weeks in the second or subsequent pregnancies. However, many women experience fetal movements earlier than these times and others may succeed in reaching full term without ever being aware of movements.

Occasionally, an abnormal desire for a particular food may occur and this is known as **pica**.

Symptoms of pregnancy

- Secondary amenorrhoea
- Nausea and vomiting
- Frequency of micturition
- Breast tenderness
- Lassitude

Pseudocyesis

All of these symptoms and many of the signs may develop in the absence of pregnancy, giving rise to a condition known as **pseudocyesis**.

An intense desire for or fear of pregnancy may cause stimulation of the hypothalamus and release of gonadotrophic hormones. The condition may be particularly difficult to diagnose because the physical signs of early pregnancy will often be apparent.

Biochemical confirmation that pregnancy has not occurred will usually convince the patient but subsequent sympathetic support will be necessary to resolve the anxieties associated with the condition.

Previous obstetric history

The term **gravidity** is the same as pregnancy and a gravida is a woman who is pregnant. A primigravida is a woman who is pregnant for the first time and a multigravida is a woman who has been pregnant several times (Fig. 1.2A).

This term must be distinguished from **parity**, which is a description of having given birth to an

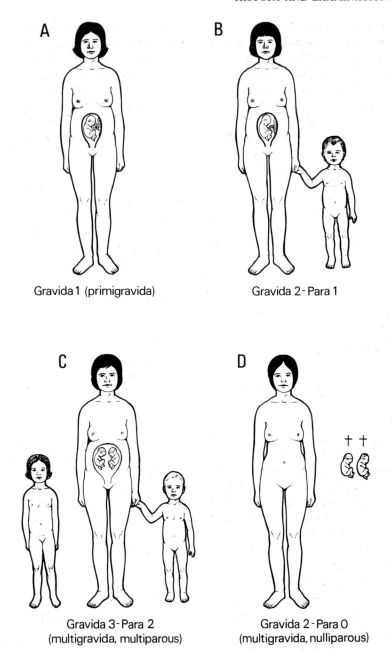

Fig. 1.2 **(A)** Gravidity refers to the number of times a woman has been pregnant; **(B)** parity refers to the number of times she has delivered potentially viable children; **(C)** an example of multigravidity and multiparity; **(D)** a multigravid but nulliparous woman who has miscarried twice.

infant, alive or dead, with a birth weight of 500 g or more (Fig. 1.2B). Thus, a primipara is a woman who has given birth to one or more infants as a result of one pregnancy. Multiple pregnancies are counted as singleton as far as the term parity is concerned. A multipara is a woman who has given birth on two or more occasions to infants weighing 500 g or more (Fig. 1.2C).

A nulliparous woman has not given birth to a viable infant (Fig. 1.2D). A grand multipara has given birth to viable infants on five or more occasions. Thus, a pregnant woman who has given birth to three viable singleton pregnancies and has had two miscarriages would be described as a gravida 6, para 3 — a multigravid multiparous woman.

A parturient is a woman in labour and a puerpera has given birth to a child during the preceding 42 days.

A record should be made of all previous pregnancies, including details of previous miscarriages and the length of gestation. In particular, it is important to note any previous antenatal complications, details of induction of labour, the length of labour, and the method of delivery. Complications of the puerperium, such as postpartum haemorrhage, infections of the genital tract and urinary system, a history of deep vein thrombosis and perineal complications may all have relevance to future pregnancies. The condition of each infant at birth and the birth weight, presentation at delivery and sex should be noted.

Previous medical history

Various medical conditions will have a significant bearing on pregnancy. Thus, it is important to note a history of diabetes, renal disease, hypertension, cardiac disease and thyrotoxicosis. Tuberculosis, syphilis and liver disease may all affect pregnancy, as may the drugs employed in the treatment of any of these conditions.

Family history

A wide variety of conditions which are genetically transmitted may have importance in the family history. In practical terms, most women will be aware of the family history of any major disorders and it is not necessary to list a catalogue of these diseases. An enquiry as to whether there are any known inherited conditions in the family will usually be sufficient, except where one or both partners are adopted and are not aware of their family histories.

Meticulous attention to the family history and past obstetric history, maternal age and medical condition may allow the precise risk of fetal abnor-

mality to be estimated, and the appropriate prenatal screening tests to be implemented.

OBSTETRIC EXAMINATION

At the initial visit a complete physical examination should be undertaken.

Height is recorded as it may provide the first indication of a small pelvis. Weight is recorded at the first and all subsequent visits.

Blood pressure is recorded with the patient supine and in the lateral supine position in late pregnancy to avoid compression of the inferior vena cava (Fig. 1.3). Apart from the effect this has on the blood pressure, the direct supine position may produce syncope and nausea in the mother, a condition which is known as the **supine hypotensive syndrome**. Blood pressure should always be recorded in the same way to give comparable measurements. Diastolic blood pressure should be taken on the fourth Korotkov sound as the point at which the sound disappears is often difficult to determine in pregnancy.

Fig. 1.3 Blood pressure recording standardized in the left lateral supine position

Head and neck

Many women develop pigmentation over the forehead and cheeks particularly when the complexion is dark and there is frequent exposure to sunlight. This is known as **chloasma** (Fig. 1.4).

Fig. 1.4   'Chloasma' — facial pigmentation over the forehead and cheeks

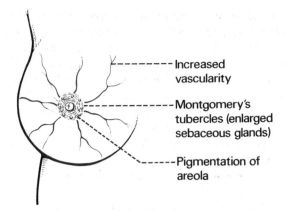

Increased vascularity

Montgomery's tubercles (enlarged sebaceous glands)

Pigmentation of areola

Fig. 1.6   Physiological changes in the breast in early pregnancy

The colour of mucosal surfaces such as those of the mouth and conjunctivae should be examined for pallor, and the general state of dentition should be noted. Pregnancy is often associated with hypertrophic gingivitis. Dental caries should be treated and appropriate advice given in dental hygiene. Some degree of thyroid enlargement is normal in pregnancy, but abnormal thyroid enlargement associated with tachycardia should arouse suspicion of hyperthyroidism.

Heart and lungs

A careful examination of the heart should be made to exclude organic murmurs. Flow murmurs are common in pregnancy and are of no significance (Fig. 1.5). Occasionally a mammary souffle may be heard arising from the internal mammary arteries, which can be confused with a systolic murmur. The sound is audible in the second intercostal space and will disappear with pressure from the stethoscope.

Breasts

The breasts show characteristic changes in pregnancy, which are apparent within the first 8 weeks (Fig. 1.6). The breasts should be examined to exclude the presence of any lumps and to note the condition of the nipples. Inverted nipples may give

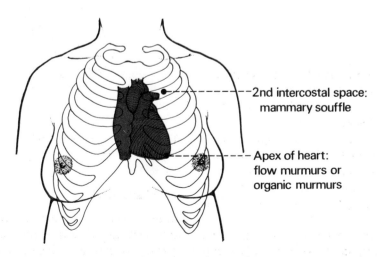

2nd intercostal space: mammary souffle

Apex of heart: flow murmurs or organic murmurs

Fig. 1.5   Flow murmurs in normal pregnancy

rise to difficulties with breast feeding and may be helped by the use of breast shields.

Abdomen

Examination of the abdomen commonly shows the presence of stretch marks or **striae gravidarum**. Marks from previous pregnancies have a silvery-white appearance, whereas recent striae are a purplish red. The striae follow the lines of stress in the skin of the abdominal wall and may also occur on the lateral aspect of the thighs and the breasts. Hepatosplenomegaly should be excluded as well as any renal enlargement. The uterus does not become palpable as an abdominal organ until after 12 weeks gestation. The linea alba often becomes pigmented and is known as the **linea nigra**. This pigmentation persists after the first pregnancy.

Limbs

The legs should be examined for evidence of varicose veins. Also, note should be made of any shortening and of any skeletal abnormalities and, in particular, of evidence of any kyphosis or lordosis (Fig. 1.7). Normal pregnancy is associated with an increase in lumbar lordosis, which frequently causes lumbar backache.

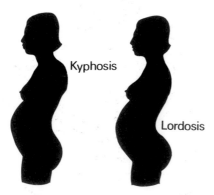

Fig. 1.7 Postural changes in pregnancy: with enlargement of the gravid uterus, there is an increased lumbar lordosis and a tendency to some degree of kyphosis

Pelvic examination

Three functions are served by pelvic examination in early pregnancy at the first attendance. The examination should confirm the presence of a pregnancy, exclude any pelvic tumours and enable a preliminary assessment of the size and shape of the bony pelvis.

Signs of pregnancy

The mother should be examined resting comfortably in the supine position with her knees drawn up and heels resting together on the examination couch.

The vulva should be examined to exclude any abnormal lesions and to assess the state of the perineum in relation to any damage sustained during previous pregnancies. Varicosities of the vulva are common and may become worse during pregnancy.

Having completed the external examination, the next important stage is the internal examination. The essential point to remember about pelvic examination is that it should be performed with the greatest gentleness. Rough and painful examination reduces the amount of information obtained as the pelvic floor and abdominal wall musculature will be tensed and the mother will lose confidence in the examiner.

Speculum examination is performed with the mother supine or in the left lateral position. If the left lateral position is employed, a Sim's speculum is used, but if the patient is examined in the supine position, a bivalve duckbill speculum is employed (Fig. 1.8). It is important to remember that the vagina runs posteriorly towards the sacrum and that the canal is widest transversely with an H-shaped cavity.

The blades of the speculum should be carefully smeared on the external surfaces with a thin layer of lubricant. The inferior blade of the speculum should be gently applied to the introitus and pressure applied towards the anus. The blades are then introduced in the line of the vagina, and when the blades are fully inserted they should be opened to expose the cervix. Remember also that the largest part of the vagina is the vaginal vault so that the speculum should not be withdrawn until the blades are closed.

The vaginal walls become more rugous as the stratified epithelium thickens with an increase in the glycogen content of the epithelial cells. There is

Fig. 1.8 Insertion of a bivalve speculum enables examination of the cervix and vaginal walls

Non-parous   Parous   Parous with tear

Fig. 1.10 Appearances of the cervical os in relation to parity

a marked increase in vascularity of the paravaginal tissues so that the appearance of the vaginal walls becomes purplish red. There is an increase in vaginal secretions associated with vaginal transudation, increased shedding of epithelial cells and some contribution from the cervical mucus.

The cervix becomes softened and shows signs of increased vascularity. Enlargement of the cervix is associated with an increase in vascularity and oedema of the connective tissues, and cellular hyperplasia and hypertrophy. The glandular content of the endocervix increases to occupy half the substance of the cervix and produces a thick plug of viscoid mucus, occluding the cervical os (Fig. 1.9).

The cervix should be examined to exclude any evidence of pathology and of previous evidence of cervical damage. The nulliparous external cervical os is circular, while the parous os is a transverse slit

and this sometimes extends into the lateral vaginal fornix where cervical damage is sustained during childbirth (Fig. 1.10). A cervical smear is taken as a routine procedure in all women and the speculum is then removed.

A digital examination is now performed. The middle finger of the examining hand should be introduced into the vaginal introitus and pressure applied towards the rectum (Fig. 1.11). As the introitus opens, the index finger is introduced as well. The cervix is palpated and feels softened.

The size and shape of the uterus is palpated bimanually. The abdominal hand compresses the uterus onto the vaginal hand. In early pregnancy the uterus feels soft and becomes globular in shape. It is palpable abdominally by 12 weeks gestation. Care is also taken to exclude uterine and ovarian tumours.

Increased vascularity

Mucus plug

Fig. 1.9 Cervical changes in pregnancy include increased glandular content and a thick mucus plug

Fig. 1.11 Bimanual examination of the pregnant uterus

Assessment of the bony pelvis

The shape and size of the bony pelvis are critical determinants in the outcome of labour. The bony

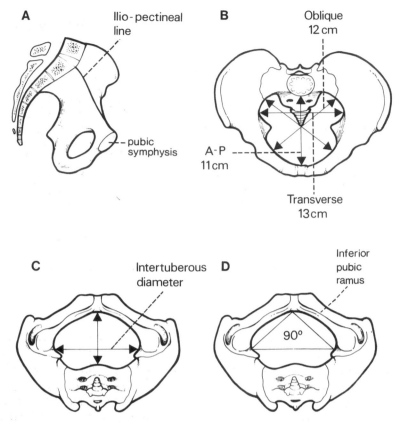

Fig. 1.12   (**A** & **B**) Inlet of the true pelvis bounded by the sacral promontory, ilio-pectineal line, pubic rami and pubic symphysis; (**C** & **D**) pelvic outlet bounded by the inferior pubic rami, the ischial tuberosities and the sacro-sciatic ligament; the inferior pubic rami should form an angle of 90°

pelvis consists of the sacrum, the coccyx and two innominate bones. The pelvic area above the iliopectineal line is known as the **false pelvis** and the area below the pelvic brim is known as the **true pelvis**. This is the important section in relation to childbearing and parturition. Thus, the wall of the true pelvis is formed from the sacrum posteriorly, the ischial bones, the sacro-sciatic notches and ligaments laterally, and anteriorly by the pubic rami, the obturator fossae and membranes, the ascending rami of the ischial bones and the pubic bones (Fig. 1.12). The shape and the dimensions of the true pelvis are best understood by consideration of the four planes of the pelvis.

The **plane of the pelvic inlet** or **pelvic brim** is bounded posteriorly by the sacral promontory, laterally by the ilio-pectineal line and anteriorly by the superior pubic rami and upper margin of the pubic symphysis. The plane is almost circular in

the normal female or gynaecoid pelvis but is slightly larger transversely than antero-posteriorly.

The true conjugate or antero-posterior diameter of the pelvic inlet is the distance between the midpoint of the sacral promontory and the superior margin of the pubic symphysis anteriorly (Fig. 1.13). The diameter measures approximately 12.75 cm. The shortest diameter, the one of greatest clinical significance, is the obstetric conjugate diameter. This is the distance between the midpoint of the sacral promontory and the nearest point on the posterior surface of the pubic symphysis. It is not possible to measure either of these diameters by clinical examination and the only diameter at the pelvic inlet that is amenable to clinical assessment is the distance from the inferior margin of the pubic symphysis to the midpoint of the sacral promontory. This is known as the diagonal conjugate diameter and is approximately 1.5 cm greater than the

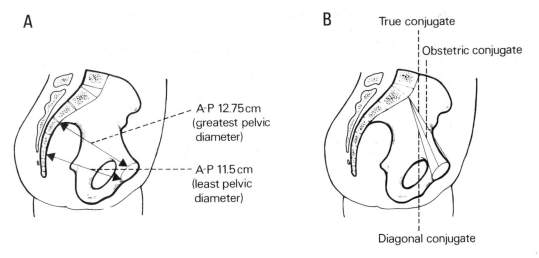

Fig. 1.13 (**A**) Antero-posterior diameters of the mid-cavity and pelvic outlet;
(**B**) conjugate diameters of the pelvic inlet

obstetric conjugate diameter. In practical terms, it is not usually possible to reach the sacral promontory on clinical examination and the highest point that can be palpated is the second or third piece of the sacrum. If the sacral promontory is easily palpable, the pelvic inlet is contracted (Fig. 1.14).

The **plane of greatest pelvic dimensions** has little clinical significance and has an anteroposterior and transverse diameter of approximately 12.75 cm. The antero-posterior diameter extends from the midpoint of the posterior aspect of the pubic symphysis to the junction of the second and third pieces of the sacrum. The transverse diameter passes laterally through the middle of the acetabuli. The only indication of the shape of the pelvis at this level is the curvature of the sacrum and the shape of the sacro-sciatic notch which should subtend an angle of 90°.

The **plane of least pelvic dimensions** represents the level at which impaction of the fetal head is most likely to occur. The antero-posterior diameter extends from the inferior margin of the pubic symphysis and transects the line drawn between

Fig. 1.14 (**A** Clinical assessment of the ischial spines and the plane of least pelvic dimensions.
(**B**) assessment of the pelvic inlet

the ischial spines or the transverse diameter of the mid pelvis. Both the transverse (interspinous) and the antero-posterior diameter can be assessed clinically, and the interspinous diameter is the narrowest space in the pelvis (10 cm). The ischial spines should be palpated to see if they are prominent and also to estimate the distance between them (Fig. 1.14A).

The **outlet of the pelvis** consists of two triangular planes. Anteriorly, the triangle is bounded by the area under the pubic arch, which should normally subtend an angle of 90°, and the transverse diameter, which is the distance between the ischial tuberosities, or intertuberous diameter (11 cm). The posterior triangle is formed anteriorly by the intertuberous diameter and postero-laterally by the tip of the sacrum and the sacro-sciatic ligaments. Clinically, the intertuberous diameter can be assessed by placing the knuckles of the clenched fist between the ischial tuberosities. The subpubic angle can be assessed by placing the index fingers of both hands along the inferior pubic rami, or by inserting two fingers of the examining hand under the pubic arch.

Obstetric examination at booking

- Height and weight
- Blood pressure
- Dentition
- Heart sounds
- Breasts/nipples
- Abdominal palpation
- Pelvic examination (smear)
- Legs
- Urinalysis

Obstetric examination at routine visits

At all antenatal visits, the blood pressure should be recorded and urine tested for glucose, protein and ketone bodies. Maternal weight should increase by an average of half a kilogram per week from 16 weeks gestation and the weight gain results from both fetal and maternal contributions. Maternal factors include contributions from breast enlargement, myometrial hypertrophy, an expansion of blood volume, retention of tissue water and deposition of fat and protein. The fetal contribution arises from the placenta and membranes, the weight of amniotic fluid and the weight of the fetus.

Rapid and excessive weight nearly always indicates abnormal fluid retention and is often associated with pitting oedema of the legs, abdominal wall and fingers. Static weight or weight loss may indicate intra-uterine fetal growth retardation.

ABDOMINAL EXAMINATION

Palpation of the uterine fundus

The estimation of gestational age is the first step in examination of the abdomen in the pregnant woman; there are several methods employed to assess the size of the fetus. The ulnar border of the left hand is placed on the uterine fundus (Fig. 1.15). The uterus first becomes palpable suprapubically at 12 weeks gestation, and by 20 weeks gestation it has reached the level of the umbilicus. At 36 weeks gestation the uterine fundus is palpable at the level of the xiphisternum and then tends to remain at this height until term, or to fall as the head enters the pelvic brim. All methods of clinical assessment of gestational age and fetal size are subject to considerable inaccuracies. The fundal height may also be described in relation to the xiphisternum.

Measurement of girth provides an alternative

Fig. 1.15 Palpation of the uterine fundus: measurement of the fundus-symphysis height is a useful method of assessing gestational age

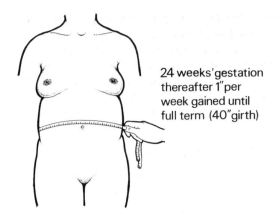

24 weeks'gestation thereafter 1"per week gained until full term (40"girth)

Fig. 1.16 Estimation of girth circumference at the level of the umbilicus

method of assessment (Fig. 1.16). Assuming that the average girth measurement in the non-pregnant state is 24 inches, no significant increase will occur until 24 weeks gestation. Thereafter, the girth should increase by 1 inch with each week of gestation so that at full term the girth will be 40 inches. If the non-pregnant girth is greater or less than 24 inches, appropriate allowance must be made. Thus, a woman with a normal 26-inch girth would have a girth measurement of 38 inches at 36 weeks.

Measurement of symphysial-fundal height

A further method of assessing gestational age is based on the measurement of symphysial-fundal height. The distance between the uterine fundus and the top of the symphysis pubis is measured in centimetres. The mean fundal height measures approximately 20 cm at 20 weeks gestation and increases to approximately 36 cm by 36 weeks gestation. Thereafter the distance tends to plateau until full term. Using two standard deviations from the mean, it is possible to describe the 10th and 90th centile values. Using this technique on a serial basis, approximately 75% of all small-for-dates infants can be detected, and the maximum accuracy detection occurs at 32 to 33 weeks gestation. It will be appreciated that accuracy is considerably less if the measurement is made after 36 weeks gestation.

The predictive value is lower for large-for-dates infants and is stated to be lowest in approximately

65% of these infants. The technique is simple and easily applicable in routine antenatal care. It is particularly useful where other more precise measurements such as those from ultrasound cephalometry are not available routinely.

Palpation of fetal parts

Fetal parts are not usually palpable before 24 weeks gestation. When palpating the fetus, it must be remembered that the presence of amniotic fluid necessitates the use of 'dipping' movements with flexion of the fingers at the metacarpo-phalangeal joints. The purpose of palpation is to describe the relationship of the fetus to the maternal trunk and pelvis (Fig. 1.17).

Fig. 1.17 Palpation of fetal parts necessitates bimanual palpation of the uterus

Lie

The term **lie** describes the relationship of the long axis of the fetus to the long axis of the uterus (Fig. 1.18). Facing the feet of the mother, the examiner's left hand is placed along the left side of the abdomen and the right hand is placed along the right lateral aspect of the uterus. Systematic palpation towards the midline will reveal either the firm resistance of the fetal back or fetal limbs.

If the lie is **longitudinal**, the head or breech will be palpable over the pelvic inlet. If the lie is **oblique**, the long axis lies at an angle of 45° to the long axis of the uterus and the presenting part will be palpable

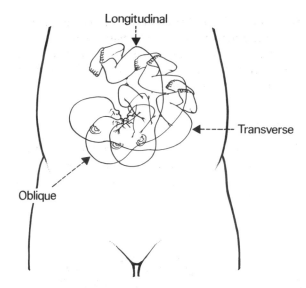

Fig. 1.18 Fetal lie describes the relationship of the long axis of the fetus to the long axis of the mother

Fig. 1.19 The normal attitude of the fetus is one of flexion

in the iliac fossa. In a **transverse** lie, the fetus lies at right angles to the mother and the poles of the fetus are palpable in the flanks.

Having ascertained the lie and the position of the fetal back, it is important now to feel for the head and breech by firm pressure with alternate hands. The head is hard, round and discreet. It can be 'bounced' between the examining hands and is described as being ballotable. The buttocks are softer and more diffuse and the breech is not ballotable. The head should be sought in the lower abdomen or in the uterine fundus. Facing the mother's feet, firm pressure is applied over the presenting part. If the head is presenting, note is made of whether it is easily palpable or whether it is necessary to apply deep pressure.

The normal attitude of the fetus is one of flexion (Fig. 1.19) but, on occasions, it may exhibit an attitude of extension.

Presentation

In a longitudinal lie, the presenting part may be the head (cephalic) or the breech (podalic). In a transverse lie, the presenting part is a shoulder.

Depending on the degree of flexion or deflexion, various parts of the head will present to the pelvic inlet. Where the head is well flexed, the presenting part is the **vertex** — the area which lies between the anterior and posterior fontanelles. If the head is completely extended, the **face** presents to the pelvic inlet (face presentation), and if it lies between these two attitudes the **brow** area presents (brow presentation). The brow is defined as the area between the base of the nose and the anterior fontanelle. The diameter of presentation for the

Fig. 1.20 Diameters of presentation of the mature fetal skull

Table 1.1 Diameters of presentation

Presenting part	Diameter	Size
Vertex	Sub-occipito-bregmatic	9.5 cm
Brow	Vertico-mental	13.5 cm
Face	Sub-mento-bregmatic	9.5 cm
Deflexed vertex	Occipito-frontal	11.7 cm

vertex is the sub-occipito-bregmatic diameter (Table 1.1, Fig. 1.20). If the head is deflexed, the occipito-frontal diameter presents. With a brow presentation, the vertico-mental diameter presents

to the pelvic inlet. Presentation and position can be accurately determined only by vaginal examination when the cervix has dilated and the suture lines and fontanelles can be palpated, and this situation pertains only in labour.

Position

Position must be differentiated from presentation as the term describes the relationship of a denominator of the presenting part to the right or left side of the maternal pelvis:

Left occipito-anterior   Left occipito-transverse   Left occipito-posterior

Right occipito-anterior   Right occipito-transverse   Right occipito-posterior

Left mento-anterior   Right mento-anterior   Right mento-posterior

Fig. 1.21 Positions of the head in vertex and face presentation

Presenting part	*Denominator*
Vertex	Occiput
Face	Chin (mentum)
Breech	Sacrum

Thus, in a vertex presentation, six different positions are described (Fig. 1.21). Viewed from below the pelvis these include right and left occipito-lateral, anterior and posterior positions. Except in advanced labour, it is very rare for a direct anterior or posterior position to be adopted. With a face presentation, the prefix **mento** is included (Fig. 1.21), and with a breech presentation the prefix is **sacro**. No such description is given to a brow presentation as it has no mechanism of labour and cannot be delivered vaginally.

The position can be determined from abdominal palpation by palpating the anterior shoulder of the fetus. If this is near the midline and easily palpable, the position is anterior. If it is not easily palpable and the limbs are prominent, it is probably posterior. The position of the presenting part can be accurately determined only by direct palpation of the suture line or the buttocks through the dilated cervix.

The degree of flexion of the head can also be determined. A deflexed head tends to feel large and the nuchal groove between the occiput and back is deep.

Station and engagement

The station of the head is also described in fifths above the pelvic brim (Fig. 1.22). Thus, a head that is only two-fifths palpable is engaged and is usually fixed in the pelvis. This is not invariably the case as a small head may be mobile when it is engaged and a large head may be fixed but not engaged.

At the simplest level, a head that is easily palpable abdominally is not engaged, whereas a head that is presenting and is deeply engaged is difficult to palpate. This can be checked by vaginal examination as the leading part of the engaged head is palpable at the level of the ischial spines.

Auscultation

Auscultation of the fetal heart is usually performed with a Pinard fetal stethoscope (Fig. 1.23). The instrument is placed over the anterior shoulder or in the midline in a posterior position and counter pressure is exerted with one hand on the opposite side of the abdomen.

Fig. 1.23 Auscultation of the fetal heart

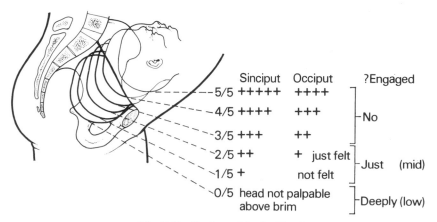

Fig. 1.22 Stations of the fetal head

With a cephalic presentation, the low frequency sound is best heard about 8 cm above the pubic symphysis, but with a breech presentation it is best heard at the level of the umbilicus. The rate and rhythm of the heart beat should be noted.

Abdominal examination of gravid uterus

- Fundal height in cm approximates to gestation in weeks after 20 weeks
- Lie
- Position
- Relation of presenting part to pelvic brim
- Auscultation of fetal heart

2. History and examination in gynaecology

Gynaecology is the study of diseases and disorders of the genital tract in women. In practice, the specialty now covers problems of reproduction in general, many of which do not fall within the realm of disease or disorder but have a social content such as therapeutic abortion, sterilization and contraception.

HISTORY

Details of name, age, marital status and occupation should always be recorded at the beginning of a consultation.

The history should be comprehensive, but not intrusive in a manner that is not relevant to the patient's problem. For example, whilst it is essential to obtain a detailed sexual history from a young couple presenting with subfertility, it would be both irrelevant and distressing to ask the same questions of an 80-year-old widow with a prolapse. The history must, therefore, be geared to the presenting symptom. It should be remembered that the presenting symptom may not always be related to the main anxiety of the patient and that some time and patience may be required to uncover the various problems that bring the patient to seek medical advice.

The patient's complaint

The patient should be asked to describe the nature of her problem, and a simple statement of the presenting symptoms should be made in the case notes. A great deal can be learnt by using the actual words employed by the patient. It is important to ascertain the time-scale of the problem and, where appropriate, the circumstances surrounding the

onset of symptoms and their relationship to the menstrual cycle. It is also important to discover the degree of disability experienced for any given symptom. In many situations, reassurance that there is no serious underlying pathology will provide sufficient 'treatment' because the actual disability may be minimal.

A social history is important with all problems but is particularly relevant where the presenting difficulties relate to abortion or sterilization. For example, a 15-year-old female requesting a termination of pregnancy may be put under substantial pressure by her parents to have an abortion and yet may not really be happy about following this course of action.

Previous medical history

A detailed history of previous serious illnesses and operations — either general or gynaecological procedures — must be recorded. This description should take particular account of any endocrine disorders and any previous episodes of pelvic inflammatory disease. Chronic lung disease and disorders of the cardiovascular system are highly relevant where any surgical procedure is likely to be necessary. It is also important, where possible, to obtain any records of previous gynaecological surgery. Many women are uncertain of the precise nature of their operations. A family history of diabetes, tuberculosis and carcinoma of the genital tract should be noted.

Menstrual history

The first question that should be asked in relation to the menstrual history is the date of the last

17

menstrual period. Omission of this one question may lead to serious errors in subsequent management.

The time of onset of the first period, **the menarche**, commonly occurs at 12 years of age and can be considered to be abnormally delayed over 16 years or abnormally early at 9 years. The term should be distinguished from the **pubarche**, which is the onset of the first signs of sexual maturation. Characteristically, the development of breasts and nipple enlargement predates the onset of menstruation by approximately 2 years.

The length of the menstrual cycle is the time between the first day of one period and the first day of the following period. Whilst there is usually an interval of 28 days, the cycle length may vary between 21 and 42 days in normal women and may only be significant where there is a change in menstrual pattern. It is important to be sure that the patient does not describe the time between the last day of one period and the first day of the next period as this may give a false impression of the frequency of menstruation. Absence of menstruation is known as **amenorrhoea** and frequent periods are known as **polymenorrhoea** or **epimenorrhoea** (Fig. 2.1). **Oligomenorrhoea** is the term used to describe infrequent menstruation.

The amount and duration of the period may change with age but may also provide a useful indication of a disease process. Normal menstruation lasts from 4 to 7 days and normal blood loss varies between 30 and 120 millilitres. A change in pattern is often more noticeable and significant than actual time and volume of loss. In practical terms, excessive menstrual loss is best assessed on the history of the number of pads or tampons used during a period and the presence or absence of clots. Excessive regular periods are described by the term **menorrhagia**, and irregular acyclic heavy bleeding is known as **metrorrhagia**. Periods that are both frequent and excessive are known as **epimenorrhagia** or **polymenorrhagia**.

The cessation of periods at the end of menstrual life is known as the **menopause**.

A history of irregular vaginal bleeding or blood loss that occurs after coitus should be noted, as should bleeding after the menopause.

Vaginal discharge is a common presenting symptom and the colour, odour and relationship to the periods should be noted. It may also be associated with vulval pruritus, particularly in the presence of specific infections.

Another common presenting symptom is abdominal pain, and the history must include details

Fig. 2.1 Normal and abnormal patterns of menstruation: the large blocks represent excessive menstrual loss

of the time of onset, the distribution and radiation of the pain, and the relationship to the periods.

The presence of an abdominal mass may be noted by the patient or may be detected during the course of a routine examination. Symptoms may also result from pressure of the mass on adjacent pelvic organs, such as the bladder and bowel.

Vaginal and uterine prolapse are associated with symptoms of a mass protruding through the vaginal introitus or difficulties with micturition and defaecation.

Urinary symptoms

Common presenting urinary symptoms include frequency of micturition, pain or dysuria, incontinence and the passage of blood in the urine, or haematuria.

The sexual history

The history should include reference to the coital frequency, the occurrence of pain during intercourse, **dyspareunia**, and functional details relating to libido, sexual satisfaction and sexual problems.

Gynaecological history

- Presenting complaint
- Previous gynaecological history and pregnancies
- Urinary symptoms
- Menstrual history
- Sexual/contraceptive history
- Medical history
- Social history
- Date of last cervical smear

A detailed obstetric history and a history of the patient's contraceptive practice, as previously described, should always be included.

THE GYNAECOLOGICAL EXAMINATION

A general examination should always be performed at the first consultation, including assessment of blood pressure and routine urine analysis. Careful note should be taken of any signs of anaemia. The distribution of facial and body hair is often important as hirsutism may be a presenting symptom of various endocrine disorders. Body weight and height should also be recorded.

Breast examination

The opportunity should always be taken to examine the breasts, both in relation to endocrine changes and for the presence of any tumours (Fig. 2.2) The breast reflects the endocrine status of the woman and the signs of pregnancy as have previously been described in Chapter 1. The presence of the secretion of milk at times not associated with pregnancy, known as **galactorrhoea**, may indicate abnormal endocrine status. Systematic palpation with the flat of the hand should be undertaken to exclude the presence of any nodules in the breast or axillae.

Examination of the abdomen

Inspection of the abdomen may reveal the presence of a mass. The distribution of body hair should be noted and the presence of scars, striae and hernias. Percussion of the abdomen may be used to outline

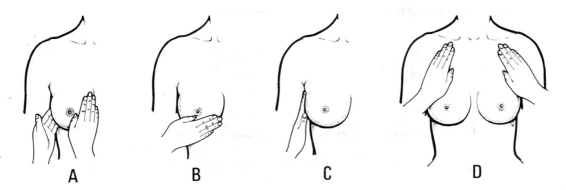

Fig. 2.2 Systematic examination of the four quadrants of the breasts

the limits of a tumour, to detect the presence of a full bladder or to recognise the presence of tympanitic loops of bowel. Free fluid in the peritoneal cavity will be recognised by the presence of dullness to percussion in the flanks and resonance over the central abdomen (Fig. 2.3).

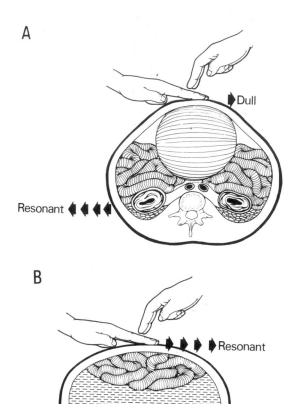

Fig. 2.3 (**A**) Percussion over a large ovarian cyst — central dullness and resonance in the flanks; (**B**) percussion in the presence of ascites — dullness in the flanks and central resonance

Palpation of the abdomen should take account of any guarding and rebound tenderness. It is important to ask the patient to outline the site and radiation of any pain in the abdomen, and palpation for enlargement of the liver, spleen and kidneys should be carried out. Auscultation of bowel sounds is important where obstruction or ileus is suspected.

Pelvic examination

The patient should be examined resting supine with knees drawn up and separated, or in stirrups in the lithotomy position. Systematic inspection of the vulva should take note of the clitoris, urethral meatus, vulval and labial skin, the fourchette and hymen, and evidence of scarring or distortion of the perineum (Fig. 2.4). The patient should be asked to cough or strain to demonstrate stress incontinence and descent of the vaginal walls. The presence of any ulceration or discharge should also be noted.

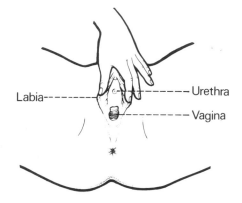

Fig. 2.4   Inspection of the external genitalia

Speculum examination

Speculum examination should be performed before digital examination to avoid any contamination with lubricant. A bivalve or Cuscoe's speculum is most commonly used and enables a clear view of the cervix to be obtained (Fig. 2.5). Where vaginal wall prolapse is suspected, a Sims' speculum should be used as it provides a clearer view of the vaginal walls.

The instrument is inserted in the direction of the vagina and the blades are opened after full insertion of the instrument. Having noted the appearance of the cervix, a cervical smear is taken with an Ayre's spatula. The spatula is gently scraped across the epithelial surface of the cervix and the smear is applied to a labelled glass slide, which is immediately placed in preservative fluid. The presence and nature of any vaginal discharge are recorded and a swab is taken for culture where appropriate.

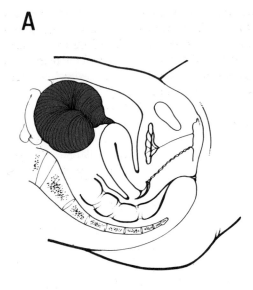

Fig. 2.5 Insertion of a Cuscoe's speculum (left) and collection of a cervical smear (right)

Fig. 2.6 Examination in the lateral semiprone position with a Sims' speculum enables inspection of the vaginal walls

Fig. 2.7 Differentiation between an adnexal mass (**A**) and a pedunculated fibroid (**B**) may be difficult.

Where the Sims' speculum is used, it is preferable to examine the patient in the semiprone or Sims' position (Fig. 2.6).

Bimanual examination is performed as previously described in the obstetric section. It must be remembered that the abdominal hand is used to compress the pelvic organs on to the examining vaginal hand.

The size, shape, consistency and position of the uterus must be noted. The uterus is commonly pre-axial or anteverted but will be postaxial or retroverted in some 10% of women. Provided the retroverted uterus is mobile, the position is rarely significant. It is important to feel in the Pouch of Douglas for the presence of thickening or nodules, and then to palpate laterally in both fornices for the presence of any ovarian or tubal masses. An attempt should be made to differentiate between adnexal and uterine masses, although this is often not possible. For example, a pedunculated fibroid may mimic an ovarian tumour, whereas a solid ovarian tumour, if adherent to the uterus, may be impossible to distinguish from a uterine fibroid (Fig. 2.7). The ovaries are usually palpable in the normal pelvis but the Fallopian tubes are only palpable if they are significantly enlarged.

In a child or in a woman with an intact hymen, it may be necessary to perform a single finger vaginal examination or a rectal examination. It should always be remembered that a rough or painful examination rarely produces any useful information and, in certain situations such as tubal ectopic pregnancy, may be dangerous.

Gynaecological examination

- Cardiovascular system
- Breast examination
- Abdominal palpation
- Pelvic examination

3. Physiological changes in pregnancy

The recognition of abnormal events in pregnancy demands a clear understanding of the normal processes of maternal adaptation. In all mammalian species, there are extensive biochemical, physiological and structural changes during pregnancy and the puerperium.

From a teleological point of view, there are two main reasons for these changes:

1. To provide a suitable environment for the nutrition, growth and development of the fetus.
2. To prepare the mother for the process of parturition and subsequent support of the newborn infant.

The changes that occur in pregnancy in order to achieve these objectives are both visible and subtle.

MATERNAL WEIGHT GAIN

Of the physical changes that occur, the most obvious are the enlargement of the abdomen and the increase in body weight. There are no reliable data available for weight gain in the first 12 weeks of pregnancy, but in normal pregnancy the average gain is 0.3 kg/week up to 18 weeks, 0.45 kg/week from 18 to 28 weeks and thereafter a slight reduction with a rate of 0.36 to 0.41 kg/week until term (Fig. 3.1). Failure to gain weight and sometimes slight weight loss may occur in the last 2 weeks. The average weight gain for primigravidae for the whole pregnancy is 12.5 kg and is probably about 0.9 kg less for multigravidae. Acute excessive weight gain is commonly associated with abnormal fluid retention.

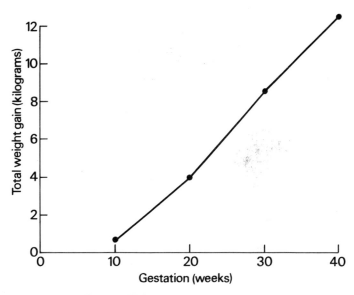

Fig. 3.1 Weight gain in normal pregnancy

Contributions to weight gain

The individual components affecting weight gain are derived from both maternal and feto-placental factors (Fig. 3.2). Pregnancy is an anabolic state and thus results in an increase in body fat, the growth of the breasts and the uterus and an expansion of blood volume and extracellular fluid. The contribution to maternal weight gain from the conceptus comes from fetal weight, amniotic fluid and the placenta. Poor weight gain is therefore associated with an increased incidence of low birth weight infants, but the range of weight gain in normal pregnancy may vary from almost zero to twice the mean weight gain.

Although there have been conflicting reports about the status of protein storage in the human, it now seems likely that no more protein is laid down than can be accounted for by fetal and placental growth and by the increase in size in specific target organs such as the uterus and breasts. An increase in fat storage occurs in normal pregnancy, with the deposition of fat occuring principally over the back, upper thighs and abdomen.

Surprisingly, there is a poor correlation between maternal weight gain and caloric intake and it is generally not advisable to inhibit weight gain (or, indeed, to reduce weight) in pregnancy — it often results in simultaneous restriction of essential nutrients, and this may have undesirable effects on fetal growth and development.

CHANGES IN BREASTS

As mentioned earlier, some of the first signs of pregnancy are recognised in the breast with an increase in size, enlargement of the nipples, increased vascularity and pigmentation of the areola.

Breast structure

The breast contains 10–20 lactiferous ducts which branch into a series of ducts and ductules terminating in multiple clusters of milk-secreting alveoli. The alveoli are surrounded by band-like myoepithelial cells which squeeze milk into the duct. The ducts and alveoli are surrounded by fat cells, connective tissue, blood vessels and lymph ducts. The ducts grow under the stimulus of high oestrogen levels and the alveoli develop as a result

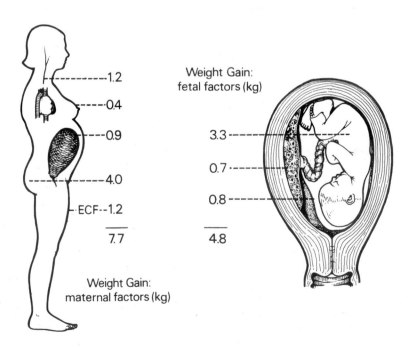

Fig. 3.2   Maternal (left) and fetal (right) contributions to weight gain at term (ECF = extracellular fluid)

Fig. 3.4 Decussation of muscle fibres in the various layers of the human uterus

Fig. 3.3 Factors regulating milk production and expulsion

The uterus is divided functionally and morphologically into three sections, namely the cervix, the isthmus (later to develop into the lower uterine segment) and the main body of the uterus (corpus uteri).

of the action of progesterone and prolactin. From 3–4 months onwards, a thick, glossy protein rich fluid, known as **colostrum**, can be expressed from the breast. Prolactin stimulates the cells of the alveoli to secrete milk by inducing the production of enzymes needed to synthesize milk proteins and lactose (Fig. 3.3).

This effect is blocked during pregnancy by the peripheral action of oestrogen and progesterone, but shortly after delivery the sudden fall in these hormones enables prolactin to act in an uninhibited manner on the breast and hence lactation begins. Suckling stimulates the release of both prolactin and oxytocin via neurological pathways between the nipple and the hypothalamus, and oxytocin stimulates contraction of the myoepithelial cells and, hence, ejection of milk.

THE UTERUS

During pregnancy, the uterus undergoes a 20-fold increase in weight from 50 g to 1100 g at term. The uterus consists of bundles of smooth muscle cells separated by thin sheets of connective tissue. The muscle cells are arranged as an innermost longitudinal layer, a middle layer with bundles running in all directions and an outer layer of both circular and longitudinal bundles (Fig. 3.4).

The cervix

The cervix is predominantly a fibrous organ whose principal function is to retain the conceptus (Fig. 3.5). Eighty per cent of the total protein consists of collagen. In pregnancy it becomes

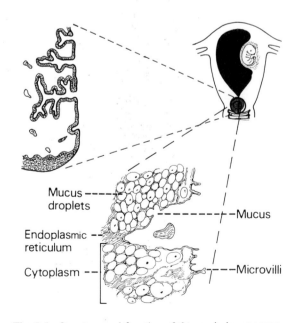

Fig. 3.5 Structure and function of the cervix in pregnancy

softened, hypertrophied and oedematous and the changes are characterized by:

1. Changes in stroma.
2. Hypertrophy of the cervical glands.
3. Changes in cervical secretions.

The connective tissue undergoes hypertrophy and hyperplasia with loosening and dissociation of the fibrils. There is a decrease in the amount of collagen and an alteration in ground structure, which enables the stretching and dilatation of the cervix. Hypertrophy of the cervical glands leads to the production of profuse cervical mucus and to the formation of a thick mucus plug or operculum which acts as a barrier against infection.

The isthmus

The isthmus of the uterus is the junctional area between the cervix and the body of the uterus. It joins the muscle fibres of the corpus to the dense connective tissue of the cervix and constitutes a transitional zone both functionally and structurally. It subsequently develops into the lower uterine segment and becomes more clearly defined from 28 weeks gestation.

Corpus uteri

The body of the uterus has to enlarge to accommodate the growing conceptus and then, at the appropriate time, commence a pattern of rhythmic contractions which will result in expulsion of the fetus. The uterus therefore adapts to these needs by a series of changes:

1. An increase in the size, shape, position and consistency of the uterus. In the latter months of pregnancy, enlargement predominantly occurs in the uterine fundus so that the round ligaments tend to emerge from a relatively caudal point in the uterus. The cavity of the uterus expands from some 4 ml to 4000 ml.
2. Hypertrophy of blood vessels and increased uterine blood flow associated with increased oxygen consumption in both the uterus and the utero-placental bed. Uterine blood flow has been shown to increase from approximately 50 ml/min at 10 weeks gestation to 500–700 ml/min at term (Fig. 3.6).

Uterine blood flow: 50 ml ——————— 500–700 ml/min
at term

Fig. 3.6 Changes in uteric blood flow in pregnancy

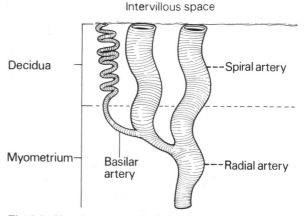

Intervillous space

Decidua

Myometrium

Basilar artery

Spiral artery

Radial artery

Fig. 3.7 Vascular structure in the utero-placental bed

The blood supply to the uterus is derived from the uterine and ovarian arteries and branches of the superior vesical arteries (Fig. 3.7). All of these vessels undergo massive hypertrophy. Control of blood flow in the arterial tree is dependent on arteriolar vasomotor control, both from the action of the autonomic nervous system and from the direct effect of vasoconstrictor and vasodilator humoral agents. The major control is exerted at an arteriolar level remote from the terminal arterioles which are invaded by trophoblast and become more passive channels with little regulatory function.

Uterine contractility

Myometrial growth is almost entirely due to muscle hypertrophy, although some hyperplasia may occur during early pregnancy. The stimulus for

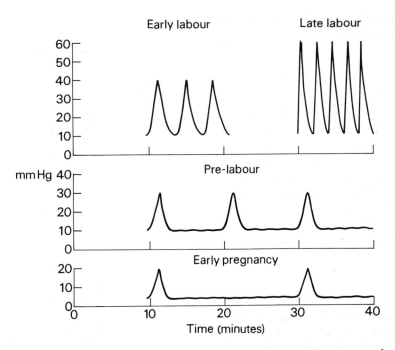

Fig. 3.8 Intra-amniotic pressure reflecting uterine contractions at different stages of gestation

myometrial growth and development is derived from direct effects of the growing conceptus and from the effect of oestrogens and progesterone produced by the ovary and the placenta.

The pregnant myometrium has a much greater compliance than the non-pregnant myometrium in response to distension. Thus, although the uterus becomes distended by the growing conceptus, intra-uterine pressure does not increase although the uterus maintains the capacity to develop maximal active tension.

The continuation of a successful pregnancy depends on the fact that the myometrium remains quiescent until the fetus is mature and capable of sustaining extra-uterine life. Progesterone appears to be the major hormone responsible and it achieves this effect by increasing the resting membrane potential of myometrial cells whilst at the same time impairing the conduction of electrical activity, and hence limits muscle activity to small clumps of cells.

Development of myometrial activity

Uterine activity occurs throughout pregnancy and is measurable as early as 7 weeks gestation when contractions may occur every 20–30 minutes, but reaching a pressure of less than 10 mmHg (Fig. 3.8). This pattern gradually changes to one of low frequency and higher amplitude so that by the third trimester contractions may occur every 10–15 minutes with an amplitude of 20–40 mmHg. These contractions often become noticeable as painless 'tightenings' known as **Braxton-Hicks contractions**. With the onset of labour, the contractions become increasingly more frequent and more painful, eventually reaching amplitudes of up to 100 mmHg in the last phase of the first stage of labour and occurring every 2–3 minutes.

THE VAGINA

The vagina is lined by stratified squamous epithelium which becomes markedly hypertrophic during pregnancy (Fig. 3.9). At the same time, the musculature in the vaginal walls becomes hypertrophied and the vagina increases in capacity and length. The rich venous vascular network in the connective tissue surrounding the vaginal walls

Cytology

Increase in stratified epithelium

Fig. 3.9 Changes in the vaginal epithelium during pregnancy

becomes engorged with blood and gives rise to the slightly bluish appearance of the vagina.

The three layers of superficial, intermediate and basal epithelial cells change their relative proportions so that the intermediate cells predominate and can be seen in the cell population of normal vaginal secretions. The intermediate cells have a tendency to clump together and curl at the edges and the epithelial cells generally multiply and enlarge and become filled with vacuoles rich in glycogen. High oestrogen levels stimulate glycogen synthesis and deposition, and the action of lactobacilli on the glycogen in these vaginal cells results in the production of lactic acid. The high acidity of the vagina, with a pH of 3.5–4, provides an acid environment which serves to keep the vagina relatively free of any bacterial pathogens.

CHANGES IN SKIN

Reference has already been made to the development of pigmentation on the face, nipples and abdominal wall in pregnancy. The development of stretch marks or striae gravidarum varies markedly in different populations and in different women. These marks, which often have a distinctly purplish colour in the first pregnancy and later adopt a silvery, thin appearance, represent the effects of disruption of collagen fibres in the subcuticular zone. Although they predominantly occur in the lines of stress of the abdominal wall, they also occur on the lateral aspect of the thighs and breasts and are as much related to the effect of increased production of adrenocortical hormones in pregnancy as they are

to actual stress in the skin folds associated with expansion of the abdomen.

THE CARDIOVASCULAR SYSTEM

Major changes occur in the cardiovascular system in pregnancy, the most significant changes taking place within the first 12 weeks. Although the longer term needs of maternal adaptation are met by alterations in the activity of the cardiovascular system, these changes tend to occur well before the physiological needs of the system arise.

Cardiac output

Cardiac output increases by 40% over the first 14 weeks of gestation and thereafter remains constant (Fig. 3.10). Thus an absolute increase of 1.5 l/min occurs at rest — from 4.5 to 6.0 l/min — under

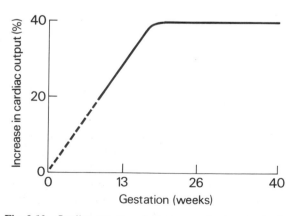

Fig. 3.10 Cardiac output undergoes a massive increase in the first trimester of pregnancy

standardised conditions of posture and time. During labour, contractions may increase cardiac output by 2 l/min. It has been suggested that this change results from injection of blood from the distended intervillous space. Normally, cardiac output increases because of an increase in both heart rate and stroke volume. As the heart rate increases by 10–15%, the remainder is the result of an increase in stroke volume. Pregnancy is known to proceed normally even when the mother has an artificial cardiac pacemaker, where compensation must occur entirely from increased stroke volume.

Cardiac position and size

With increasing enlargement of the uterus, the diaphragm is pushed upwards and the heart is correspondingly displaced so that the apex beat moves upwards and laterally (Fig. 3.11). The heart enlarges during pregnancy by an increase in volume of 70–80 ml and this enlargement results both from increased diastolic filling and muscle hypertrophy. Myocardial contractility is increased in association with lengthening of myocardial muscle fibres.

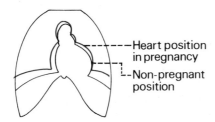

Fig. 3.11 Progressive enlargement of the uterus results in upward displacement of the heart and diaphragm

Arterial blood pressure

Posture has a profound effect on blood pressure in pregnancy so that blood pressure is higher when taken with the mother sitting up, lower when she is lying down, and lowest when lying on her side. Longitudinal studies in pregnancy have shown that blood pressure falls during mid pregnancy, but the fall is most noticeable in diastolic pressure (Fig. 3.12) Profound falls in blood pressure may occur in late pregnancy when the mother lies supine on her back and this phenomenon has previously been described

Fig. 3.12 A longitudinal study of the effect of posture on blood pressure in pregnancy

as the **supine hypotensive syndrome.** This results from compression of the inferior vena cava. It must be remembered that aortic compression may also occur and this will result in a conspicuous difference between brachial and femoral blood pressures in pregnancy. Thus, when the woman turns from a supine to a lateral supine position, the blood pressure may fall by some 10–15% (Fig. 3.12). Changes in venous pressure are dramatic in some areas. Although central venous pressure remains constant in pregnancy, venous pressure in the arms also remains constant but pressure from the uterus and fetal presenting part results in a marked increase in femoral venous pressure.

Peripheral resistance

In parallel with the increase in cardiac output, peripheral resistance falls to nearly 50% of the non-pregnant values. The factors controlling peripheral resistance are not clearly understood, although there is evidence to suggest that increased production of vasodilator prostaglandins may provide the principal mechanism. The regulation of blood pressure in pregnancy and the development of pregnancy-induced hypertension are determined by the balance of vasoconstrictor and vasodilator factors regulating peripheral resistance.

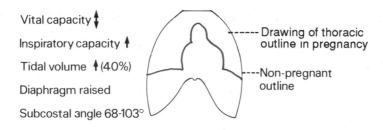

Fig. 3.13 Change in respiratory function in pregnancy

RESPIRATORY FUNCTION

Alterations to the configuration of the thorax occur in pregnancy. The level of the diaphragm rises and the intercostal angle increases from 68° in early pregnancy to 103° in late pregnancy and, because of these changes, breathing tends to be diaphragmatic rather than costal (Fig. 3.13).

Vital capacity is a measure of the maximum amount of gas that can be expired after maximum inspiration. Some pregnant women increase their vital capacity, but this does not always occur. It appears to be related to body build and the increase is not apparent in obese women.

Inspiratory capacity is a measure of tidal volume plus inspiratory reserve volume and is increased in late pregnancy. This change appears to occur progressively throughout pregnancy.

Respiratory rate does not change during pregnancy, whereas tidal volume, a measurement of the volume of gas inspired and expired in each respiration, does rise by approximately 40%. Minute ventilation therefore also increases. Thus, the resting pregnant woman increases her ventilation by breathing more deeply and not more frequently.

CHANGES IN BLOOD

Plasma volume

Sequential studies on plasma volume in pregnancy show a progressive rise until it reaches a plateau at about 32 weeks gestation. Where measurements have been made in the supine position, there is an apparent fall in plasma volume in late pregnancy, which is probably due to poor mixing of dye because of obstructed venous return from the legs. In general terms, multiple pregnancy is associated with a significantly higher increase in plasma volume (Fig. 3.14). Pregnancies exhibiting intrauterine fetal growth

Fig. 3.14 Changes in plasma volume and red cell mass in: A: quadruplets, B: triplets, C: twins, D: healthy multigravidae E: healthy primigravidae and F: intra-uterine growth retardation; the effect of iron supplement in singleton pregnancy is also shown

retardation are also associated with a poor increase in plasma volume. The actual increase in a singleton pregnancy is approximately 1250 ml from a non-pregnant mean of 2600ml.

Red cell mass is a measurement of the total volume of red cells in the circulation, and a steady increase occurs throughout pregnancy. The increase appears to be linear, and the discrepancy between the rate of increase of plasma volume and that of red cell mass results in a decline in haemoglobin concentration, haematocrit and red cell count during pregnancy and, in particular, in the second trimester. At the same time, mean corpuscular haemoglobin concentration remains constant.

The white cells

The total **white cell count** rises during pregnancy, and this increase is mainly due to an increase in neutrophil polymorphonuclear leucocytes, which reaches its peak at 30 weeks (Fig. 3.15).

A further massive neutrophilia occurs during labour with a fourfold increase in the number of polymorphs. Furthermore, there is an increase in the metabolic activity of granulocytes during pregnancy, which may be an effect of oestrogen stimulation.

Eosinophils, basophils and **monocytes** appear to remain relatively constant during pregnancy, but there is a profound fall in eosinophils during labour, and they are virtually absent at delivery. The lymphocyte count remains constant, and the number of T and B cells does not alter. However, lymphocyte function and cell-mediated immunity are profoundly depressed by a factor in maternal serum, and this suppression is associated with a lowered resistance to viral infection.

Platelets

Platelet counts decrease slightly during pregnancy, but studies on platelet function have shown no convincing evidence of any significant change.

Changes in plasma and serum

Plasma osmolality falls abruptly during the first 8 weeks of pregnancy, and this change is associated with a resetting of the osmoreceptor system to preserve the new low level of osmolality. The ability to excrete a water load is significantly affected by posture, with the upright posture being more antidiuretic than in non-pregnant subjects.

Changes in plasma proteins

Total protein concentration falls from about 7 to 6 g/100 ml during the first trimester and remains reduced throughout pregnancy. This fall is largely due to the fall in albumin concentration. On the other hand, globulins show a small rise in concentration,

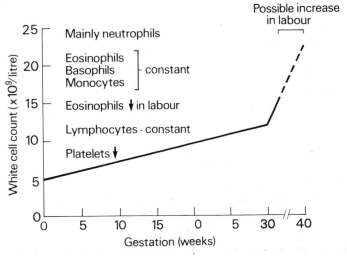

Fig. 3.15 Pregnancy is associated with an increased white cell count; the increase occurs predominantly in polymorphonuclear leucocytes

but there are marked differences in various globulin fractions. Lipoproteins are classified according to their density into four groups, namely, very low density lipoprotein, intermediate density lipoprotein, low density lipoprotein and high density lipoprotein. α-lipoproteins generally lie in the high density fraction, and β-lipoproteins in the low density fraction. Within the very low density and intermediate density lipoprotein fractions, three- to fourfold increases occur in triglyceride, cholesterol and phospholipid concentrations.

Amino acids

With the exception of alanine and glutamic acid, amino acid levels in plasma decrease below levels found in the non-pregnant state.

Free fatty acids

Levels of free fatty acids (non-esterified fatty acids) are extremely labile in pregnancy and are highly sensitive to fasting, exertion, emotional stress and smoking. Levels of free fatty acids in late pregnancy, however, are consistently elevated above non-pregnant and early pregnancy levels.

Clotting factors in pregnancy

Pregnancy is associated with an increased tendency towards blood clotting, and, in a situation where haemorrhage from the uterine vascular bed may be sudden and life threatening, this increased coagulability has an essential protective and life-saving function. Most clotting factors either remain constant or increase during pregnancy, and this particularly applies to fibrinogen, which exhibits a substantial increase in concentration. The increased tendency to clot in pregnancy is potentiated to some degree by a decrease in plasma fibrinolytic activity. This decrease disappears within 1 hour of delivery, and it seems likely that it is mediated from the placenta. There is also an increase in circulating fibrin degradation products in the plasma in normal pregnancy.

IMMUNOLOGY OF PREGNANCY

Maternal tolerance

The fetus constitutes an allograft and if it is not to be rejected, it requires the presence of maternal tolerance. The mother continues to respond to and destroy other foreign antigens and confers passive immunity in the newborn, but does not normally reject the fetus. The mechanism by which this apparent anomaly occurs is not completely understood.

The fetus expresses paternal antigens and these are capable of stimulating the production of maternal antibodies. Although pregnancy may induce blocking antibodies, these do not appear to be vital to the continuation of pregnancy. The placenta is not an impermeable immunological barrier as shown by the presence of maternal antibodies in the fetus. The uterus is not an immunologically privileged site as shown by the fact that other tissues implanted there are rejected.

Cell surface antigens

The major histocompatibility complex for cell surface antigens is encoded on chromosome 6. These antigens are central to transplant and cytotoxic responses. They are absent on trophoblast which is central to the feto-maternal interface. Fetal stem vessels and Hofbauer cells are able to bind maternal immunoglobulin and may therefore act as a filter.

In addition, the fetus has a less well–defined local immunoregulatory capacity, signalling the maternal immune system not to attack via special HLA-like surface antigens expressed by elements of the cytotrophoblast.

Decidual response

The leucocyte response on the decidua is unusual in that lymphoid cells do not appear to be activated and may act as suppressor cells by inhibiting the action of lymphokines essential for cytotoxic and natural killer cell action.

In summary, the fetus appears to avoid attack by the maternal immune system by a combination of having a relatively non–immunogenic interface with the maternal circulation, filtering out harmful antibodies in the placenta and by a locally mediated manipulation of the maternal immune response.

CHANGES IN THE LYMPHATIC SYSTEM AND THE THYMUS GLAND

Although it is difficult to measure changes in the thymus gland in human pregnancy, there is evidence from animal data that the thymus involutes markedly in pregnancy, probably as a result of the direct action of progesterone on the thymus. At the same time, the lymph nodes draining the uterus increase in size. The number of circulating T cells probably remains constant, but the number of B lymphocytes appears to increase. Maternal humoral responses are generally enhanced in pregnancy with increased antibody synthesis in the IgG fraction. Antibodies to fetal components are frequently found in maternal plasma but marked variations occur within and between pregnancies. As far as cellular immunity is concerned, the situation is confused, but current evidence suggests that a specific cellular blockade occurs, which is due to immunological enhancement of suppressor cell activity.

RENAL FUNCTION IN PREGNANCY

In line with the increase that occurs in cardiac output, renal blood flow increases by 30–50% in the first trimester and remains elevated throughout pregnancy. The change in renal blood flow is

Increased GFR

Glycosuria

Change in proximal tubule reabsorption

Blood flow ↑

Effective renal plasma flow ↑

Serum creatinine and urea ↓

Uric acid clearance ↑

Fig. 3.16 Changes in renal function in pregnancy

associated with an increase in both glomerular filtration rate (GFR) and effective renal plasma flow (Fig. 3.16). These changes are in fact apparent soon after conception and are fully developed by the end of the first trimester. There is evidence that a slight decline in glomerular filtration rate may occur between 26 and 36 weeks gestation. The increase in glomerular filtration rate is not associated with any substantial increase in production of creatinine and urea and therefore plasma levels fall during pregnancy.

Renal tubular function

Renal tubular function also undergoes significant change. Uric acid clearance increases from 6–12 ml/min to 12–20 ml/min with a consequent reduction in plasma uric acid levels. Net tubular reabsorption of uric acid is reduced. With progression of the pregnancy, the filtered load of uric acid increases whilst excretion remains constant, and plasma levels therefore return to non-pregnant values. Glycosuria is a common feature of normal pregnancy and it exhibits considerable variability from day to day. Glucose reabsorption is not solely dependent on tubular function, although it is linked with proximal tubular reabsorption of sodium and bicarbonate ions. Glomerular filtration rate also plays a significant role in glucose loss through the glomerulus.

The renin-angiotensin system

The renin-angiotensin system shows an early and persistent increase in activity. Renin is a proteolytic enzyme which acts on a substrate of α-2-globulin to produce angiotensin I. Under the action of converting enzyme produced predominantly in the lungs, but also in the placenta, angiotensin I is converted to angiotensin II, which is a potent vasoconstrictor, and also stimulates the release of aldosterone. Renin is produced in the kidney, and also in the uterus and chorion (Fig. 3.17). Approximately 70% of renin in the circulation in pregnancy is biologically inactive. A two-and-a-half-fold increase occurs in plasma renin concentration in the first 12 weeks and then tends to fall slightly as pregnancy progresses. Renin substrate increases gradually throughout pregnancy and appears to be

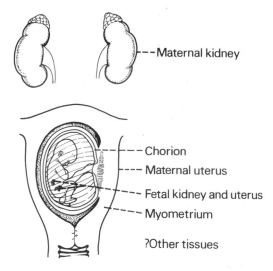

Fig. 3.17 Sources of renin in mother (above) and fetus (below)

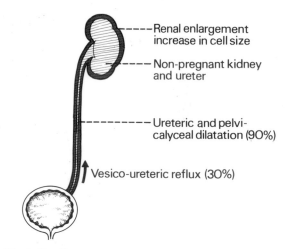

Fig. 3.18 Changes in the urinary tract include renal enlargement and ureteric dilatation

under control of oestrogen stimulation. The changes are of particular interest in pregnancy because there is a selective loss of vascular sensitivity to angiotensin II, which does not appear to be the case with adrenaline and noradrenaline.

Aldosterone levels rise gradually throughout pregnancy, but correlate poorly with plasma concentrations of both renin and angiotensin II. There are increasing data to show that tissue prostaglandins provide the mechanism which blocks vascular reactivity to angiotensin II in pregnancy, and the renin–angiotensin system in the genital tract may play an important role in regulating uterine blood flow.

Other changes in the urinary system

Apart from the functional changes in the kidney, various anatomical changes occur in the urinary tract (Fig. 3.18). There is marked dilatation of the calyces and renal pelvis and of the ureters. The changes appear in the first trimester of pregnancy and it is unlikely that they are due to back pressure. However, the ureters do not exhibit actual hypotonicity and hypomotility and there is hypertrophy of the ureteral smooth muscle and hyperplasia of the connective tissue. Vesicoureteric reflux occurs sporadically, and the combination of reflux and ureteric dilatation is associated with a high incidence of urinary stasis and an increased tendency to urinary tract infection.

THE ALIMENTARY SYSTEM

Heartburn is a common disorder of pregnancy and this has generally been ascribed to reflux oesophagitis. However, it is known that reflux also occurs in women without any symptoms of heartburn. With increased intra–abdominal pressure, there is commonly displacement of the lower oesophageal sphincter through the diaphragm, but this is not necessarily the cause of heartburn. The predominant factors appear to be decreased sphincter tonus and a decreased sphincter response to raised intra-abdominal pressure.

Gastric secretion is reduced in pregnancy and gastric motility is low. As a consequence gastric emptying tends to be delayed. Reduced motility also occurs in both the small bowel and the large bowel and there is also evidence that absorption of sodium and water is increased in the large bowel. This may account for the increased tendency to constipation that characterizes pregnancy.

ENDOCRINE CHANGES

Massive production of sex steroids by the placenta tends to dominate the endocrine picture; these changes will be described in a subsequent chapter

Fig. 3.19 Thyroid function in pregnancy.

on placental function. Significant alterations occur in all maternal endocrine organs.

The pituitary gland

The pituitary gland enlarges in normal pregnancy and the increase is largely due to changes in the anterior lobe. Prolactin-secreting cells increase in number whilst the number of gonadotrophin cells decreases. Prolactin levels increase substantially, probably as a result of oestrogen stimulation of the lactotrophe. Gonadotrophin secretion is inhibited. The secretion of growth hormone is inhibited whilst plasma adrenocorticotrophic hormone (ACTH) levels increase. Thyrotrophin levels remain constant. The major role of the posterior pituitary lies in the release of oxytocin and this principally occurs during the first stage of labour and during suckling. Very little is known of vasopressin release.

Thyroid function

The thyroid gland enlarges in up to 70% of all pregnant women and was relied on by the ancient Egyptians as a sign of pregnancy. There is increased urinary excretion of iodine and this leads to a relative deficiency in plasma iodide.

The thyroid gland triples its uptake of iodide from the blood. Thus, the relative iodine deficiency is probably responsible for the compensating follicular enlargement of the gland.

Thyroxine binding globulin (TBG) is doubled by the end of the first trimester and remains elevated throughout pregnancy (Fig. 3.19). As a result, total T_3 and T_4 increase in pregnancy, although free T_3 and T_4 rise early in pregnancy and then fall to remain within the normal non-pregnant range. Thyroid stimulating hormone (TSH) may increase slightly but tends to remain within the normal range. T_3 and T_4 and TSH do not cross the placental barrier and there is therefore no direct relationship between maternal and fetal thyroid function. However, iodine and antithyroid drugs cross the placenta, as does long–acting thyroid stimulator (LATS). Hence, the fetus may be affected by the level of iodine intake and by the presence of auto-immune disease in the mother.

The adrenal gland

Plasma cortisol increases throughout pregnancy, and much of this rise is due to binding to corticosteroid-binding globulin. However, the mean unbound cortisol is also elevated in normal pregnancy. Sex hormone-binding globulin also rises so that plasma testosterone and androsterone levels rise. 11-deoxycorticosterone (DOC) shows the greatest percentage increase of all adrenal steroids, and aldosterone, which is predominantly bound to albumin, also increases substantially in normal pregnancy.

Medullary function remains surprisingly constant with little change in plasma levels of adrenaline and noradrenaline.

Changes in maternal physiology in pregnancy

- Weight gain (12.5 kg at 0.4 kg/week; 1/3 fetal)
- Breast; ducts stimulated by oestrogen, alveoli by progesterone and prolactin
- Uterus increases ×20 in weight, ×10 blood flow
- Hypertrophy of lower genital tract
- Plasma volume increases by 50%
- Cardiac output up 40%
- Increase in tidal volume
- Plasma osmolality falls
- Renal blood flow and GFR increase; creatinine and urea fall
- Ureteric and pelvicalyceal dilatation and reflux
- Reduced bowel motility and sphincter tone
- Endocrine changes in pituitary, thyroid and adrenal glands

BIBLIOGRAPHY

Hytten F, Chamberlain G 1980 Clinical physiology in obstetrics. Blackwell Scientific Publications, Oxford
Philipp E E, Barnes J, Newton M 1986 Scientific Foundations of obstetrics and gynaecology. Heinemann Medical Books, London
Rodin A 1989 Thyroid disease in pregnancy. British Journal of Hospital Medicine 41:234–242
Studd J 1975 The plasma proteins in pregnancy. In: Hytten F E (ed) Clinics in Obstetrics and Gynaecology, Physiological adjustments in pregnancy, 2:285

4. Antenatal care

The concept that the general well-being and reproductive performance of a woman might be improved by antenatal supervision is surprisingly recent and was first introduced in Edinburgh in 1911. In many societies, antenatal care is not available and for social or religious reasons is not used when it is available.

The basic aims of antenatal care are:

1. To ensure optimal health of the mother throughout her pregnancy.
2. To detect and treat disorders arising during pregnancy which relate to the welfare of both mother and fetus and to ensure that the pregnancy results in a healthy mother and healthy infant.

The ways by which these objectives are achieved vary in relation to the efficiency of clinical observation at any given time and to the value of current screening tests, which are designed to detect maternal or fetal problems.

Antenatal examinations are performed at regular intervals and the recommended timing for visits (Fig. 4.1) is:

1. Monthly visits for the first 28 weeks.
2. Bimonthly visits from 28 to 36 weeks.
3. Weekly visits for the remaining weeks.

These recommendations clearly apply only to apparently normal pregnancies and need to be modified where circumstances indicate an increased risk to mother or fetus.

ROUTINE CLINICAL EXAMINATIONS

The details of antenatal history and routine clinical examinations have been discussed in Chapter 1. The importance of clinical assessment cannot be overemphasized. Routine assessment of blood

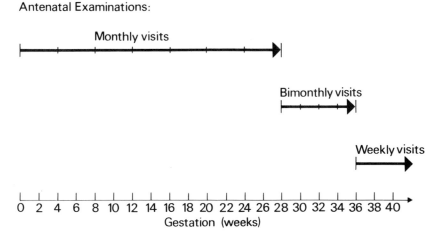

Fig. 4.1 Timing of antenatal visits

Fig. 4.2   Schedules for routine tests of haemoglobin estimation and detection of Rhesus antibodies

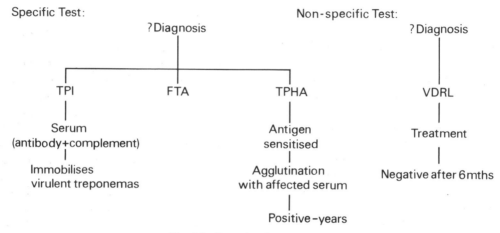

Fig. 4.3   Screening for syphilis

pressure, urine and body weight and estimates of fetal growth and size form the basis of good antenatal care.

LABORATORY TESTS

At the first visit to clinic, the following routine haematological and urinary investigations are recommended:

1. Haemoglobin concentration and, where indicated, a complete blood picture. This should be repeated on at least two subsequent occasions at 28 weeks and 36 weeks gestation. Estimates of total red cell mass would be more reliable indi-

cators of anaemia but are generally impracticable in most clinics.

2. Determination of blood groups (ABO and Rh) should be routinely performed and include screening for Rh antibodies in Rh negative women. If no antibodies are detected, the test should be repeated at 32 weeks gestation. If antibodies are detected, the titre is determined and subsequent samples taken for further titre estimations at appropriate intervals (Fig. 4.2).

3. **Wasserman reaction.** Routine screening for syphilis is recommended practice because of the importance of early detection of the disease in pregnancy (Fig. 4.3). The yield is small and the value of the procedure is debatable. There are numerous serological tests available for syphilis,

some of which are non-specific, such as the Wasserman reaction, and some of which are specific.

Non-specific tests. The Wasserman reaction, which is a complement fixation test, was the first successful serological test. This test is dependent on the presence of treponemal antibodies in the serum which then unite with a colloidal suspension of lipoids to produce visible flocculation. A similar flocculation test that is widely used is the **venereal disease research laboratory test** (VDRL) which employs a cardiolipin antigen.

The difficulty with these tests is that they may give a false positive reaction in association with malaria or virus pneumonia, or in auto-immune conditions, such as lupus erythematosus, haemolytic anaemia, Hashimoto's disease or rheumatoid arthritis.

Specific tests. Where there is doubt about the diagnosis, specific tests should be employed. The *Treponema pallidum* **immobilisation test** (TPI) is the most specific test available and is based on the fact that the serum from syphilitic patients contains an antibody which, in the presence of complement, immobilises virulent treponemas. Positive tests are also found in patients with yaws and other treponemal diseases. Other tests include the **fluorescent treponemal antibody test** (FTA) and the *Treponema pallidum* **haemagglutination test** (TPHA). In the TPHA, the antigen consists of a suspension of turkey red blood cells in formalin and tannin which have been sensitized by contact with virulent treponemas. Positive tests are characterized by agglutination of the sensitized cells on contact with affected serum. The test is easy to perform and is highly specific. The VDRL usually becomes negative within 6 months of treatment, whereas the TPHA remains positive for many years. The VDRL, therefore, assumes the most important role in monitoring treatment.

4. **Screening for HIV infection.** The basis of tests for the detection of HIV infection is the detection of Human Immunodeficiency Virus (HIV) antibodies. The virus can be isolated and grown but this is difficult. The virus has a predilection for the T helper subset of lymphocytes. There is an altered T helper/T suppressor ratio.

All of these tests can be normal, even with the presence of infection. The most important clinically confounding variable is that HIV antibodies may be absent in the incubation phase. Seropositive mothers always have seropositive babies, but this may not indicate AIDS in the baby. However, 30–50% of babies have AIDS.

Screening necessitates taking a serum blood sample and repeating after 6 months. Screening is indicated if there are risk factors, i.e. intravenous drugs, a sexual partner who is a drug abuser, or from a high-risk area or who is bisexual, and haemophiliacs. Testing for HIV in an unselected population gives a false positive for every true positive so caution must be exercised. If screening is limited to high-risk groups, selection is much better.

5. **Serum alphafetoprotein.** Neural tube defects form one of the commonest fetal abnormalities with an incidence that varies between 3 and 8 per 1000 depending on the geographic environment. In 1972, Brock & Sutcliffe described an increase in the concentration of alphafetoprotein in amniotic fluid in the presence of open neural tube defects. It is, of course, impossible to screen an obstetric population by routine amniocentesis as this involves puncturing the amniotic sac and carries hazards in its own right (Fig. 4.4). Where there is a previous history of one affected infant, the risk of a subsequent abnormal child is 1 in 20. This risk is 1 in 10 after two children and 1 in 5 after three children. Under these circumstances, routine amniocentesis is justified. However, total population screening is now undertaken on serum measurements.

Blood samples should be taken between 16 and 19 weeks gestation; where there is doubt about the gestational age, ultrasound assessment should be performed and the serum measurement repeated. If the serum values of alphafetoprotein are abnormally elevated, amniocentesis should be performed and the level of alphafetoprotein in the amniotic fluid measured. An abnormal value usually indicates an open neural tube defect — either a major degree of spina bifida or anencephaly. At 2.5 times the normal median, 80% of anencephalic fetuses and 74% of open spina bifida fetuses will be detected, but 3.3% of normal fetuses will also be included. The precision of

Serum alphafetoprotein →
abnormally elevated

Abnormal value =
open neural tube defect

Amniocentesis

(3-8/1000)

	Risk:	Blood Samples:
Previous history of one affected infant	1 in 20	16 and 19 weeks'
After 2 children	1 in 10	gestation
After 3 children	1 in 5	

Fig. 4.4 Screening for neural tube defects

diagnosis is much greater where amniotic fluid is used and it is therefore necessary to proceed to amniocentesis and further ultrasonography where an abnormal serum level is found. Several other conditions, including multiple pregnancy, threatened abortion, intrauterine death, congenital nephrosis, exomphalos and duodenal or oesophageal atresia, have been found to be associated with raised levels of serum aplhafetoprotein; in particular it is essential to exclude multiple pregnancy. Where a multiple pregnancy is demonstrated, it is better not to proceed to amniocentesis. Even if one fetus is abnormal, it is doubtful that it is valid to terminate the pregnancy and, in any case, results from amniotic fluid may be misleading as the sac of the unaffected fetus may be sampled, thereby giving a false indication of fetal normality. The specificity of the diagnosis can also be enhanced by the measurement of acetylcholinesterase in amniotic fluid. Elevated levels occur specifically in the presence of exposed CNS tissue.

Recent studies on data obtained from low values of maternal serum alphafetoprotein have shown an increased incidence of Down's syndrome. If the first 16-week test is 0.5 multiples of the normal median and the maternal age is greater than 35 years, then the risk of Down's syndrome is 1 in 172. If this measurement is combined with the measurement of unconjugated oestriol and human chorionic gonadotrophin measurement, the accuracy of prediction is enhanced.

SCREENING FOR RUBELLA

In 1970, the Department of Health and Social Security in the United Kingdom recommended that rubella vaccination should be offered to all girls between their 11th and 14th birthdays in an attempt to reduce the incidence of congenital rubella defects. However, many women still remain at risk because they have declined, or have not been offered, immunisation and it has been estimated that approximately 10–15% remain susceptible to the disease at the time of pregnancy. The presence of rubella antibodies in serum is determined by using a technique of radial haemolysis or the haemagglutination inhibition test. The former test is favoured for mass screening programmes.

All women attending antenatal clinics should have serum taken for rubella antibodies unless immunity is already established. Seronegative women should be offered rubella vaccination in the immediate puerperium unless they do not intend to have any further children. Vaccination is performed with a live attenuated rubella virus with vaccines such as Almevax® and involves a single dose of 0.5 ml injected subcutaneously. Although there is little evidence to suggest any significant abnormality rate in women who have conceived immediately before or following rubella vaccination, it is generally recommended that pregnancy should be avoided for 2 months after vaccination.

The diagnosis of rubella during pregnancy can be made on the clinical manifestations of the infection which include a fine macular rash, lymphadenopathy

Mild pyrexia

Fine macular rash

Lymphadenopathy

throat swab or
blood culture
–virus isolation

diagnosis by
determination of
level of antibodies
in mother

Cord blood
measurements show
similar antibody titres
to mother

Fig. 4.5 Clinical manifestations of rubella infection

in the cervical region and a mild pyrexia (Fig. 4.5). The diagnosis can be confirmed in the acute phase by virus isolation from a throat swab or from blood culture, but usually the diagnosis is established by determination of the level of antibodies in the mother. A fourfold rise in antibody titre in consecutive blood samples taken 2 weeks apart constitutes evidence of recent rubella infection in the mother. In the infant, cord blood measurements will show similar antibody titres to the mother. However, the presence of raised levels of IgM strongly suggests infection acquired in utero.

SCREENING FOR URINARY TRACT INFECTION

Culture of urine is now used as a routine screening procedure. The presence of pathogenic organisms in excess of 10^4 organisms/ml indicates significant bacteriuria, and there is evidence to show that the treatment of asymptomatic bacteriuria of this type will produce a significant reduction in subsequent urinary tract infection.

Clinical examinations and laboratory tests

- Blood pressure, weight, urinalysis
- Abdominal palpation and auscultation
- Hb, Rh antibodies, hepatitis
  syphilis and rubella
- Detailed scan of fetus
- Serum alphafetoprotein

ANTENATAL EDUCATION

An important part of antenatal care is the preparation for childbirth and the subsequent care of the child. Antenatal education should, ideally, start before pregnancy as part of school education and it should continue throughout pregnancy and the puerperium. Whatever approach is considered preferable, there is a common need to inform the mother of the changes she can expect during pregnancy and of the nature of labour and delivery. The education programme should also include parentcraft and the advice on care of the child should be continued in the puerperium.

DIETARY ADVICE

Diet in pregnancy

There is ample evidence that the outcome of pregnancy can be influenced by dietary intake. Gross malnutrition is known to result in intra-uterine growth retardation, anaemia, prematurity and fetal malformation.

Lesser degrees of malnutrition may also be associated with increased frequency of fetal malformation and it is therefore important to identify those mothers who have poor dietary intake and provide advice for all mothers during pregnancy. There is also some evidence to suggest that mothers who have experienced complications in a previous pregnancy may benefit from appropriate dietetic advice which may prevent the development of abnormalities. However, this hypothesis remains to be proved.

Caloric intake

A total caloric intake of 2000–2500 Calories a day is optimal during the last two trimesters and this requirement may increase to 3000 Calories per day in the puerperium in lactating women.

Protein

First class protein is expensive and therefore is most likely to be deficient in the diet. An average of 60–80 g per day is desirable, and the diet is particularly likely to be deficient in lower socio-economic group and in association with vegetarian diets. Animal

Table 4.1 (a)   Common dietary sources of protein and iron

Sources of protein		Sources of iron	
16 g sources		*5 mg sources*	
Beef, chicken, pork, fish		Liver, kidney	2 oz
cheddar cheese	2 oz	Beef heart	3 oz
Cottage cheese	½ cup	Beans, cooked dry	1 cup
Dried beans (cooked)	1 cup	*3 mg sources*	
Peanuts	½ cup	Beef, pork	3 oz
8 g sources		Spinach, greens	½ cup
Milk (whole, skim, dried)	1 cup	*2 mg sources*	
Peanut butter	2 table sp.	Peaches or apricots, dried	
Egg	1 large	cooked; raisins, prunes,	
Peas (split, dry, cooked)	½ cup	green peas	½ cup
4 g sources		Chicken	3 oz
Macaroni, rice, oatmeal	¾ cup	*1 mg sources*	
Coconut, shredded (fresh) or		Egg, sweet potato	1 medium
2 cups dried, shredded	1½ cup	Broccoli, oatmeal, enriched	
Bread	2 slices	macaroni, winter squash	½ cup
		Orange	1 large
		Bread — enriched	2 slices

protein is obtained from meat, poultry, fish, eggs and cheese. Vegetable protein occurs in nuts, lentils, beans and peas (Table 4.1a).

Fats

The importance of fats, particularly essential fatty acids, has been underestimated and, indeed, essential fatty acids may play an important role in preventing the development of hypertension during pregnancy. Fats are an important source of calories and they provide fat soluble vitamins, including vitamins A, D and K.

Animal fats are found in meat, eggs and dairy produce, which contain a high percentage of saturated fats. Vegetable fats are also important as they contain unsaturated fats such as linolenic and linoleic acids.

Carbohydrates

Carbohydrates are a major source of calories and energy. Our present understanding of fetal bio-chemistry suggests that there is a close correlation between maternal and fetal blood glucose levels and that glucose is a major source of energy for the fetus.

Minerals and vitamins

The requirements for iron, calcium, iodine and various trace elements such as magnesium and zinc

Table 4.1 (b)   Dietary sources of calcium

Sources of calcium	
0.30 g sources	
Milk	1 cup
Cheddar cheese	1¼ oz
0.15 g sources	
Canned salmon (with bones), cottage	
cheese, broccoli	½ cup
0.05 g sources	
Dried raisins, cooked beans: pinto, kidney	½ cup
Orange	1 medium
Sweet potato	1 medium
Bread — enriched	2 slices

all increase in pregnancy. These elements are found in lean meat, various stone fruits, beans and peas, dairy produce and seafoods (Table 4.1(b)).

Vitamins A and B are found in kidney, liver and dark green vegetables. Vitamin B_2 is found in whole grain and cereals, and vitamin B_5 in fish, lean meat, poultry and nuts (Table 4.2).

Ascorbic acid is essential for normal fetal growth and maternal health, and is found in citrus fruits, Brussels sprouts and broccoli. Vitamin D and folic acid are also important, although it is very rare now to see any signs of vitamin D deficiency. Folic acid deficiency is still relatively common and is associated with the development of megaloblastic anaemia in the mother. Green vegetables, nuts and yeast are all rich sources of folic acid and it is common practice to give specific supplements during pregnancy.

Table 4.2 General advice on foodstuffs recommended in pregnancy (portions given per day unless otherwise stated)

Foodstuff	Quantity
Dairy	
Milk	600–1000 ml
Butter	150 g
Cheese	1 serving
Meat	
Chicken, pork or beef	2 servings
Liver	Once/week or more
Fish	*Once or twice/week*
Vegetables	
Potato	1–2 servings
Other	1–2 servings
Salads	Freely
Fruit	
Citrus	1
Other	2–3
Cereals	
Wheat, corn, rice, macaroni, spaghetti	4 servings

1 serving = ½ cup

EXERCISE IN PREGNANCY

Pregnant women should be encouraged to undertake reasonable activity. This will be limited with advancing gestation by the physical restrictions imposed by the pregnancy but during early pregnancy there is no need to restrict sporting activities beyond the commonsense limits of avoiding excessive exertion and fatigue. Swimming is helpful, particularly in late pregnancy.

COITUS IN PREGNANCY

There is no contraindication to coitus in pregnancy at any stage of gestation, other than the physical difficulties imposed by the changes in abdominal size. It is, however, sensible to advise against coitus where there is evidence of threatened abortion or a history of recurrent abortions. It is also generally contraindicated where there is a history of antepartum haemorrhage or premature rupture of the membranes.

SOCIAL HABITS
Smoking in pregnancy

Smoking has an adverse effect on fetal growth and development. These adverse effects derive principally from two major effects:

1. **The effect of carbon monoxide on the fetus.** Carbon monoxide has an affinity for haemoglobin 200 times greater than oxygen. Fresh air contains up to 0.5 parts per million (p.p.m.) of carbon monoxide, but in cigarette smoke values as high as 60 000 p.p.m. may be detected. Carbon monoxide shifts the oxygen dissociation curve to the left in both fetal and maternal haemoglobin. Maternal carbon monoxide saturation may rise to 8% in the mother and 7% in the fetus, so that there is specific interference with oxygen transfer.

2. **The effect of nicotine on the uteroplacental vasculature as a vasoconstrictor.** Animal studies on the effect of infusions of nicotine on cardiac output and uteroplacental blood flow have shown that high-dose infusions produce a fall in cardiac output and uteroplacental blood flow. However, at levels up to 5 times greater than those seen in smokers, there are no measurable effects and it is unlikely that nicotine exerts any adverse effects by reducing uteroplacental blood flow.

Fig. 4.6 Smoking during pregnancy has adverse maternal and fetal effects

The effect on perinatal mortality

Smoking during pregnancy reduces the birth weight of the infant, and also reduces the crownheel length.

It is also now generally agreed that the perinatal death rate is increased as a direct effect of smoking and this increased risk has been quantified at 20% for those women smoking up to 20 cigarettes per day, and 35% in excess of one packet per day. Mothers should be advised to stop smoking during pregnancy.

Alcohol intake in pregnancy

Excessive alcohol intake is associated with a specific syndrome, the fetal alcohol syndrome. The features in the infant include growth retardation, various structural defects, various facial defects, multiple joint anomalies and cardiac defects. However, these problems arise in women who consume 30–60 ml of absolute alcohol per day.

There is no evidence to show that such problems arise in association with modest social drinking, so that the occasional glass of wine has not been shown to be associated with risk.

BREAST CARE

Breast feeding should be encouraged in all women unless there is any specific contraindication which would make breast feeding excessively difficult, such as grossly inverted nipples or previous damage to the breasts. It must also be remembered that, although breast feeding is desirable, the reality is that children tend to grow and develop equally satisfactorily on artificial feeding. It is, therefore,

Care of nipples

Manual expression of colostrum

Fig. 4.7 Nipple care and breast preparation

wise to do no more than encourage women to breast feed, rather than apply any coercion, and the mother's desire must be taken into account.

In the antenatal period, the breasts should be washed daily and carefully dried. The nipples should be massaged with an appropriate cream and the nipple drawn with the fingers if there is any evidence of retraction (Fig. 4.7). The breasts should be supported with an appropriate maternity brassiere. Manual expression of colostrum should be taught and practised from 36 weeks gestation.

COMMON MINOR DISORDERS OF PREGNANCY

Vomiting in pregnancy

Minor degrees of nausea and vomiting are very common in early pregnancy. Nevertheless, this is a symptom complex which appears to have become less significant in recent years. Although it is commonly described as 'morning sickness' it does not always occur in the morning and is often triggered by the smell of food and conditions of stress. The use of anti-emetic drugs has generally fallen into disrepute because of anxiety over taking drugs in early pregnancy. Even a drug such as Debendox®, which has been extensively used and investigated in early pregnancy and where there is no evidence of any increase in congenital malformations, has now been withdrawn from the market. There is some evidence to suggest that untreated nausea and vomiting in early pregnancy, with the associated dietary restrictions, may carry risks in their own right.

Most vomiting diminishes or stops by 12–14 weeks gestation and can often be relieved by frequent small meals and the avoidance of highly spiced foods. It also helps to have a sweetened drink before starting activities in the morning. Sometimes the severity of vomiting necessitates hospital admission and intravenous therapy. Reassurance and continued support are essential requirements in management.

Abdominal pain

Very few women manage to experience an entire pregnancy without an episode of abdominal pain.

Most of these episodes are transitory and unaccompanied by any signs of systemic disorder. Nevertheless, it is important to distinguish these from organic disorders such as appendicitis, and yet to avoid unnecessary interference and surgery which may, in themselves, produce disastrous results. The cause for most episodes is never determined.

Heartburn

With the enlargement of the uterus and displacement of the gut, reflux of gastric juices occurs in many women, with resultant heartburn. This is particularly noticeable when the woman is supine and can, to some degree, be avoided by raising the head with pillows when resting and the use of antacids.

Constipation

The increased levels of progesterone in pregnancy appear to reduce bowel motility so that constipation is a common problem. This is sometimes intractable until the pregnancy is completed, but can be helped by increasing dietary fibre intake with bran and green vegetables and by the use of bulk-forming laxatives, or stimulants such as Senokot® and milk of magnesia.

Backache

Pregnancy is associated with changes in posture and with increasing lumbar lordosis. The increased laxity of pelvic ligaments induced by high circulating levels of sex steroids also results in some instability of the bony pelvis. Lumbar and sacral backache are therefore very common in pregnancy. Occasionally the pain may be incapacitating and associated with sciatic pain. It may be lumbar or sacro-iliac. In rare cases, it is associated with disc protrusion and the symptoms may persist after delivery. However, in most women no obvious cause is identified and the pain disappears after delivery. Pregnant women should be advised to lift objects by flexing their knees and thighs, and not their backs. Sometimes, a supportive corset may be necessary, and rest on a well-supported bed is advisable.

Syncopal episode

'Fainting' in pregnancy is very common and it is surprising how rarely serious injury ensues. Presumably most pregnant women have sufficient warning signs to avoid dangerous situations. There is little that can be done except to reassure the woman that this is a common problem associated with the general vascular instability of pregnancy and to encourage them to avoid potentially hazardous situations.

Varicosities

Varicose veins and haemorrhoids almost invariably become worse during pregnancy and women should be advised that this is the case. Local support with elastic hosiery can significantly relieve symptoms. In the case of haemorrhoids, constipation should be avoided, and replacement and bed rest recommended where the haemorrhoids have prolapsed. Appropriate vasoconstrictor suppositories should be used.

Common minor disorders of pregnancy

- Vomiting
- Acid reflux
- Constipation
- Backache
- Syncope
- Varicosities
- Carpal tunnel syndrome

Carpal tunnel syndrome

Compression of the median nerve with tingling and paraesthesia in the distribution of the median nerve involving the thumb and the lateral two-and-a-half fingers occurs as a complication of pregnancy (Fig. 4.8). It is sometimes relieved by diuretics and occasionally requires splinting of the wrist to produce symptomatic relief. It rarely appears to result in any residual neurological damage and always disappears in the puerperium.

In summary, numerous minor disorders occur in pregnancy. Provided they are recognised as short-term problems, they rarely require more than symptomatic relief and reassurance that the condition will improve with the completion of the pregnancy.

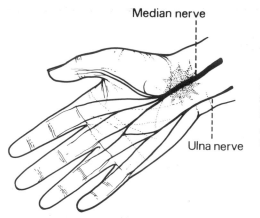

Median nerve

Disturbance of
sensation in skin
Pain on flexion of wrist
Atrophy of thenar muscles
Swelling of fingers

Ulna nerve

Fig. 4.8 Carpal tunnel syndrome is a common complication of pregnancy

BIBLIOGRAPHY

Brock D J H 1982 Early diagnosis of fetal defects. Churchill Livingstone, Edinburgh

Brock D J H, Sutcliffe R G 1972 Alphafetoprotein in the antenatal diagnosis of anencephaly and spina bifida. Lancet ii: 197–199

Harley J M G (ed) 1982 Pre-pregnancy counselling in obstetrics. Clinics in Obstetrics and Gynaecology 9:1. W B Saunders, Eastbourne

Ferguson-Smith M A 1984 Pre-natal diagnosis. Wiley Medical Publications, Chichester

Jordan J, Symonds E M 1978 The diagnosis and management of neural tube defects The Royal College of Obstetricians and Gynaecologists

McClure Browne J C, Dixon G, 1978 Antenatal care. Churchill Livingstone, Edinburgh

Rayburn W F, Zuspan F P 1982 Drug therapy in obstetrics and gynaecology. Appleton-Century-Crofts

5. Conception and nidation

OOGENESIS

Primordial germ cells originally appear in the yolk sac and can be identified by the fourth week of fetal development (Fig. 5.1). The cells migrate through the dorsal mesentery of the developing gut and finally reach the genital ridge between 44 and 48 days. Migration occurs into a genital tubercle, consisting of mesenchymal cells, which appears over the ventral part of the mesonephros. The germ cells form sex cords and become the cortex of the gonad. The sex cords break up into separate clumps of cells and by 16 weeks these clumps of cells become primary follicles which incorporate central germ cells. These cells undergo rapid mitotic activity and by 20 weeks of intra-uterine life there are about 7 million cells known as oogonia. After this time, no further cell division occurs and no further ova are produced. At birth, the oogonia have begun the first

meiotic division and have become primary oocytes. The number of oocytes falls to one million by birth and half a million by puberty.

Meiosis

The chromosome number of the gametes is half that of normal cells. With the fusion of egg and sperm, the chromosome complement is returned to the normal count of 46 chromosomes. In meiosis, two cell divisions occur in succession, each of which consists of a prophase, metaphase, anaphase and telophase (Fig. 5.2). At the end of the first meiotic prophase, the double chromosomes undergo synapsis producing a group of four homologous chromatids called a tetrad. The two centrioles move to opposite poles, a spindle forms in the middle and the membrane of the nucleus disappears. As the cell enters the metaphase of the first meiotic division,

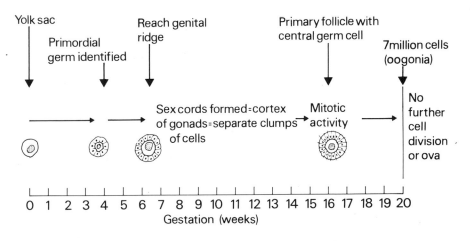

Fig. 5.1 Embryonic and fetal development of oogonia

Prophase   Metaphase   Anaphase   Telophase   Meiosis

Fig. 5.2 Nuclear events in oogenesis associated with meiosis

the tetrads line up around the equator of the spindle. Primary oocytes remain in suspended prophase until sexual maturity is reached. Meiotic division resumes as each individual follicle begins to mature and is completed about the time of ovulation. In anaphase, the daughter chromatids separate and move towards opposite poles. The centrioles divide again and the haploid number of double chromosomes lines up on the equator of each spindle. The chromosomes separate and move to appropriate poles. In the telophase of the second meiotic division, 23 chromosomes arrive at each pole.

Thus, the nuclear events in oogenesis are the same as in spermatogenesis but cytoplasmic division is unequal, resulting in one secondary oocyte. This small cell consists almost entirely of a nucleus and is known as the first polar body. As the ovum enters the Fallopian tube, the second meiotic division occurs and a secondary oocyte forms with the development of a small second polar body.

Oogenesis

- Primordial germ cells at 4th week
- Migrate to genital ridge by 48th day
- Primary follicles by 16 weeks
- Oogonia by 20 weeks
- Meiosis starts
- Oocytes by birth
- Follicles mature 11–50 years later
- Meiosis completed by ovulation to give secondary oocyte (haploid)

THE STRUCTURE OF THE MATURE OVARY

The mature ovary in the reproductive era is 3–5 cm in length and weighs 5–8 g. The ovary is suspended from the uterus by the ovarian ligament attached to its medial end. The ovary has a free margin and a

hilus through which the blood vessels and lymphatics enter. The ovary is attached to the dorsal aspect of the broad ligament by a fold of peritoneum known as the mesovarium, and to the lateral pelvic wall by the suspensory or infundibulo-pelvic ligament, which contains the ovarian artery and vein. The blood supply to the ovaries comes from the ovarian arteries, which anastomose with the uterine arteries (Fig. 5.3). Both ovarian arteries arise directly from the aorta from a point immediately below the origin of the renal arteries. The right ovarian vein drains into the inferior vena cava and accompanies the right ovarian artery. The left ovarian vein drains into the left renal vein. The lymphatic capillary plexus accompanies the ovarian vessels and therefore drains to the middle lumbar lymph nodes and along the uterine vessels to the sacral nodes.

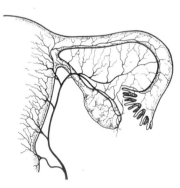

Fig. 5.3 Blood supply to the ovaries formed by anastomosis of uterine and ovarian arteries and veins

Innervation

The ovary receives innervation from both sympathetic and parasympathetic fibres (Fig. 5.4). The sympathetic fibres arise predominantly from

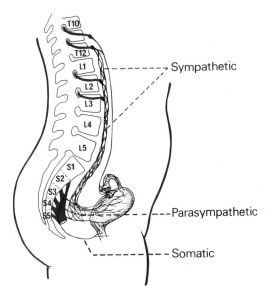

Fig. 5.4 Innervation of the ovaries arises from the lumbar and sacral autonomic outflow

the tenth and eleventh thoracic segments and from the lumbo-sacral region. Parasympathetic fibres from the lumbo-sacral region enter the ovary along the vessels of the utero-tubal anastomosis. Sensory fibres to the ovary arise in the lower thoracic area (T10).

The nerves supplying the smooth muscles of intra-ovarian vessels and fibres also terminate in the theca interna and around Graafian follicles, which are surrounded by structures resembling smooth muscle cells. The nerve supply does not penetrate the basement membrane of follicles.

Contractions occur around the follicles and are mediated by adrenergic α-receptors, whereas relaxation is mediated by β-receptors. The function of the nerve supply remains uncertain but it should be remembered that the suspensory ligaments of the ovary also contain smooth muscle fibres and that contraction of the fibres in the infundibulo-pelvic fold draw the infundibulum of the tube and the ovary together, thus facilitating oocyte entrapment.

Structure of the ovary

- Length 3–5 cm, weight 5–8 g
- Attached to dorsal aspect of broad ligament
- Blood supply from the ovarian artery
- Left ovarian vein drains into left renal vein
- Middle lumbar lymph nodes
- Sympathetic supply from T10 and T11, parasympathetic S2–5, sensory T10

FOLLICULAR DEVELOPMENT IN THE OVARY

The surface of the ovary is covered by a single layer of cuboidal epithelium. The cortex of the ovary contains a large number of oogonia surrounded by follicle cells which become granulosa cells. The remainder of the ovary consists of a mesenchymal core. Most of the ova in the cortex never reach an advanced stage of maturation and become atretic early in follicular development. At any given time, follicles can be seen in various stages of maturation and degeneration (Fig. 5.5). The first stage of development is characterized by enlargement of the

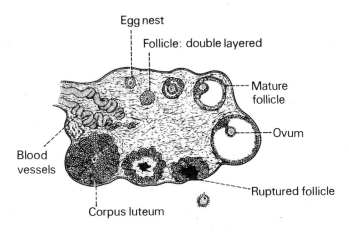

Fig. 5.5 Maturation of the Graafian follicle

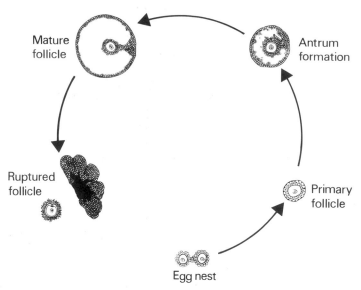

Fig. 5.6   Ovulation and maturation of the corpus luteum

ovum and proliferation of granulosa cells around the ovum with the aggregation of stromal cells to form the thecal cells. The innermost layers of granulosa cells adhere to the ovum and form the **corona radiata.** A fluid-filled space develops in the granulosa cells and a clear layer of gelatinous material collects around the ovum forming the **zona pellucida.** The ovum becomes eccentrically placed and the Graafian follicle assumes its classical mature form. The mesenchymal cells around the follicle become differentiated into two layers forming the **theca interna** and **theca externa.**

As the follicle enlarges, it bulges towards the surface of the ovary and the area under the germinal epithelium thins out. The ovum, with its surrounding investment of granulosa cells, escapes through this area at the time of ovulation.

The cavity of the follicle often fills with blood but, at the same time, the granulosa cells and the theca interna cells undergo changes of luteinization to become filled with yellow carotenoid material. The corpus luteum in its mature form shows intense vascularization and pronounced vacuolization of the theca and granulosa cells, with evidence of hormonal activity. This development reaches its peak approximately 7 days after ovulation and thereafter the corpus luteum regresses unless implantation occurs. This degeneration is characterized by

increasing vacuolization of the granulosa cells and increased quantities of fibrous tissue in the centre of the corpus luteum; which finally develops into a white scar known as the **corpus albicans** (Fig. 5.6).

HORMONAL EVENTS ASSOCIATED WITH OVULATION

The maturation of oocytes, ovulation and the endometrial and tubal changes of the menstrual cycle are all regulated by a series of interactive hormonal changes (Fig. 5.7). The process is initiated by the release of luteinizing hormone-releasing hormone (LH-RH) which is a major neurosecretion produced in the median eminence of the hypothalamus. LH-RH has been isolated in many sites in the central nervous system and may act as a neurotransmitter. The hormone is a decapeptide and is released from axon terminals into the pituitary portal capillaries. It stimulates the release of both follicle-stimulating hormone (FSH) and luteinizing hormone (LH) and can, therefore, be properly designated as **gonadotrophin-releasing hormone** (GnRH) (Fig. 5.7A). The hormone is released in episodic fluctuations but there is no definite association with these surges and LH release. However, there is an increase in the number of surges associated with the higher levels of plasma

Fig. 5.7   The hormonal regulation of ovulation: (**A**) GnRH stimulates the release of gonadotrophins from the pituitary; blood levels of (**B**) gonadotrophins (= LH, FSH), (**C**) oestradiol and (**D**) oestradiol and (**D**) progesterone in the menstrual cycle

LH and there is evidence of a decline in the LH-RH content of the hypothalamus in mid-cycle in women.

The three major hormones involved in reproduction are produced by the anterior lobe of the pituitary gland or adenohypophysis, and include FSH, LH and prolactin. Blood levels of both FSH and LH appear to remain at a relatively constant level in the first half of the cycle. There is a marked surge of LH 24–36 hours before ovulation and a smaller coincidental FSH peak (Fig. 5.7B). Recent detailed studies suggest that the LH surge is composed of two closely proximate surges. A peak

in plasma oestradiol precedes the LH surge and may be the factor that stimulates the hypothalamus to release LH-RH (Fig. 5.7C). Plasma LH and FSH levels are slightly lower in the second half of the cycle than in the pre-ovulatory phase. Pituitary gonadotrophins influence the activity of the hypothalamus by a short-loop feedback system.

Prolactin is secreted by lactotrophs in the anterior pituitary gland. Prolactin levels rise at mid-cycle and remain elevated during the luteal phase, and tend to follow the changes in plasma oestradiol-17β. Prolactin tends to control its own secretion through

Fig. 5.8   Factors regulating the release of prolactin

a short-loop feedback on the hypothalamus, which produces the prolactin-inhibiting factor, dopamine, and probably by the production of a hypothalamic-releasing factor (Fig. 5.8). Oestrogen appears to stimulate prolactin release, and various neuro-transmitters such as serotonin, noradrenaline, histamine, morphine and encephalins also to stimu-late prolactin release by a central action in the brain. Antagonists to dopamine, such as phenothiazine, reserpine and methyl-tyrosine, also stimulate the release of prolactin, whereas dopamine agonists such as bromocriptine have the opposite effect.

THE ACTION OF GONADOTROPHINS

FSH stimulates follicular growth and development and binds exclusively to granulosa cells in the growing follicle. Of the 30 or so follicles that begin to mature in each menstrual cycle, one becomes pre-eminent. The granulosa cells produce oestrogen, which feeds back on the pituitary to suppress FSH release. At the same time, FSH stimulates receptors for LH.

LH stimulates and sustains development of the corpus luteum, and receptors to LH are found in theca and granulosa cells and in the corpus luteum. There is a close interaction between FSH and LH in follicular growth and maturation. The corpus luteum produces progesterone until the structure begins to deteriorate in the late luteal phase (see Fig. 5.6). Prolactin appears to exert a direct effect

on the follicle and to have a role in the initiation and maintenance of luteinization. It stimulates the development of LH receptors and thereby supports the production of high levels of progesterone.

THE ENDOMETRIAL CYCLE

The normal endometrium responds in a cyclical manner to the fluctuations in ovarian steroids. The endometrium consists of three zones and it is the two outer zones that are shed during menstruation (Fig. 5.9).

The basal zone (**zona basalis**) is the thin layer of compact stroma that interdigitates with the myometrium and shows little response to hormonal change. It is not shed at the time of menstruation. The next adjacent zone (**zona spongiosa**) contains the endometrial glands which are lined by columnar epithelial cells surrounded by loose stroma. The surface of the endometrium is covered by a compact layer of epithelial cells (**zona compacta**), which surrounds the ostia of the endometrial glands. The endometrial cycle is divided into four phases:

1. **Menstrual phase.** This occupies the first 4 days of the cycle and results in shedding of the outer two layers of the endometrium. The onset of menstruation is preceded by segmented vaso-constriction of the spiral arteries. This leads to necrosis and shedding of the functional layers of the endometrium. The vascular changes are

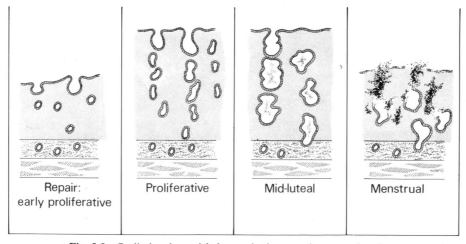

Fig. 5.9 Cyclical endometrial changes in the normal menstrual cycle

associated with a fall in both oestrogen and progesterone levels but the mechanism by which these vascular changes are mediated is still not understood.

2. The **phase of repair.** This phase extends from day 4 to day 7 and is associated with the formation of a new capillary bed arising from the arterial coils, and with regeneration of the epithelial surface.

3. The **follicular, or proliferative phase.** This is the period of maximal growth of the endometrium and is associated with elongation and expansion of the glands, and with stromal development. This phase proceeds from day 7 until the time of ovulation on day 14.

4. The **luteal** or **secretory phase.** This follows ovulation on day 14 and continues until day 28 when menstruation starts again. During this phase the endometrial glands become convoluted and 'saw-toothed' in appearance. The epithelial cells exhibit basal vacuolation, and by day 20 of the cycle there is visible secretion in the cells. The secretion subsequently becomes inspissated and as menstruation approaches there is oedema of the stroma and a pseudodecidual reaction. Within 2 days of menstruation, there is infiltration of the stroma by leucocytes.

It is now clear that luteinization of the follicle can occur in the absence of release of the oocyte. This condition is described as **entrapped ovulation** and is associated with progesterone production and with a normal ovulatory cycle. Histological examination of the endometrium generally enables precise dating of the menstrual cycle and is particularly important in providing evidence of ovulation.

Follicular development/ovulation

- 30 follicles begin development under influence of FSH
- Ovum enlarges, granulosa proliferates and thecal cells formed
- Innermost granulosa cells form corona radiata, separated from others by zona pellucida
- Proliferative phase of endometrial cycle
- Plasma oestradiol peaks (stimulating LH-RH release)
- LH(FSH) surge 24–36 hours prior to ovulation
- Follicle ruptures becoming corpus luteum under influence of LH and prolactin
- Luteal phase of endometrial development

SPERMATOGENESIS

The testis provides a dual function of spermatogenesis and androgen secretion. FSH is predominantly responsible for the stimulation of spermatogenesis and LH for the stimulation of Leydig cells and the production of testosterone (Fig. 5.10). The full maturation of spermatozoa takes 16 days and all phases of maturation can be seen in the testis. The spermatogonia divide and give rise to primary spermatocytes which have a diploid number of chromosomes. These cells undergo maturation division to secondary spermatocytes and finally reduction division to form the haploid spermatids which develop into the mature spermatozoa.

Structure of the spermatozoon

The spermatozoon consists of a head, neck and tail (Fig. 5.11). The entire structure is enveloped in a plasma membrane. The head is flattened and ovoid

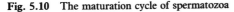

Fig. 5.10 The maturation cycle of spermatozoa

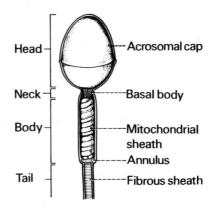

Fig. 5.11 Structure of the mature spermatozoon

in shape and is covered by the acrosomal cap, which contains lysins.

The nucleus is densely packed with the genetic material of the sperm. The neck contains two centrioles which form the beginning of the tail while the body contains a coiled helix of mitochondria which provides the 'power house'. The tail consists of a central core of two longitudinal fibres. This structure is surrounded by nine pairs of fibres which terminate at various points until a single ovoid filament remains. These contractile fibres propel the spermatozoa.

Seminal plasma

Spermatozoa carry little nutritional reserve and therefore depend on seminal plasma for nutritional support. Seminal plasma originates from the prostate, seminal vesicles, the epididymis, the vas deferens and the bulbo-urethral glands. There is a high concentration of fructose, which is the major source of energy for spermatozoa. The plasma also contains high concentrations of amino acids, particularly glutamic acid, and several unique amines such as spermine and spermidine. The seminal plasma also contains high concentrations of prostaglandins, which have a potent stimulatory effect on the uterine musculature. Normal semen clots shortly after ejaculation but reliquefies within 30 minutes due to fibrinolytic activity during this period.

Spermatogenesis

- Maturation of spermatozoa takes 16 days
- Spermatogonia form primary (diploid) spermatocytes
- Secondary spermatocytes form (haploid) spermatids
- Spermatids form spermatozoa

FERTILIZATION

The process of fertilization involves the fusion of the male and female gametes to produce the diploid genetic complement from the genes of both partners.

Sperm transport

Following the deposition of semen near the cervical os migration of sperm occurs rapidly into the cervical mucus. The speed of this migration depends on the presence of receptive mucus in mid-cycle. During the luteal phase, the mucus is not receptive to sperm invasion and therefore very few spermatozoa reach the uterine cavity. Under favourable circumstances, sperm migrate at a rate of 6 mm/min. This is much faster than could be explained by the motility of the sperm and must therefore also be dependent on active support within the uterine cavity. Only motile spermatozoa reach the fimbriated end of the tube.

Capacitation

During their passage through the Fallopian tube the sperm undergo the final stage in maturation (capacitation), which enables penetration of the zona pellucida. It seems likely that these changes are enzyme-induced and enzymes such as β-amylase or β-glucuronidase may act on the membranes of the spermatozoa to expose receptor sites involved in sperm penetration. In addition, various other factors that may be important in capacitation have been identified such as the removal of cholesterol from the plasma membrane, and the presence of α- and β-adrenergic receptors on the spermatozoa. Until recently, it was thought that capacitation occurred only in vivo in the Fallopian tube. However, it can also be induced in vitro by apparently non-specific effects of relatively simple culture solutions.

Inhibitory substances in the plasma of the cauda epididymis and in seminal plasma can prevent capacitation, and these substances also occur in the lower reaches of the female genital tract. It seems likely that these substances protect the sperm until shortly before fusion with the oocyte.

Fertilization

A small number of spermatozoa reach the oocyte in the ampulla of the tube and surround the zona pellucida. The adherence of the sperm to the oocyte initiates the **acrosome reaction**, which involves the loss of plasma membrane over the acrosomal cap (Fig. 5.12A). This process allows the release of lytic enzymes which facilitate penetration of the oocyte membrane. The nucleus of the head passes into the cytoplasm of the oocyte — a process known as **syngamy** (Fig. 5.12B). Fertilization is usually monospermic and the second polar body is expelled

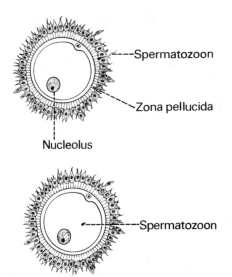

Fig. 5.12 (**A**) Adherence of the sperm to the oocyte initiates the acrosome reaction; (**B**) Syngamy involves the passage of the nucleus of the sperm head into the cytoplasm of the oocyte, with the formation of the zygote

from the **zygote** as soon as the sperm enters the egg. The fusion of maternal and paternal chromosomes is followed almost immediately by the first cleavage division.

During the 36 hours after fertilization, the conceptus is transported through the tube by muscular peristaltic action. The egg undergoes cleavage and at the 16-cell stage becomes a solid ball of cells known as a **morula** and then a fluid-filled cavity develops to form the **blastocyst** (Fig. 5.13). Six days after ovulation, the embryonic pole of the blastocyst attaches itself to the endometrium, usually near to the midportion of the uterine fundus. By the seventh day, the blastocyst has penetrated deeply into the endometrium.

Endometrial cells are destroyed by the cytotrophoblast and the cells are incorporated by fusion and phagocytosis into the trophoblast. The endometrial stromal cells become large and pale and this is known as the **decidual reaction**. Thus, the process of fertilization and implantation is now complete.

Fertilization

> - Sperm migration inhibited by luteal phase cervical mucus
> - Sperm undergo capacitation in the tube
> - Adherence of sperm to oocyte initiates acrosome reaction
> - Chromosomes fuse and second polar body expelled
> - First cleavage division occurs

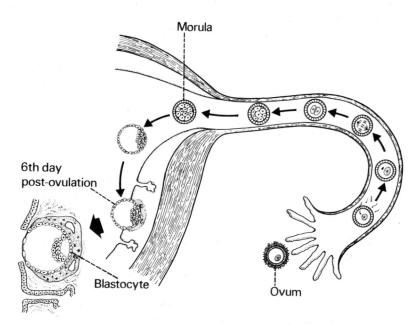

Fig. 5.13 Stages of development from fertilization to implantation

THE PHYSIOLOGY OF COITUS

Normal sexual arousal has been described in four levels in both men and women. These levels consist of excitement, plateau, orgasmic and resolution phases. In the male, the excitement phase results in compression of the venous channels of the penis resulting in erection which is mediated through the parasympathetic plexus through S2 and S3. During the plateau phase, the penis remains engorged and the testes increase in size with elevation of the testes and scrotum. Secretion of the bulbo-urethral glands results in the appearance of a clear fluid at the urethral meatus. These changes are accompanied by general systemic features including carpopedal spasm, increased skeletal muscle tension, hyper-ventilation and tachycardia (Fig. 5.14).

The orgasmic phase is induced by stimulation of the glans penis and by movement of penile skin on the penile shaft. There are reflex contractions of the bulbocavernosus and ischiocavernosus muscles and ejaculation of semen in a series of spurts. Specific musculo-skeletal activity occurs, which is charac-terized by penile thrusting. The systemic changes of tachycardia and rapid respiration persist.

During the resolution phase, penile erection rapidly subsides as does the hyperventilation and tachycardia. There is a marked sweating reaction in some 30–40% of individuals. During this phase, the male becomes refractory to further stimulation. The plateau phase may be prolonged if ejaculation does not occur.

In the female, the excitement phase involves nipple and clitoral erection, vaginal lubrication, which results partly from transudation through the vaginal walls and partly from secretions from Batholin's glands, thickening and congestion of the labia majora and the labia minora and engorgement of the uterus. Stimulation of the clitoris and the labia results in progression to the orgasmic platform with narrowing of the outer third of the vagina and ballooning of the vaginal vault. The vaginal walls become congested and purplish in colour and there is a marked increase in vaginal blood flow. During orgasm, the clitoris retracts behind the pubic symphysis and a succession of contractions occur in the vaginal walls and pelvic floor approximately every second for several seconds. At the same time, there is an increase in pulse rate, hyperventilation and specific skeletal muscular contractions. Blood pressure rises and there is some diminution of consciousness. Both intravaginal and intra-uterine pressure rise during orgasm. The plateau phase may be sustained in the female and result in multiple

Fig. 5.14 Pulse rate changes during coitus

orgasm. Following orgasm, resolution of the congestion of the pelvic organs occurs rapidly although the tachycardia and hypertension accompanied by a sweating reaction may persist.

Factors which determine human sexuality are far more complex than the simple process of arousal by clitoral or penile stimulation. Although the frequency of intercourse and orgasm declines with age, this is in part mediated by the loss of interest in the partners. The female remains capable of orgasm until late in life but this behaviour is substantially determined by the interest of the male partner. Sexual interest and performance also declines with age in the male and the older male requires more time to achieve excitement and erection. Ejaculation may become less frequent and forceful.

Common sexual problems will be discussed in a separate chapter.

6. Placental and fetal growth and development

EARLY PLACENTAL DEVELOPMENT

After fertilization and egg cleavage, the morula is transformed into a blastocyst by the formation of a fluid-filled cavity within the ball of cells.

The outer layer of the blastocyst consists of primitive cytotrophoblast, and by day 7 the blastocyst penetrates the endometrium as a result of trophoblastic invasion (Fig. 6.1). The outer layer of trophoblast becomes a syncytium. In response to contact with the syncytiotrophoblast, the endometrial stromal cells become large and pale, a process known as the decidual reaction, and endometrial cells are phagocytosed by the trophoblastic cells.

The nature and function of the decidual reaction remain uncertain but it seems likely that the decidual cells both limit the invasion of trophoblastic cells and serve an initial nutritional function for the developing placenta.

During development of the placenta, cords of cytotrophoblast or Langhans' cells grow down to the basal layers of decidua and penetrate some of the endometrial venules and capillaries. The formation of lacunae filled with maternal blood presages the development of the intervillous space.

The invading cords of trophoblast form the primary villi, which later branch to form secondary villi and, subsequently, free-floating tertiary villi. The central core of these villi is penetrated by a column of mesoblastic cells which become the capillary network of the villi. The body stalk, which attaches the developing fetus to the placenta, forms the umbilical vessels, which advance onto the villi to join the villous capillaries and establish the placental circulation.

Although trophoblastic cells surround the original blastocyst, the area which develops into the placenta becomes thickened and extensively branched and is known as the **chorion frondosum**. However, in the area which subsequently expands to form the outer layer of the fetal membranes, the villi become atrophic and the surface smooth; this structure forms the **chorion laeve** (Fig. 6.2). The decidua underlying the placenta is known as **decidua basalis** and the decidua between the membranes and the myometrium as **decidua capsularis**.

Endometrium

Inner cell mass

Trophoblast

Blastocyst cavity

Fig. 6.1 Implantation of the blastocyst

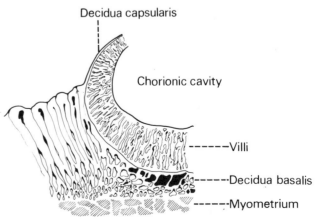

Decidua capsularis

Chorionic cavity

Villi

Decidua basalis

Myometrium

Fig. 6.2 Development of early placentation

FURTHER PLACENTAL DEVELOPMENT

By 6 weeks after ovulation, the trophoblast has invaded some 40–60 spiral arterioles. Blood from the maternal vasculature pushes the free-floating secondary and tertiary capillaries into a tent-shaped 'maternal cotyledon'. The tents are held down to the basal plate of the decidua by anchoring villi, and the blood from arterioles spurts towards the chorionic plate and then returns to drain through maternal veins in the basal plate. There are eventually about 12 large maternal cotyledons and 40–50 smaller ones.

Placental development

- Blastocyst penetrates endometrium by day 7
- Primary villi formed by cords of cytotrophoblast invading decidua
- The chorion frondosum and underlying decidua basalis form the placenta
- The chorion laeve forms the membranes

THE VILLUS

Despite the arrangement of villi into maternal cotyledons, the functional unit of the placenta remains the stem villus or fetal cotyledon (Fig. 6.3). There are initially about 200 stem villi arising from the chorion frondosum. About 150 of these struc-

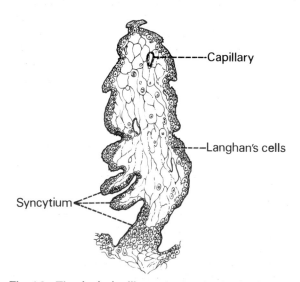

Fig. 6.3 The chorionic villus as the functional unit of the placenta

tures are compressed at the periphery of the major maternal vascular units and become relatively functionless, leaving a dozen or so large cotyledons, and 40–50 smaller ones are left as the active units of placental function.

The estimated surface area of the chorionic villi in the mature placenta is approximately 11 square metres. The surface area is enlarged by the presence of numerous microvilli. The core of the villus consists of a stroma of closely packed spindle-shaped fibroblasts and branching capillaries (Fig. 6.5B). The stroma also contains phagocytic cells known as Hofbauer cells. In early pregnancy, the villi are covered by an outer layer of syncytiotrophoblast and an inner layer of cytotrophoblast. As pregnancy advances, the cytotrophoblast disappears until only a thin layer of syncytiotrophoblast remains. The formation of clusters of syncytial cells, known as **syncytial knots,** and the reappearance of cytotrophoblast in late pregnancy, is probably the result of hypoxia.

STRUCTURE OF THE UMBILICAL CORD

The umbilical cord contains two arteries and one vein (Fig. 6.4). The two arteries carry deoxygenated blood from the fetus to the placenta and the oxygenated blood returns to the fetus via the umbilical vein. Absence of one artery occurs in about 1 in 200 deliveries and is associated with a 10–15% incidence of cardiovascular anomalies. The vessels are surrounded by a hydrophilic mucopolysaccharide known as Wharton's jelly, and the outer layer covering the cord consists of amniotic epithelium. Cord length varies between 30 and 90 cm. The vessels grow in a helical shape, which has the functional advantage of protecting the patency of the vessels by absorbing torsion without the risk of kinking or snarling of the vessels. The few measurements that have been made of cord pressures in situ indicate that the arterial pressure is around 70 mmHg systolic and 60 mmHg diastolic, and the venous pressure is exceptionally high at approximately 25 mmHg. This high pressure also tends to preserve the integrity of cord blood flow and indicates that pressure within the villus capillaries must be in excess of the cord venous pressures. The cord vessels often contain a false knot consisting of a refolding of the arteries; occasionally, blood flow is threatened by a

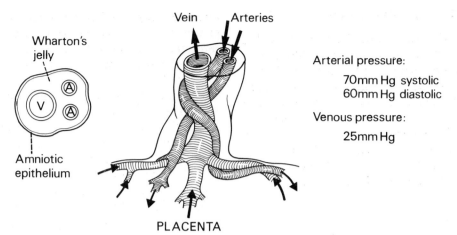

Fig. 6.4 Vascular structure of the umbilical cord: transverse section (left) shows two arteries carrying de-oxygenated blood and one vein carrying oxygenated blood

true knot. In a full-term fetus, the blood flow in the cord is approximately 350 ml/min.

PLACENTAL BLOOD FLOW

Trophoblasts invade the maternal arterioles early in pregnancy. Blood enters the intervillous space from the uterine arterioles and spurts towards the chorionic

Fig. 6.5 (**A**) Venous and arterial circulation in the chorio-decidual vascular bed; (**B**) branching of capillary in a terminal villus

plate and then returns to the uterine venous openings in the placental bed (Fig. 6.5A). The pressure in the intervillous space is estimated at 10 mmHg. Assessments of uterine blood flow indicate values of 500–750 ml/min.

FACTORS WHICH INFLUENCE UTERINE BLOOD FLOW

The regulation of uterine blood flow is of critical importance to the welfare of the fetus and chronic impairment of flow leads to growth retardation and, in severe circumstances, may result in fetal death. Factors which adversely influence uterine blood flow include haemorrhage, uterine contractions, adrenaline and noradrenaline. Angiotensin II increases uterine blood flow in physiological levels as a result of the direct effect on placental tissue in promoting the local release of vasodilator prostaglandins. In high concentrations it produces vasoconstriction.

Lying in the supine position in late pregnancy may also reduce uterine blood flow by producing compression of the aorta and inferior vena cava.

The placenta

- Stem villi or fetal cotyledons form the functional unit (40–50)
- Surface area 11 m^2
- Blood flow through the cord is 350 ml/min with an arterial pressure of 70/60 mmHg
- Glucose is the main energy source

PLACENTAL TRANSFER

The placenta plays an essential role in growth and development in the fetus and in regulating maternal adaption to pregnancy.

Transfer of materials across the placental membrane is governed by molecular weight, solubility and the ionic charge of the substance involved. Actual transfer is achieved by simple diffusion, facilitated diffusion, active transport and pinocytosis (Fig. 6.6).

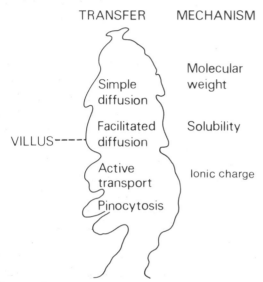

TRANSFER   MECHANISM

Simple diffusion

Molecular weight

Facilitated diffusion

Solubility

VILLUS

Active transport

Ionic charge

Pinocytosis

Fig. 6.6 Factors which determine transfer of nutrients and gases across the placenta.

Simple diffusion

Transfer between maternal and fetal blood is regulated by the trophoblast, and it must be remembered that the lining of the chorionic villus is not a simple semipermeable membrane but consists of a metabolically active cellular layer.

Although there are exceptions, small molecules generally cross the placenta by simple diffusion and movement is determined by chemical or electrochemical gradients. The quantity of solute transferred is described by the Fick diffusion equation:

$$\frac{Q}{t} = \frac{KA\,(C^1 - C^2)}{L}$$

where Q/t is the quantity transferred per unit time,

K is a diffusion constant for the particular substance, A is the total surface area available and C^1 and C^2 indicate the difference in concentrations of solute; L represents the thickness of the membrane. This method is applicable particularly to transfer of gases although the gradient of oxygen, for example, is substantially increased by the fact that oxygen is extracted by the placenta and myometrium.

Facilitated diffusion

Some compounds are transported across the placenta at rates that are considerably enhanced above the rate that would be anticipated by simple diffusion. Transport always occurs in favour of the gradient but at an accelerated rate. This system pertains to glucose transport and can only be explained on the basis of a specific transport system.

Active transport

Transfer against a chemical gradient occurs with some compounds and must involve an active transport system which is energy dependent. This process occurs with essential amino acids and water-soluble vitamins and can be demonstrated by the presence of higher concentrations of the compound in fetal blood as compared with maternal blood. Such transfer mechanisms can be inhibited by cell poisons and are stereo specific.

Pinocytosis

Transfer of large molecular weight compounds is known to occur and involves ingestion or engulfing of microdroplets of material into the cytoplasm of the trophoblast. This process applies to the transfer of globulins, phospholipids and lipoproteins and is of particular importance in the transfer of immunologically active material. The major source of materials for protein synthesis and for nutrition in the fetus comes from the transfer of amino acids.

Transport of intact cells

Fetal red cells are commonly seen in the maternal circulation, particularly following delivery. Although some maternal red cells may be found in the fetal circulation, this is much less common, as the pressure gradient favours movement from the relatively high pressure of the fetal capillaries to the low pressure environment of the intervillous space.

PLACENTAL FUNCTION

The placenta has three major functions:

1. Gaseous exchange
2. Fetal nutrition and removal of waste products
3. Endocrine function

1. Gaseous exchange

As the transfer of gases occurs by simple diffusion, the major determinants of gaseous exchange are the efficiency of the fetal and maternal circulations, the surface area of the placenta and the thickness of the placental membrane.

Oxygen transfer

The average difference in oxygen tension across the placenta is about 20 mmHg and this gradient favours the transfer of oxygen from maternal to fetal circulation. Fetal haemoglobin has a higher affinity for oxygen than does adult haemoglobin, and haemoglobin concentration is higher in the fetus. All these factors favour the rapid uptake of oxygen by the fetus at relatively low oxygen tensions. The extent to which haemoglobin can be saturated by oxygen is affected by hydrogen ion concentration, the increase of which in deoxygenated blood favours the release of maternal oxygen in the feto-placental bed. The oxygen dissociation curve is shifted to the right by increases in H^+ ion concentration, pCO_2 and temperature, and this is known as the **Bohr effect.** Oxygen is predominantly transported in the form of oxyhaemoglobin as there is little free oxygen in solution in blood.

Carbon dioxide transfer

Carbon dioxide is readily soluble in blood and transfers rapidly across the placenta. The partial pressure difference is about 5 mmHg. Transport of carbon dioxide may occur in solution as either bicarbonate or carbonic acid. It is also transported as carbaminohaemoglobin. The binding of CO_2 to haemoglobin to form carbaminohaemoglobin is affected by factors which influence oxygen release and, thus, an increase in carbaminohaemoglobin results in the release of oxygen. This is known as the **Haldane effect.**

2. Fetal nutrition and removal of waste products

Carbohydrate metabolism

Glucose transferred from the maternal circulation provides the major substrate for oxidative metabolism in the placenta. Facilitated diffusion allows for rapid transfer of glucose across the placenta. Animal studies have shown that transfer of sugars is selective; generally, glucose and the monosaccharides cross the placenta readily whereas the placenta is virtually impermeable to disaccharides such as sucrose, maltose and lactose. The placenta is also impermeable to the sugar alcohols such as sorbitol, mannitol, deleitol and meso-inositol.

In the fasting, normal pregnant woman, blood glucose achieves a concentration of approximately 70 mg/100 ml in the maternal venous circulation and 60 mg/100 ml in the fetal cord venous blood. Infusion of glucose into the maternal circulation results in a parallel increase in both maternal and fetal blood glucose levels until the fetal levels reach 190 mg/100 ml, when no further increase occurs regardless of the values in the maternal circulation.

The hormones that are important in glucose homeostasis, namely insulin, glucagon, human placental lactogen and growth hormone, do not cross the placenta and maternal glucose levels appear to be the major regulatory factor in fetal glucose metabolism. The placenta itself utilizes glucose and may retain as much as half of the glucose that enters the tissues. In mid-pregnancy, approximately 70% of this glucose is metabolized by glycolysis, 10% via the pentose phosphate pathway, and the remainder is stored by glycogen and lipid synthesis. By full term, the rate of placental glucose utilization has fallen by 30%. Glycogen storage occurs in the placenta and in the fetal liver, muscle and heart. Glycogen levels in the fetal liver increase steadily throughout pregnancy and are twice the adult levels at full term. A rapid fall to adult levels occurs within the first few hours of life.

The reserves are of particular importance in providing an energy source in the asphyxiated fetus when anaerobic glycolysis is activated.

Fat metabolism

Fats are insoluble in water and are therefore transported in blood either as free fatty acids bound to albumin, or as lipoproteins consisting of triglyceride attached to other lipids or proteins, and packaged in chylomicra.

The fetus needs fatty acids for cell membrane construction and for deposition in the adipose tissue. This is particularly important as a source of energy in the immediate neonatal period.

There is evidence that free fatty acids cross the placenta and that this transfer is not selective. Essential fatty acids are also transferred from the maternal circulation and evidence suggests that the placenta has the ability to convert linoleic acid to arachidonic acid. Starvation of the mother increases mobilization of triglycerides in the fetus.

Protein metabolism

Fetal protein is synthesized by the fetus from free amino acids transported across the placenta against a concentration gradient. The concentration of free amino acids in the fetus is higher than in the maternal circulation.

The placenta takes no part in the synthesis of fetal proteins although it does synthesize some protein hormones which are transferred into the maternal circulation, namely, chorionic gonadotrophin and human placental lactogen. By full term, the human fetus has accumulated some 500 g of protein.

Immunoglobulins are synthesized by fetal lymphoid tissue and IgM first appears in the fetal circulation by 20 weeks gestation, followed by IgA and finally IgG. IgG is the only gammaglobulin to be transferred across the placenta and this appears to be selective for homologous IgG. There is no evidence of placental transfer of growth-promoting hormones.

Urea and ammonia

Urea concentration is higher in the fetus than in the mother by a margin of about 0.5 mmol/l and the rate of clearance across the placenta is approximately 0.54 (mg/min)/kg fetal weight at term. It has been suggested that protein provides about 25% of the energy source for the fetus. Ammonia transfers readily across the placenta and it is believed that maternal ammonia may provide a source of some fetal nitrogen.

3. Placental hormone production

The placenta plays a major role as an endocrine organ and is responsible for the production of both protein and steroid hormones. The fetus is also involved in many of the processes of hormone production and in this capacity the conceptus functions as a feto-placental unit.

Protein hormones

Chorionic gonadotrophin. Human chorionic gonadotrophin (hCG) is produced by trophoblast and has a structure which is chemically very similar to that of luteinizing hormone. It is a glycoprotein with two non-identical alpha and beta subunits. hCG reaches a peak in maternal urine and blood between 7 and 8 weeks of pregnancy. A small subpeak occurs between 32 and 36 weeks. The beta subunit of hCG can be detected in plasma within 7 days of conception.

The only known function of the hormone appears to be the maintenance of the corpus luteum of pregnancy. The hormone is measured by agglutination inhibition techniques using coated red cells or latex particles and forms the basis of the standard pregnancy test. This will be positive in urine by 2 weeks after the period is missed in 97% of pregnant women.

Human placental lactogen. Human placental lactogen (hPL) or chorionic somatomammotrophin is a peptide hormone with a molecular weight of 22 000 which is chemically similar to growth hormone. It is produced by syncytiotrophoblast, and plasma hPL levels rise steadily throughout pregnancy (Fig. 6.7). The function of the hormone remains uncertain although it does appear to reduce blood glucose levels and to increase levels of free fatty acids and insulin.

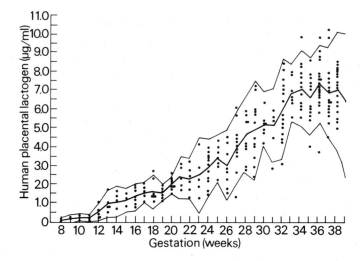

Fig. 6.7 Human placental lactogen levels in plasma in relation to gestational age: the graph shows the mean and two standard deviations

Plasma hPL levels have been extensively used in the assessment of placental function. In the last 2 weeks of gestation the levels in serum fall. The hormone is measured by radioimmunoassay.

Steroid hormones

Progesterone. The placenta becomes the major source of progesterone production by the 17th week of pregnancy and the biosynthesis of progesterone is mainly dependent on the supply of maternal cholesterol. In maternal plasma, 90% of progesterone is bound to protein and is metabolized in the liver and kidneys. Some 10 to 15% of progesterone is excreted in urine as pregnanediol. The placenta produces about 350 mg progesterone per day by full term, and plasma progesterone levels increase throughout pregnancy to achieve values around 150 mg/ml by full term. The measurement of urinary pregnanediol or plasma progesterone has been used as a method of assessing placental function but has not been proved to be particularly useful as the scatter of hormonal values is so wide that the assessment of abnormality is obscured.

Oestrogens. Over 20 different oestrogens have been identified in the urine of pregnant women but the major oestrogens are oestrone, oestradiol-17 and oestriol. The largest increase in oestrogen excretion occurs in oestriol. Whereas oestrone excretion increases one-hundred-fold, urinary

Fig. 6.8 Formation of oestriol by the feto-placental unit

oestriol increases one-thousand-fold. The ovary makes only a minimal contribution to this increase as the placenta is the major source of oestrogen in pregnancy. The substrate for oestriol production comes from the fetal adrenal gland (Fig. 6.8). Dehydroepiandrosterone (DHEA) synthesized in the fetal adrenal cortex passes to the fetal liver where it is 16 (OH) hydroxylated. Conjugation of these precursors with phospho-adenosyl phospho-sulphate aids solubility, and active sulphatase activity in the placenta results in the release of free oestriol. Oestradiol and oestrone are directly synthesized by the syncytiotrophoblast. Urinary and plasma oestriol levels increase progressively throughout pregnancy until 38 weeks gestation when some fall occurs. Oestriol excretion falls as a result of fetal adrenal suppression. This will occur following the administration of corticosteroid to the mother, or in the absence of the fetal adrenal gland as seen in anencephaly. It may also occur in the presence of placental failure, and excretion therefore forms the basis of a placental function test.

Corticosteroids. There is little evidence that the placenta produces corticosteroids. In the presence of Addison's disease or following adrenalectomy, 17-hydroxy-corticosteroids and aldosterone disappear from the maternal urine. In normal pregnancy, there is a substantial increase in cortisol production and this is at least partly due to the raised levels of transcortin in the blood, so that the capacity for binding cortisol increases substantially.

Placental function

- Oxygen transfer to fetus occurs by simple diffusion promoted by a 20 mmHg difference in O_2 tension, the higher O_2 affinity of fetal Hb and the Bohr effect
- Carbon dioxide transfer to mother by simple diffusion
- Glucose transport by facilitated diffusion
- Fats transported by pinocytosis of free fatty acids-albumin or as lipoproteins
- Amino-acids by active transport
- Synthesis of some fatty acids
- Immunoglobulin transfer (IgG only) by pinocytosis
- Hormone production including hCG, progesterone and various oestrogens (with the fetus)

FETAL DEVELOPMENT

Growth

Up to 10 weeks gestation, a massive increase in cell numbers occurs in the developing embryo but the actual gain in weight is small. Thereafter, a rapid increase occurs until the full-term fetus achieves a weight of about 3.5 kg (Figs 6.9 and 6.10). Protein accumulation occurs in the fetus throughout pregnancy but fetal adipose tissue does not reach significant levels in the subcutaneous and intra-abdominal stores until after 28 weeks. There is reduction in the fetal growth rate towards term. Actual growth rate is determined by a variety of factors including the efficiency of the placenta, the adequacy of the utero-placental blood flow and inherent genetic factors in the fetus.

Cardiovascular system

The heart develops initially as a single tube and by 4–5 weeks gestation a heartbeat is present at a rate of 65 beats per minute. The definitive circulation has developed by 11 weeks gestation and the heart rate increases to around 140 beats per minute. In the mature fetal circulation, about 40% of the venous

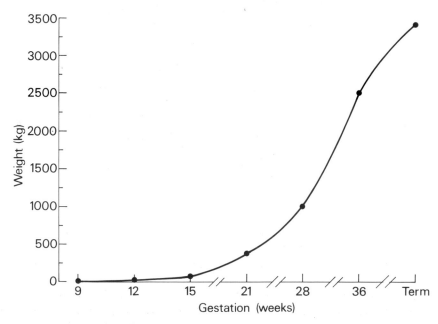

Fig. 6.9 Fetal weight and gestational age

Fig. 6.10 Fetal crown-rump (C-R) length and gestational age

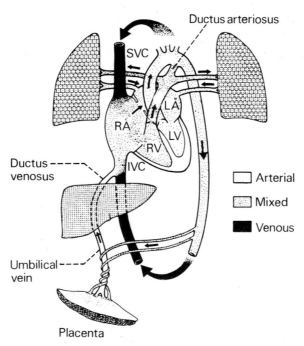

Fig. 6.11 Fetal circulation showing the distribution of arterial, venous and mixed blood

return entering the right atrium flows directly into the left atrium through the foramen ovale (Fig. 6.11). Blood pumped from the right atrium into the right ventricle is expelled into the pulmonary artery where it passes either into the aorta via the ductus arteriosus or into the pulmonary vessels.

The fetal cardiac output is estimated to be 200 ml/kg body weight per minute. Unlike the adult, fetal cardiac output is entirely dependent on heart rate and not on stroke volume. Autonomic control of the fetal heart matures during the third trimester and parasympathetic vagal tonus tends to reduce the basal fetal heart rate.

The fetal respiratory system

There is evidence that fetal respiration is present from 12 weeks onwards and that, by 34 weeks gestation, respiration occurs at a rate of 40–60 movements/minute with intervening periods of apnoea. These respiratory movements are shallow but occasional gasps occur which result in a larger flow of fluid into the bronchial tree. Fetal breathing is stimulated by hypercapnia but hypoxia tends to reduce breathing movements whilst increasing gasping behaviour. Fetal respiration is inhibited by maternal smoking.

The fetal pulmonary alveoli are lined by two main types of alveolar epithelial cells. Gaseous exchange occurs across the type I cells and the type II cells secrete phospholipid surfactant, which is necessary to prevent the collapse of the alveoli in neonatal life (Fig. 6.12). The principal surfactants are lecithin and sphingomyelin and production of lecithin begins to increase at about 36 weeks gestation. Measurement of lecithin in amniotic fluid provides a useful method of assessing fetal lung maturity.

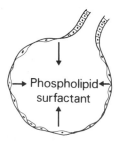

Fig. 6.12   Secretion of phospholipid into the alveoli determines lung expansion at birth

Fetal gastrointestinal tract

Mucosal glands appear in the gut by 16–20 weeks gestation, and by 26 weeks most of the digestive enzymes are present. Amylase does not appear until after birth. The fetus swallows amniotic fluid and peristaltic gut movement is established by mid-pregnancy. The digestion of cells and protein in amniotic fluid results in the formation of fetal faeces or meconium. Meconium normally remains in the gut and appears in the amniotic fluid only under conditions of fetal stress and asphyxia.

The fetal kidney

Functional renal corpuscles first appear in the juxta-glomerular zone of the renal cortex at 22 weeks gestation and filtration begins at this time. The formation of the kidney is complete by 36 weeks gestation. Glomerular filtration increases towards term as the number of glomeruli increase and the fetal blood pressure rises.

In the fetus, only 2% of the cardiac output perfuses the kidneys. The fetal renal tubules are capable of active transport before any glomerular filtrate is received and thus some urine may be produced within the tubules before glomerular filtration starts. The efficiency of tubular reabsorption is low and glucose in the fetal circulation spills into fetal urine at levels as low as 4.2 mmol/1.

Fetal urine makes a significant contribution to the formation of amniotic fluid.

Special senses

The fetus will respond to sound by movement of the limbs and trunk, and by the alteration of fetal heart rate. Visual perception is more difficult to assess but it seems likely that some perception to light develops in late pregnancy.

Fetal development

- 5 weeks: fetal heartbeat present
- 11 weeks: fetal circulation developed
- 12 weeks: fetal respiratory movements
- 20 weeks: mucosal glands appear in gut, peristalsis established
- 22 weeks: functional renal corpuscles and filtration
- 26 weeks: most digestive enzymes present
- 28 weeks onwards: autonomic control starts to slow basal heart rate
- 36 weeks: lecithin rises

AMNIOTIC FLUID

The formation of amniotic fluid

The amniotic sac develops early in pregnancy and has been identified in the human embryo as early as 7 days. The first signs of the development of the amniotic cavity can be seen in the inner cell mass of the blastocyst.

Early in pregnancy, amniotic fluid is probably a dialysate of fetal and maternal extracellular compartments. There is some evidence, for example, that up to 24 weeks gestation, when keratinization begins, significant transfer of water may occur across fetal skin. In the last half of pregnancy, fetal urine provides a significant contribution to amniotic fluid volume. Certainly, the absence of kidneys, renal agenesis, in the fetus is invariably associated with minimal amniotic fluid volume — **oligohydramnios.**

The role of the fetus in regulation of amniotic fluid volume is poorly understood, but the fetus swallows amniotic fluid, absorbs it in the gut and later excretes urine into the amniotic sac (Fig. 6.13). Congenital abnormalities which impair the ability to swallow are commonly associated with excessive amniotic fluid volume or **polyhydramnios.**

In summary, amniotic fluid is formed by secretion of fluid from amnion and fetal skin and from the passage of fetal urine into the amniotic sac. Circulation of amniotic fluid occurs by reabsorption of fluid through the fetal gut, skin and amnion.

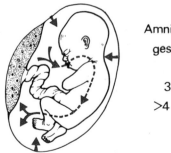

Amniotic fluid volume:	
gestation	ml
8 weeks	5-10
38 weeks	1000
>42 weeks	<300

Fig. 6.13 Amniotic fluid secreted in the amnion is swallowed by the fetus, absorbed through the gut and excreted in fetal urine

Amniotic fluid volume

By 8 weeks gestation, 5–10 ml of amniotic fluid has accumulated; thereafter the volume increases rapidly in proportion to fetal growth and gestational age to a maximum volume of 1000 ml at 38 weeks gestation. Subsequently, serial diminution in the amount of fluid takes place, so that after 42 weeks the mean volume falls below 300 ml.

Clinical significance of amniotic fluid volume

The fetus exerts a large influence on this fluid space through urine production and swallowing.

Diminution of amniotic fluid volume is associated with reduced placental function, and this is seen particularly in pre-eclampsia and essential hypertension.

Polyhydramnios, or excessive fluid, is commonly associated with oesophageal or duodenal atresia and with central nervous system abnormalities such as anencephaly and hydrocephaly, which interfere with swallowing. In approximately 30% of all cases of polyhydramnios there is a significant congenital anomaly. The distribution of such anomalies is as follows in order of frequency:

- Anencephaly
- Oesophageal atresia
- Duodenal atresia
- Iniencephaly
- Hydrocephaly
- Diaphragmatic hernia

Cells of the amniotic fluid

Amniotic fluid contains two distinct types of cells. The first group is derived from the fetus, the second from the amnion. Cells of fetal origin are larger and more likely to be anucleate. Those originating from the amnion are smaller, with a prominent nucleolus contained within the vesicular nucleus, and are found in proportionately greater numbers prior to the 32nd week (Fig. 6.14).

In addition to these groupings by cellular morphological criteria, two other distinct populations of cells in the amniotic fluid are differentiated by haematoxylin and eosin staining. The relative numbers of each cell type vary depending upon the duration of pregnancy. Cells which stain with eosin are most prominent early in gestation, but after the 38th week compose less than 30% of the total cell

Prominent nucleus   Microtubules on surface   Smooth and microtubular surfaces

Fig. 6.14   Scanning electron microscope image of amniotic fluid cells showing prominent nuclei and surface microtubules

population. These are probably the cells derived from the amnion.

Basophilic cells increase in number as pregnancy progresses but also tend to decrease after the 38th week. The presence of these cells in large numbers has been correlated with the female fetus, and the fetal vagina is felt to be a possible source.

After 38 weeks gestation, a large number of eosinophilic anucleate polygonal cells appear. These cells stain orange with Nile blue sulphate and are thought to be derived from maturing fetal sebaceous glands.

Clinical value of tests on amniotic fluid

Both the biochemical and cytological components of amniotic fluid are used for a variety of clinical estimations. Amniotic fluid can be obtained after

Fig. 6.15   Amniotic fluid is obtained by amniocentesis under ultrasound control

16 weeks gestation by **amniocentesis**, which involves the insertion of a fine needle through the anterior abdominal wall into the amniotic sac and the withdrawal of amniotic fluid (Fig. 6.15). This is performed under local anaesthetic, after localization of the placenta by ultrasound in order to avoid any damage from the procedure. The following diagnostic procedures are currently employed in clinical practice.

Prenatal diagnosis

Alphafetoprotein can be measured in amniotic fluid and this is useful in the prenatal diagnosis of neural tube defects — particularly anencephaly and open spina bifida. Elevated levels may also be associated with other abnormalities, such as exomphalos, ectopia vesicae and fetal nephrotic syndrome.

Chromosomal abnormalities and sex-linked diseases

The fetal karyotype can be determined on cells cultured from amniotic fluid. This can reveal chromosome abnormalities such as Down's syndrome, trisomy 21, and will also reveal the sex of the fetus which may be useful in the management of patients with sex-linked disorders such as haemophilia and muscular dystrophy.

Metabolic disorders

There are a large number of metabolic disorders, all fairly rare, such as Tay Sach's disease and galactosaemia, which can be diagnosed in utero from tests on amniotic fluid cells.

Rhesus isoimmunization

A spectrophotometric peak at 450 nm representing unconjugated bilirubin is present in amniotic fluid throughout normal pregnancy, the peak becoming smaller and disappearing at about 36 weeks gestation. During pregnancy complicated by rhesus (Rh) incompatibility, the height of the 450 nm peak has been correlated with the severity of the fetal anaemia resulting from intravascular haemolysis.

This discovery has significantly altered the clinical management of Rh disease. When there is evidence of Rh incompatibility, a sample of amniotic fluid is collected at 32 weeks gestation by amniocentesis. The height of the peak at 450 nm gives an indication of the severity of the disease and from this measurement a decision can be made concerning the optimal time for induction of labour, or whether, in very severe disease, intra-uterine transfusion of the fetus is necessary (Fig. 6.16).

Amniotic fluid

- Produced by amnion, fetal skin and fetal urine
- Volume up to 1000 ml at 38 weeks
- Oligohydramnios associated with poor placental function and renal agenesis
- Polyhydramnios associated with significant congenital anomalies in 30% cases
- Contains fetal cells and cells from the amnion
- Clinical estimations of alphafetoprotein, fetal chromosomes, metabolic abnormalities, Rhesus disease and fetal maturity

Estimation of fetal maturity

After the 38th week of gestation, large numbers of eosinophilic anucleate polygonal cells appear. These cells stain orange with Nile blue sulphate and are thought to be derived from maturing fetal sebaceous glands, but may be related to the appearance of increased quantities of phospholipid at this time. After the 40th week of gestation, the orange-stained cells usually constitute more than 50% of the total cellular content of the amniotic fluid. Prior to the 38th week, only 10% or less of the total number of cells are of this type.

The measurement of lecithin or the lecithin/sphingomyelin ratio has been used to measure fetal lung maturity. Lecithin is a major part of the surfactant produced by the fetal alveolar epithelial cells

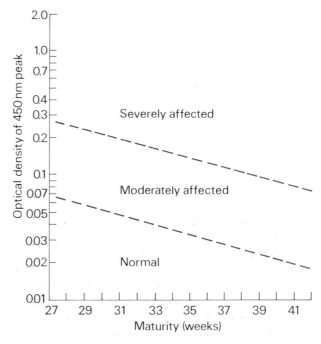

Fig. 6.16 Optical density of amniotic fluid in the prediction of rhesus isoimmunization

and the presence of concentrations of lecithin in excess of 3 mg/100 ml indicates that the fetal lungs are mature and that there is no risk of the development of respiratory distress syndrome.

The determination of creatinine may also be helpful, since a level greater than 2 mg/100 ml appears to indicate a gestation of longer than 37 weeks. However, the values may also be increased by severe pre-eclampsia, irrespective of length of gestation.

Fetal distress and placental insufficiency

Chronic fetal hypoxia commonly results in the passage of meconium into amniotic fluid. Placental insufficiency is also associated with a reduction in amniotic fluid volume.

Direct examination of the amniotic fluid can be achieved by **amnioscopy**, the passage of an amnioscope through the uterine cervix. This enables inspection of the colour of amniotic fluid, and will also give an impression of amniotic fluid volume. Amnioscopy is a useful adjunct in the management of the 'at risk' pregnancy, but can only be performed where the cervix is sufficiently dilated to allow the passage of the amnioscope. It may sometimes result in the rupture of membranes unless undertaken with care.

BIBLIOGRAPHY

Edwards R G 1980 Conception in the human female. Academic Press, London

Faber J J, Thornburg K L 1983 Placental physiology. Raven Press, New York
Klopper A, Genazzani A, Crosignani P G 1980 The human placenta, proteins and hormones. Academic Press, London
Sandler M 1981 Amniotic fluid and its clinical significance. Marcel Dekker, New York

7. Infertility

Fig. 7.1 The incidence of infertility is estimated at 1 in every 10 couples in Western European societies

The incidence of infertility varies in different countries and has been recorded to be as high as 50% in some West African communities compared with values of around 10% in Western European societies (Fig. 7.1).

It is important to differentiate between infertility, which is diminished fertility, and sterility, which is absolute infertility. Primary infertility is defined as diminished fertility throughout the reproductive years and secondary infertility infers failure to conceive after one or more successful pregnancies.

If conception does not occur after 12 months of normal sexual activity without contraception, the couple should be considered to be potentially infertile, as 75% of couples normally conceive within 1 year. It is therefore reasonable to proceed with investigations at this time.

Such a definition has to be modified by circumstances. For example, if a woman has had secondary amenorrhoea for 2 years, it would be pointless to wait for 12 months of regular sexual exposure before investigating her subfertility. At the other extreme, if the husband was away for a substantial part of the year, it would be sensible to defer intensive investigations until regular sexual exposure could be established. Both partners must be investigated, as infertility may result from male or female factors and is often associated with a combination of both factors. At the completion of all investigations, about 10% will exhibit no identifiable cause for their infertility and long–term follow-up studies on these couples have shown that only 30 – 40% will conceive over a 7-year period after investigation.

HISTORY AND EXAMINATION

Both partners should be requested to attend at the initial interview. On occasions, the male partner may be reluctant to attend and this should not be considered as a basis for refusing investigation. It should however, be apparent to the woman that the value of investigation will be seriously limited without the cooperation of the male partner.

The initial interview

The initial interview should take into account the following factors:

1. Age, occupation, religion and educational background.
2. Number of years that conception has been attempted and the previous history of contraception.
3. Previous marriages and pregnancies of either partner.
4. Whether the infertility is primary or secondary and, if necessary, the details of any complications associated with previous pregnancies.

5. Coital history including frequency of intercourse. Any history of dyspareunia or of impotence or difficulty in ejaculation may be important.
6. General medical history of any concurrent or previous serious illness and of any surgery, particularly in relation to appendicitis in the female or herniorrhaphy in the male. A history of undescended testes or of orchidopexy may be particularly important.

FEMALE CAUSES OF INFERTILITY

General factors such as the age of both partners, a history of serious systemic illness, inadequate nutrition and emotional stress may all be factors that contribute to infertility but the major defined problems are found in defects of ovulation, tubal disease and cervical hostility.

Disorders of ovulation

Disorders of ovulation are divided into five categories:

1. Primary amenorrhoea — the failure of onset of menstruation by the age of 18 years. This is rarely a presenting symptom in relation to subfertility and will be considered separately.
2. Secondary amenorrhoea — no menstruation for 6 months or more in a woman with a previous history of menstruation.
3. Oligomenorrhoea (infrequent periods) where the periods occur between 6 weeks and 6 months and may be ovulatory or anovulatory, However, even if the cycles are ovulatory, ovulation is so infrequent that fertility becomes impaired.
4. Anovulatory cycles — cycle length may be within normal limits but ovulation does not occur.
5. Ovulation appears to occur but the ovum is entrapped in the follicle. The corpus luteum may be defective and implantation does not occur.

Endocrine causes of oligomenorrhoea and secondary amenorrhoea

Anovulation is commonly, although not invari-

ably, associated with amenorrhoea or oligomenorrhoea and these conditions may occur as the result of any one of a series of changes in the hypothalamic, pituitary, ovarian axis (Fig. 7.2). Alterations in the menstrual cycle are commonly associated with periods of stress and also with excessive weight gain or obesity and, at the other extreme, with anorexia nervosa or self-inflicted starvation.

Pituitary failure, as in Sheehan's syndrome, is now a rare condition but pituitary tumours in the form of pituitary microadenomas, which are prolactin secreting, are a relatively common cause of secondary amenorrhoea.

Fig. 7.2   Endocrine factors associated with non-ovulation

Disorders of adrenal and thyroid function may not be clinically apparent if they are mild and therefore should be excluded by biochemical assessment.

Ovarian failure may occur as a result of premature menopause and the presence of streak ovaries. Polycystic ovaries associated with hirsutism, obesity and oligomenorrhoea commonly result in anovulation. This is due to an enzyme block in the conversion of androstenedione and testosterone to oestrogen and is associated with a high production rate of LH and FSH.

Anovulatory 'normal cycles'

The presence of a normal menstrual cycle does not necessarily imply that ovulation is occurring and, in recent years, it has been recognized that the oocyte may not be released from the follicle whilst luteinization of the unruptured follicle may still occur. This is known as the **luteinized unruptured follicle (LUF) syndrome** and is commonly associated with endometriosis. The diagnosis can only really be made by laparoscopic inspection of the ovary to establish whether there is any evidence of an ovulation stigma.

Abnormalities of implantation and the luteal phase

Implantation requires the presence of adequate development of the secretory phase of the endometrium. Luteal phase inadequacy results in either failure of implantation or early abortion. Diagnosis may be difficult and the aetiology is not understood but there is no doubt that the problem arises in the first half of the cycle with defective follicular development.

Tubal factors

The function of the Fallopian tubes involves both ovum pick-up and transport of the fertilized gamete. Ovum pick-up is dependent on the action of the tubal fimbriae in pulling the tubal ostium over the follicle. The action of the tubal cilia also serves to aspirate the ovum. Subsequent progress and nutrition of the zygote by the tube is determined by the muscular action of the tubal wall, by the ciliated action and secretion of the tubal epithelium and by the secretions of the tubal epithelium.

It is estimated that tubal factors account for about 20% of cases of infertility although this figure will vary considerably according to the population under consideration.

Occasionally congenital anomalies occur but the commonest cause of tubal damage is infection (Fig. 7.3).

Infection may cause occlusion of the fimbrial end of the tube with the collection of fluid, **hydrosalpinx** , or pus, **pyosalpinx** , within the tubal lumen.

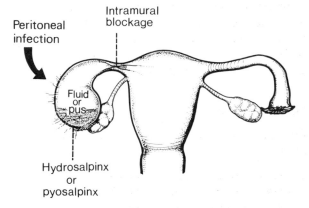

Fig. 7.3 The pathogenesis of tubal obstruction and subfertility: intramural tubal obstruction results from intra-uterine infections

Acute salpingitis results from sexually transmitted diseases such as gonorrhoea but may also result from other organisms such as *Escherichia coli* , anaerobic and haemolytic streptococci, staphylococci and *Clostridium welchii*. It may also result from infection with bacteriodes and from mycoplasma and viral infections. Tuberculosis of the tubes may occur in women with pulmonary tuberculosis but has become increasingly rare as a cause of subfertility. Infections arising from intra-uterine contraceptive devices and following abortion or termination of pregnancy and infections · in the puerperium commonly result in cornual blockage — often without any other significant change to the remainder of the tube. Pelvic infection from appendicitis associated with peritonitis results in peritubal adhesions and leaves the tubal lining unaffected.

Infections which affect the lumen of the tube result in loss of the ciliated epithelium and damage and fibrosis within the tubal wall, thus impairing the peristaltic function of the tube in promoting movement of the gamete. Therefore, even in the presence of a patent tube, damage to the wall and lumen may result in severe impairment of tubal function.

Lesions of the uterine cavity

Conditions which impinge on the uterine cavity may interfere with implantation and conception. Intramural and submucous fibroids interfere with implantation although pregnancy can occur and continue in the presence of large fibroids (Fig. 7.4).

Fig. 7.4 Submucous fibroids cause subfertility by interference with implantations or by causing recurrent abortions

Severe intra-uterine infections following pregnancy associated with retained products of conception and where uterine curettage is performed, may result in complete ablation of the uterine cavity by adhesion of the walls, or partial occlusion of the cavity by the formation of intra-uterine adhesions or synechiae. This condition is known as **Asherman's syndrome.**

Congenital abnormalities of the uterus do not interfere with conception as a rule but may result in recurrent abortions.

Cervical factors

Ejaculation occurs into the vagina and semen is deposited around the cervix. However, the cervix is effectively closed with cervical mucus and sperm migration occurs by penetration of sperm into the cervical mucus. At the time of ovulation, endocervical cells secrete copious, clear, watery mucus which has a high water content and consists of long chains of polypeptide macromolecules with occasional side chains of carbohydrate. The chains of molecules contain channels which allow a direct passage of the spermatozoa into the uterine cavity. Sperm penetration occurs within 2–3 minutes of deposition. Between 100 000 and 200 000 sperms colonise the cervical mucus and remain at this level for approximately 24 hours after coitus. Approximately 200 sperms eventually reach the Fallopian tube. The vagina is generally hostile to sperm survival and sperm in the vagina pool soon become immobilised. Mucus produced by the cervix under the influence of progesterone is hostile to sperm penetration.

Thus, poor penetration of sperm may result from cervical infection, from antisperm antibody activity in either cervical mucus or seminal plasma, from production of abnormal mucus by the cervix or from the effect of progestational agents on the mucus.

Female causes of infertility

- Disorders of ovulation
- Luteal phase failure of implantation
- Tubal occlusion or impaired cilia action
- Congenital / acquired lesion of uterine cavity
- Cervical infection, antisperm antibodies

INVESTIGATION OF THE FEMALE

The investigation of the female involves determination of three basic issues:

1. Does ovulation occur on a regular basis?
2. Is there any impairment of tubal function and of implantation?
3. Is there a cervical factor preventing sperm invasion?

Detection of ovulation

Basal temperature

An increase of 0.5 °C occurs in basal body temperature in the luteal phase of the menstrual

TEMPERATURE RECORD

Name   Address

Usual Time Between Periods..............Days.

Usual Length of Periods...................Days.

Physician   Address

Date   Telephone

Fig. 7.5 Recording basal body temperature provides an indication of the time of ovulation

cycle. The temperature should be recorded sublingually before rising each morning and provides a useful indication of the time of ovulation (Fig. 7.5). However, ovulation may occur in the absence of any temperature shift.

Cervical mucus

The production of mucus increases during the follicular phase to reach a peak at the time of ovulation with profuse production of clear, acellular mucus with low viscosity and high 'stretchability' (Spinnbarkeit) (Fig. 7.6). This mucus can be recognised by the woman herself and is the best method for self-assessment of the time of ovulation. Some women experience pain in the mid-cycle (Mittel—Schmertz) associated with ovulation

Viscosity (Spinnbarkeit)   Ferning

Fig. 7.6 Characteristics of cervical mucus: the 'stretchability' can be evaluated between two glass slides (left); mid-cycle mucus shows ferning (right)

and can therefore asses the timing of their ovulation. Mid-cycle mucus also dries on a glass slide with a characteristic fern pattern. This pattern presents a granular amorphous appearance which disappears with the influence of progesterone.

Hormonal tests

Serial measurement of FSH and LH in either blood or urine show a well-defined peak which occurs approximately 20 hours before ovulation and can therefore be used as a technique for timing ovulation. However, the practical difficulties imposed by this approach limit its value.

The measurement of daily oestrogen levels provides a useful technique in assessing follicle maturation but is of limited value in timing ovulation.

The best hormonal evidence that ovulation has occurred is the measurement of serum progesterone in the luteal phase of the cycle. The interpretation of the results depends on the day of the cycle and values in excess of 10 ng/ml indicate that ovulation has occurred. However, none of these tests are infallible.

Endometrial biopsy and vaginal cytology

Biopsy of the endometrium can be performed without anaesthesia or formal dilatation and curettage

Fig. 7.7 Endometrial biopsy can be achieved without anaesthesia using 'vabra' aspiration or simple endometrial curettage; magnified view (inset)

(Fig. 7.7). The presence of secretory phase endometrium is taken as evidence of ovulation.

Examination of vaginal squames using the Papanicolaou stain can also be employed in the assessment of hormonal status (Fig. 7.8). Vaginal cells are shed as three types of cell — parabasal, intermediate and superficial (or cornified), according to the size and staining characteristics of the cells. Progesterone causes maturation of intermediate cells, which tend to clump together, and the appearance of numerous polymorphonuclear leucocytes.

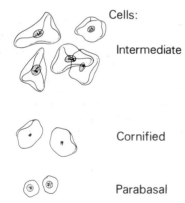

Fig. 7.8 Vaginal cytology can be useful in assessing hormone status. Cells from the vaginal epithelium include parabasal intermediate and superficial squames. The nature and staining features change with the hormonal status.

Ultrasonography

Ultrasound examination of the ovaries can be used to identify follicular growth. Follicular diameter increases from 11.5 mm 5 days before ovulation to 20 mm on the day before ovulation and decreases to approximately half this size on the day after ovulation. This is a useful and practical way of monitoring the time of ovulation.

Laparoscopy

Direct visualization of the ovary enables the observer to obtain more definite evidence of ovulation. Even this technique can be fallacious as it is sometimes difficult to be certain if follicular rupture has occurred.

In summary, there are numerous techniques which provide presumptive evidence of ovulation. In the initial assessment, basal body temperature charts and serum progesterone measurements are the most widely used techniques. The only definite proof of ovulation is pregnancy.

Investigation of non-ovulation

If there is evidence of non-ovulation, then further investigation should include measurement of:

1. Serum prolactin—to exclude hyperprolactinaemia.
2. FSH and LH levels in secondary ammenorrhoea. High levels of gonadotrophins in the presence of low levels of oestrogen indicate ovarian failure.
3. Assessment of thyroid function and TSH.
4. X-ray of the sella turcica if prolactin levels are raised to search for evidence of a pituitary prolactinoma. Tomography may be necessary if there is any sign of 'double flooring' of the pituitary fossa.

Investigation of tubal function

It is essential to establish tubal patency before embarking on prolonged drug therapy in either partner. Tubal patency is assessed by:

1. Hysterosalpingography

A radio-opaque dye, such as diodrast or urografin, is injected into the uterine cavity and Fallopian tubes. This technique can be performed without

Fig. 7.9 Hysterosalpingography enables assessment of the site of tubal obstruction and the presence of pathology in the uterine cavity. The radio-opaque dye outlines the uterine cavity and Fallopian tubes

anaesthesia provided the approach is gentle and the dye injected slowly. The dye outlines the uterine cavity and will demonstrate any filling defects. It will also show whether there is evidence of tubal obstruction and the site of the obstruction (Fig. 7.9).

2. Laparoscopy and dye insufflation

Laparoscopy enables direct visualization of the pelvic organs and, in particular, enables the diagnosis of endometriosis (Fig. 7.10). Methylene blue is injected through the uterine cavity to demon-

Fig. 7.10 Dye laparoscopy for evaluation of tubal patency

strate tubal patency. It is not always possible to be certain of the site of tubal obstruction.

3. Gas insufflation

Inflation of the tubes with CO_2 has been used to demonstrate tubal patency but involves the risk of gas embolism. It has been replaced by laparoscopy and salpingography.

Investigation of the cervical factor

It is important to determine that viable sperm penetrate the cervical mucus. A series of tests have been developed to examine this factor:

1. The postcoital test

This is the most widely used method of assessment and involves asking the couple to have intercourse and to examine the cervical mucus some 2–6 hours after intercourse. The test is best performed at the time of ovulation. The mucus is examined microscopically for the presence of progressive motile sperms. The presence of pus cells in the mucus is also noted as well as evidence of clumped or abnormal sperms.

2. In vitro sperm penetration tests

A series of in vitro tests have been developed which essentially examine the reaction between cervical mucus and semen from the husband on a slide or in a glass capillary and also the rate of sperm migration and sperm clumping or abnormal motility. Where there is a specific interaction with clumping of sperm, it is useful to test the mucus against donor semen to see if the same effect is obtained.

Investigation of the female

- Temperature chart
- FSH/LH (peaks 20 hours pre-ovulation), day 21 serum progesterone
- Endometrial biopsy
- Ultrasonography to identify follicular development
- Serum prolactin, thyroid function tests, pituitary X-ray
- Hysterosalpingography / dye laparoscopy
- Postcoital test, in vitro sperm penetration tests

INVESTIGATION OF THE MALE PARTNER

The simplest and most important investigation of the male partner is the semen analysis. Semen should be collected by masturbation into a sterile container after a period of 2 days abstinence and examined within 2 hours of collection. Special note should be made of:

1. *Volume* — 80% of fertile males ejaculate between 1 and 4 ml of semen. Low volumes may indicate androgen deficiency and high volumes abnormal accessory gland function.
2. *Sperm concentration* — the absence of all sperm (azoospermia) indicates male sterility. However, the lower limit of normality is more difficult to define. It is generally accepted that the lower limit is probably between 15–20 million sperm/ml but the findings should not be accepted on a single sample. Furthermore, abnormally high values in excess of 200 million sperm/ml may be associated with subfertility.
3. *Total sperm count* — this measurement is sometimes used as an alternative to sperm concentration. The lower limit of normal is accepted as 50 million per ejaculate.
4. *Sperm motility* — sperm motility is an important measurement of fertility and normal semen should show good motility in 60% of sperm within 1 hour of collection. The characteristic of forward progression is equally important.

The World Health Organization now grades sperm motility according to the following criteria:

Grade 1 – rapid and linear progressive motility.
Grade 2 – slow or sluggish linear or non-linear motility.
Grade 3 – non-progressive motility.
Grade 4 – immotile.

5. *Sperm morphology* — sperm morphology shows great variability even in normal fertile males. It is unusual to see a count with more than 80% normal forms. It is important to look for leucocytes as they may indicate the presence of infection. If pus cells are present, the semen should be cultured for bacteriological growth. In general terms, fertility relates poorly to abnormal sperm morphology.

In the presence of a normal semen analysis and a normal postcoital test, further tests on the male are unlikely to contribute to subsequent management. In the presence of oligospermia or azoospermia, further studies should include the following investigations:

1. *Hormone measurements.* High levels of FSH indicate severe testicular damage whereas normal levels may indicate obstructive disease. Low or undetectable levels are found in males with hypopituitarism. The presence of high FSH levels and azoospermia obviates the need for further investigation as these findings indicate irreversible failure of spermatogenesis.

    LH and testosterone levels are of limited value although low values of both hormones may indicate a pituitary or hypothalamic disorder and high levels of LH with low levels of testosterone are characteristic of Klinefelter's syndrome.

    Hyperprolactinaemia may occur in the male in association with a pituitary adenoma and may cause impotence or oligospermia.
2. *Cytogenetic studies.* Chromosome analysis in males with azoospermia may indicate the presence of a karyotype of XXY or XYY and, occasionally, autosomal translocation in the presence of oligospermia. About 2% of infertile males exhibit an abnormal karyotype.
3. *Testicular biopsy* should be undertaken only where an obstructive cause of subfertility is suspected. The advent of hormone investigations has greatly reduced the need for this investigation.

    Rarely, retrograde ejaculation may cause subfertility and this should be suspected following surgical procedures such as transurethral resection of the prostate. The diagnosis is made by detecting spermatozoa in the urine following orgasm.

Investigation of the male

- Ejaculate volume 1–4 ml
- Sperm concentration 15–200 million/ml
- Total count > 50 million
- Motility at collection 60%
- Morphology
- FSH, serum prolactin, chromosome studies if the above abnormal

TREATMENT OF SUBFERTILITY

The treatment of subfertility is the treatment of the cause.

1. Anovulation

In the presence of normal gonadotrophin and prolactin levels, the drug of choice is clomiphene or tamoxifen. These compounds are anti-oestrogens and stimulate the release of FSH and LH; they will produce ovulation in 80% of subjects. Clomiphene is administered from the fifth to the ninth day of the cycle with an initial dosage of 50 mg/day increased to 200 mg/day where necessary. It is sometimes necessary to supplement this regimen with a mid-cycle injection of hCG.

If these compounds are not effective, then it may be necessary to use human FSH prepared from human pituitary glands or extracted from the urine of menopausal woman as in preparations such as Pergonal®. These drugs must be used with great caution as they may result in ovarian hyperstimulation and multiple pregnancy. Daily monitoring of oestrogen levels in blood or urine is advisable and an injection of hCG is used to trigger ovulation. If anovulation is associated with hyperprolactinaemia, it is essential to exclude a significant pituitary lesion. If there is no major lesion present, treatment is initiated with a dopamine receptor agonist such as bromocriptine. Treatment should be initiated by taking 2.5 mg at night and can be increased to 5 mg/day, depending on the response as judged by the prolactin levels.

2. Tubal pathology

The main method of treatment is by surgical intervention. Success rates are generally poor but have been improved by the use of microsurgery.

Salpingolysis involves the freeing of adhesions around the tubes and generally carries the best prognosis (Fig. 7.11). New techniques involving laser vaporization minimize recurrence of the adhesions.

Salpingostomy in the presence of a hydrosalpinx may re-establish patency but, because of damage to the tubal wall, is successful in only 10–15% of cases (Fig. 7.12). Following all forms of tubal

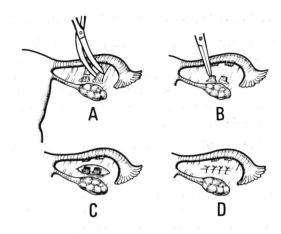

Fig. 7.11 Salpingolysis: (**A**) division of adhesions; (**B**) diathermy of adhesions; (**C & D**) reconstruction of peritoneum

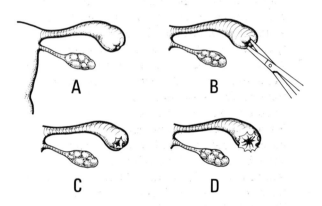

Fig. 7.12 Salpingostomy for fimbrial occlusion and hydrosalpinx: (**A**) intact hydrosalpinx; (**B-C**) opening the fimbriae; (**D**) position for suturing the opened hydrosalpinx

surgery, there is an additional risk of ectopic pregnancy. Tubal obstruction in the intramural portion of the tube is treated by re-implantation of the patent tube into the uterine cavity and localized areas of obstruction, such as pertain following sterilization procedures, can be resected and the tube re-anastomosed.

IN VITRO FERTILIZATION AND EMBRYO TRANSFER

Recent developments in extracorporeal fertilization have provided an alternative method of treatment for tubal damage. Oocytes recovered by laparoscopy are fertilized in vitro and the zygote is transferred back into the uterine cavity. Although this technique is still in the developmental stage, it carries great hope for the future. The stimulation of multiple follicular development by exogenous FSH results in the harvesting of several oocytes during each treatment cycle. Although fertilization may occur in 80–90 per cent of the oocytes, the embryos often do not 'take' in the endometrium. Success rates vary, but in good units a 20% success rate can be obtained. The technique is valid for both donor sperm and donor oocytes.

A series of variants have now been developed on this technique.

GIFT (gamete intrafallopian transfer) involves the mixing of oocytes and sperms and their replacement into the fallopian tube. It is only appropriate where the tubes are patent.

ZIFT (zygote intrafallopian transfer). In this situation, eggs are collected, fertilized in vitro and transferred back to the Fallopian tube.

TREATMENT OF CERVICAL HOSTILITY

This presents a difficult problem but may be treated by intra-uterine insemination with the husband's semen (AIH). Success rates are low and the treatment is not without complication as it may result in severe uterine pain. It is contraindicated in the presence of a normal postcoital test.

TREATMENT OF THE MALE PARTNER

Specific treatment is possible in only a small proportion of infertile males. Testicular size is important and in the presence of small testes, azoospermia and high FSH levels, it is highly unlikely that any therapy will help.

Where FSH levels are normal and testicular size is normal, ductal obstruction should be suspected and testicular biopsy performed. If normal spermatogenesis is demonstrated, then it is necessary to proceed to vasography and exploration of the scrotum. Surgical anastomosis sometimes allows the re-establishment of fertility.

Ligation of a varicocoele sometimes improves semen quality, probably as a result of reducing testicular temperatures. In the presence of idiopathic oligospermia, hCG, clomiphene and bromocriptine are used and sometimes appear to be effective but the variability in semen analysis makes assessment of efficacy of therapy difficult. Oral androgen therapy has been widely used but there is little evidence that these compounds are effective.

Case study: sub–fertility

Mr and Mrs S.J. attended their general practitioner complaining of their inability to have a child.

Mr J. had been married before, but had no children by his first wife. He was a successful businessman who worked long hours under considerable emotional and physical pressure. His wife worked part-time. She had an irregular menstrual cycle with periods every 3 or 4 months. Coitus occurred infrequently as the husband was occasionally impotent and frequently tired. The semen analysis showed evidence of oligospermia and there was evidence that the wife was anovulatory.

There was nothing abnormal to find on physical examination of either partner. The husband was advised to modify his lifestyle and after appropriate investigation, the wife was started on clomiphene. Within 3 cycles conception was successfully achieved.

Subfertility is often multifactorial.

DONOR INSEMINATION (AID)

If all evidence suggests that there is no prospect of improving the fertility of the male partner, then the question of donor insemination (AID) should be discussed with the couple.

The implications of the procedure, from both a legal and personal point of view, should be discussed in depth before accepting the woman for donor insemination. The establishment of frozen semen banks has greatly simplified the management and availability of donor insemination and, provided the emotional aspects are thoroughly explored, AID can provide a very satisfactory method of treatment.

Treatment of subfertility

Depends on cause but options include:
- Stimulation of ovulation with anti–oestrogen +/− hCG
- Treat raised prolactin with bromocriptine (having excluded pituitary lesion)
- Tubal surgery
- IVF / GIFT / ZIFT
- AIH
- AID
- Ligation of varicocoele, surgery to correct obstruction in testis

BIBLIOGRAPHY

Chamberlain G, Winston R 1982 Tubal infertility, diagnosis and treatment. Blackwell, Oxford
Hull M G M 1981 Developments in infertility practice. Clinics in Obstetrics and Gynaecology. W B Saunders, Eastbourne
Pepperell R J, Hudson B, Wood C 1980 The infertile couple. Churchill Livingstone, Edinburgh
Trounson A, Wood C 1984 Clinical in vitro fertilisation. Springer, Berlin

8. Complications of early pregnancy

Abortion, extra-uterine pregnancy and hydatidiform mole

SPONTANEOUS ABORTION

The definition of spontaneous abortion is the termination of pregnancy before the 24th week of pregnancy. In some countries, such as the USA, this definition is modified to termination of pregnancy before fetal viability or less than 500 g. Most spontaneous abortions occur in the second or third month of pregnancy and account for 10% of all pregnancies. It has been suggested that a much higher proportion of pregnancies abort at an early stage if the diagnosis is based on the presence of a significant plasma level of β-subunit hCG.

Clinical types of abortion

Threatened abortion

The first sign of an impending abortion is the development of vaginal bleeding in early pregnancy (Fig. 8.1). The uterus is found to be enlarged and the cervical os is closed. Lower abdominal pain is either minimal or absent. About 50% of women presenting with a threatened abortion will continue with the pregnancy irrespective of the method of management.

Fig. 8.1   Threatened abortion: blood loss in early pregnancy

Incomplete abortion

The threatened abortion may either settle and the pregnancy continue or proceed to abort. The patient develops abdominal pain and bleeding becomes worse. The cervix opens and eventually products of conception are passed into the vagina. However, if some of the products of conception are retained, then the abortion remains incomplete (Fig. 8.2).

Fig. 8.2   Incomplete abortion: progression to expulsion of part of the conceptus is accompanied by pain and bleeding

Complete abortion

An incomplete abortion may proceed to completion spontaneously when the pain will cease and vaginal bleeding will subside with involution of the uterus. Spontaneous completion of an abortion is more likely in abortions over 16 weeks gestation than in those between 8 and 16 weeks gestation, when retention of placental fragments is common.

Septic abortion

During the process of abortion — either spontaneous or induced — infection may be introduced into the

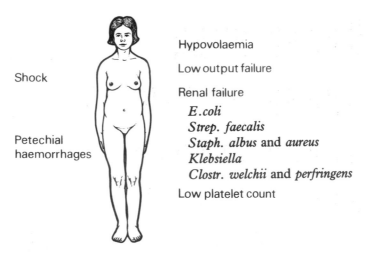

Shock

Petechial
haemorrhages

Hypovolaemia

Low output failure

Renal failure

E.coli
Strep. faecalis
Staph. albus and *aureus*
Klebsiella
Clostr. welchii and *perfringens*

Low platelet count

Fig. 8.3   Manifestation of endotoxic shock complicating septic abortion

uterine cavity. The clinical findings of septic abortion are similar to those of incomplete abortion with the addition of uterine and adnexal tenderness. The vaginal loss may become purulent and the patient pyrexial. In cases of severe overwhelming sepsis, endotoxic shock may develop with profound and sometimes fatal hypotension (Fig. 8.3). Other manifestations include renal failure, disseminated intravascular coagulopathy and multiple petechial haemorrhages. Organisms which commonly invade the uterine cavity are *E. coli*, *Streptococcus faecalis*, *Staphylococcus albus* and *aureus*, *Klebsiella*, and *Clostridium welchii* and *perfringens*.

Missed abortion

Sometimes the fetus dies in utero but is not immediately expelled. There is usually some pain and bleeding and the uterus does not increase in size. There may be bleeding into the choriodecidual space which forms a mass of clot. This becomes organized and laminated and forms what is termed a **carneous mole**.

Recurrent abortions

A patient who has three or more spontaneous abortions is known as a recurrent aborter and should be investigated for the underlying cause.

The aetiology of abortion

In the majority of cases, no definite cause can be found for the abortion.

Feto-placental factors

Genetic abnormalities. Chromosomal abnormalities are a common cause of early abortion and may result in failure of development of the embryo with formation of a blighted ovum or with later expulsion of an abnormal fetus (Fig. 8.4).

Hormone imbalance. Progesterone production is predominately dependent on the corpus luteum for the first 8 weeks of pregnancy and the function is then assumed by the placenta. Progesterone is essential for the maintenance of a pregnancy and early failure of the corpus luteum may lead to abortion. However, it is difficult to be certain when falling plasma progesterone levels represent a primary cause of abortion and when they are the index of a dying placenta.

Maternal factors

Maternal illness. Severe maternal febrile illnesses associated with infections, such as influenza, pyelitis and malaria, predispose to abortion. Other severe illnesses involving the cardiovascular, hepatic and renal systems may also result in abortion. Specific

Fig. 8.4 Karyotype of trisomy 13, an example of a chromosomal abnormality. If the fetus survives it has a grossly abnormal face and a poorly developed brain

infections such as syphilis cause abortion, particularly in the second trimester.

Abnormalities of the uterus. Congenital abnormalities of the uterine cavity, such as a bicornuate uterus or subseptate uterus, may result in abortion and sometimes recurrent abortion (Fig. 8.5). Factors which distort the uterine cavity, such as uterine fibroids and intra-uterine synechiae, interfere with implantation. Cervical incompetence may be congenital but is commonly the result of overvigorous cervical dilatation. There is premature rupture of the membranes and rapid spontaneous abortion in the second trimester of pregnancy.

Criminal abortion

Abortion induced by a variety of techniques makes up a substantial percentage of abortion in some countries. Where the indications for legal abortion are liberal, criminal abortion is infrequent, but in many countries it contributes to a high percentage of apparently spontaneous abortions.

Management

Threatened abortion should be treated by rest in bed until the bleeding subsides. Examination of the

Bicornis bicollis

Bicornis unicollis

Planiform uterus

Subseptate uterus

Fig. 8.5 Anomalies of the genital tract are sometimes a cause of recurrent abortion patient should include gentle vaginal and speculum examination to ascertain cervical dilatation. Some women may prefer not to be examined because of apprehension that the examination may promote abortion, and their wishes should be respected.

In some cases, it may be justifiable to give a progestogen such as 17α-OH progesterone caproate by intramuscular injection; 19-nor-steroids should not be used as they promote virilisation of the female fetus.

An ultrasound scan is valuable in deciding if the fetus is alive and normal and urinary chorionic gonadotrophin estimation will also provide additional useful information.

If there is pyrexia, a high vaginal swab should be taken for bacteriological culture.

Abortion may be complicated by haemorrhage and severe pain, and may necessitate blood transfusion and relief of pain with opiates.

If there is evidence that products of conception have been passed, the uterus must be evacuated by direct curettage or suction curettage as soon as possible. Products of conception should be submitted for histological examination (Fig. 8.6).

If there is evidence of infection, antibiotic therapy should be started immediately and adjusted subsequently if the organism identified in culture is not sensitive to the prescribed antibiotic.

Septic abortion complicated by endotoxic shock is treated by massive antibiotic therapy, large doses of corticosteroids and adequate, carefully controlled fluid replacement.

Complications of treatment include perforation of the uterus and continuing bleeding associated with incomplete evacuation of the uterus. Intrauterine infection may result in tubal infection and tubal obstruction with subsequent infertility. If uterine perforation is suspected and there is evidence of intraperitoneal haemorrhage or damage to the bowel, then laparotomy should be performed.

Spontaneous abortion

- Over 10% pregnancies abort under 24 weeks
- Can be threatened, incomplete, complete, septic, missed or recurrent
- Aetiology usually unknown but possible causes include chromosomal abnormalities, hormonal factors, maternal illness, uterine abnormalities and cervical incompetence
- Investigations include hCG, ultrasound and assessment of cervical dilation
- Treatment is expectant for threatened, and curettage for missed or incomplete abortion, with antibiotics, analgesia and transfusion if indicated

Fig. 8.6   Evacuation of retained products of conception

Suction curette

ECTOPIC PREGNANCY

The term ectopic pregnancy refers to any pregnancy occurring outside the uterine cavity.

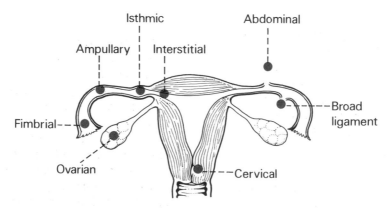

Fig. 8.7   Sites of implantation of ectopic pregnancies

The most common site of extra-uterine implantation is the fallopian tube but it may occur in the ovary as an ovarian pregnancy, in the abdominal cavity as an abdominal pregnancy, or in the cervical canal as a cervical pregnancy (Fig. 8.7).

Tubal pregnancy occurs in 1 in 200 pregnancies in the UK, although this incidence varies substantially in different populations. Tubal pregnancy may occur in the ampulla, the isthmus and the interstitial portion of the tube and the outcome will depend on the site of implantation.

Predisposing factors

The majority of cases of ectopic pregnancy have no identifiable predisposing factor, but a previous history of pelvic inflammatory disease, subfertility and the presence of an intra-uterine device all increase the likelihood of an ectopic pregnancy.

Clinical presentation

Acute presentation

The classical pattern of symptoms includes amenorrhoea, lower abdominal pain and uterine bleeding. The abdominal pain usually precedes the onset of vaginal bleeding, and may start in one side of the lower abdomen, but rapidly becomes generalized as blood loss extends into the peritoneal cavity. Subdiaphragmatic irritation by blood produces referred shoulder tip pain and syncopal episodes may occur.

The period of amenorrhoea is usually 6–8 weeks but may be longer if implantation occurs in the interstitial portion of the tube or in abdominal pregnancy. Clinical examination reveals a shocked woman with hypotension, tachycardia and signs of peritonism including abdominal distension, guarding and rebound tenderness. Pelvic examination is usually unimportant because of the acute pain and discomfort, and should be undertaken with caution. This type of acute presentation occurs in no more than 25% of cases.

Case study: acute presentation
An 18-year-old woman, para 0, was brought into casualty collapsed with lower abdominal pain. On admission she was shocked with a blood pressure of 80/40, a pulse of 120 b.p.m. and a tender, rigid abdomen. Vaginal examination revealed a slight red loss, bulky uterus and marked cervical excitation with a tender mass in the right fornix. At laparotomy, 800 ml of fresh blood were removed from the peritoneal cavity and a ruptured right tubal ectopic pregnancy was found. Subsequently, a history of recurrent pelvic infections and irregular periods was elicited.

Subacute presentation

After a short period of amenorrhoea, the patient experiences recurrent attacks of vaginal bleeding and abdominal pain. Any woman who develops lower abdominal pain following an interval of amenorrhoea should be considered as a possible ectopic pregnancy. In its subacute phase, it may be possible to feel a mass in one fornix.

Case study: subacute presentation
A 22-year-old woman, para 0, was admitted with vaginal bleeding after 8 weeks' amenorrhoea. She had had a positive home pregnancy kit test and described passing some tissue per vaginum. Ultrasound scan showed an empty uterus, although serum beta hCG was still positive. A presumptive diagnosis of incomplete abortion was made and evacuation of uterus carried out uneventfully. She was discharged the following day, but readmitted that night with lower abdominal pain; a ruptured ampullary ectopic was found at laparotomy. Some days later, histology of the original curettage was reported as 'decidua with Arias-Stella type reaction, no chorionic villi seen'.

Pathology

Implantation may occur in a variety of sites, and the outcome of the pregnancy will depend on the site of implantation.

Abdominal pregnancy may result from direct implantation of the conceptus in the abdominal cavity or on the ovary, in which case it is known as primary abdominal pregnancy, or it may result from extrusion of a tubal pregnancy with secondary implantation in the peritoneal cavity, which is known as secondary abdominal pregnancy. Implantation of the conceptus in the tube results in hormonal changes that mimic normal pregnancy.

Fig. 8.8   Penetration of the tubal wall by placental tissue (above) results in haemorrhage and extrusion of the gestational sac (below)

Fig. 8.9   Culdocentesis — aspiration of blood from the Pouch of Douglas — provides strong presumptive evidence of an ectopic pregnancy

The uterus enlarges and the endometrium undergoes decidual change. Implantation within the fimbrial end or ampulla of the tube allows greater expansion before rupture occurs, whereas implantation in the interstitial portion or the isthmic part of the tube presents with early signs of haemorrhage or pain (Fig. 8.8).

Trophoblastic cells invade the wall of the tube and erode into blood vessels. This process will continue until the pregnancy bursts into the abdominal cavity or into the broad ligament, or the embryo dies, thus resulting in a tubal mole. Under these circumstances, absorption or tubal abortion may occur. Expulsion of the embryo into the peritoneal cavity or partial abortion may also occur with continuing episodes of bleeding from the tube.

Differential diagnosis

Ectopic pregnancy should always be suspected where early pregnancy is complicated by pain and bleeding. It is often overlooked if the diagnosis is not considered and may be confused with a threatened or incomplete abortion. It may also be confused with acute salpingitis or appendicitis with pelvic peritonitis. It may sometimes be confused with rupture or haemorrhage of an ovarian cyst.

Management

Diagnosis of the acute ectopic pregnancy rarely presents a problem and blood should be taken for urgent cross-matching and transfusion. Laparotomy should be performed as soon as possible with removal of the damaged tube.

Diagnosis of tubal pregnancy in the subacute phase may be much more difficult. If sufficient blood loss has occurred into the peritoneal cavity, the haemoglobin level will be low and the white cell count will be usually normal or slightly raised. A pregnancy test may be positive but is not reliable in tubal pregnancy. Clinical examination may reveal a mass in one fornix and needle aspiration of the Pouch of Douglas (culdocentesis) will reveal a haemoperitoneum (Fig. 8.9). Ultrasound scan of the pelvis may demonstrate a tubal pregnancy but is generally more helpful in excluding an intrauterine pregnancy. Where there is any possibility of an ectopic pregnancy, laparoscopy is essential. Occasionally, there may be no clinical signs of an ectopic pregnancy but if curettings submitted for histopathology show evidence of decidual reaction and the Arias–Stella phenomenon then it is advisable to consider laparoscopy. Once the diagnosis has been established, the ectopic pregnancy must be removed by one of the following techniques:

1. *Salpingectomy* — if the tube is badly damaged the correct treatment is removal of the affected tube. If implantation has occurred in the interstitial portion of the tube, then it may be necessary to resect part of the uterine horn in addition to removing the tube.
2. *Salpingotomy* — where the ectopic pregnancy is contained within the tube, it may be possible to conserve the tube by removing the pregnancy

and reconstituting the tube. This is particularly important where the contralateral tube has been lost. However, there is an increased risk of recurrent ectopic pregnancy in the damaged tube.

3. *Tubal compression* — occasionally where the tubal pregnancy occurs in the fimbrial end of the tube it may be possible to express the conceptus without opening the tube, but it is essential to be certain that adequate haemostasis is obtained.

Management of other forms of extra-uterine pregnancy

Abdominal pregnancy

Abdominal pregnancy presents a life-threatening hazard to the mother. The placenta implants outside the uterus and across the bowel and pelvic peritoneum. Any attempt to remove it will result in massive haemorrhage which is extremely difficult to control. The fetus should be removed by laparotomy and the placenta left in situ to reabsorb or extrude spontaneously.

Cervical pregnancy

Cervical pregnancy often presents as the cervical stage of a spontaneous abortion. Occasionally, it is possible to remove the conceptus by curettage but haemorrhage can be severe, and in 50% of cases it is necessary to proceed to hysterectomy to obtain adequate haemostasis.

Ectopic pregnancy

- 1 in 200 pregnancies
- Predisposing factors are previous ectopic pregnancy, or pelvic inflammatory disease, IUCD in situ
- Acute presentation in 25% cases
- Common features are 6–8 weeks amenorrhoea, anaemia, lower abdominal pain localised to one side and vaginal bleeding
- Pitfalls in diagnosis are negative urinary hCG or ultrasonography and misdiagnosis as abortion
- Laparoscopy essential to confirm the diagnosis

TROPHOBLASTIC DISEASE

Abnormality of early trophoblast may arise as a developmental anomaly of placental tissue and

Fig. 8.10 Graph-like vesicles of a hydatidiform mole

results in the formation of a mass of oedematous and avascular villi. There is usually no fetus but the condition can be found in the presence of a fetus. The placenta is replaced by a mass of grapelike vesicles known as a **hydatidiform mole** (Fig. 8.10).

Invasion of the myometrium without systemic spread occurs in about 16% of cases of benign mole and is known as **invasive mole** or **chorioadenoma destruens**. Frankly malignant change occurs in 2.5% and is known as **choriocarcinoma**.

Incidence

The overall prevalence of this condition is about 1 in 2000 pregnancies in Western European countries but is much higher in Asia and South-East Asia. It is relatively more common at the extremes of reproductive age. Molar pregnancies are nearly all female, with occasional cases of triploidy.

Pathology

Benign mole remains confined to the uterine cavity and decidua. The histopathology exhibits a villous pattern, which is also found in the invasive mole. However, invasive molar tissue penetrates the myometrium deeply and may result in serious haemorrhage. Choriocarcinoma comprises plexiform columns of trophoblastic cells without villous patterns. Widespread blood-borne metastases are a feature of this disease which, until recent years, carried a very high mortality rate. Metastases may occur locally in the vagina but most commonly appear in the lungs. Theca lutein cysts occur in about one-third of all cases as a result of high circulating levels of hCG. These regress spontaneously with removal of the molar tissue.

Clinical presentation

Molar pregnancy most commonly presents as bleeding in the first half of pregnancy and spontaneous abortion often occurs at about 20 weeks' gestation. Occasionally, the passage of a grape-like villus heralds the presence of a mole. The uterus is larger than dates in about half the cases but this is not a reliable sign as it may sometimes be small for dates. Severe hyperemesis, pre-eclampsia and unexplained anaemia are all factors suggestive of this disorder. The diagnosis can be confirmed by ultrasound scan and by the presence of very high levels of hCG in the blood or urine.

Management

Once the diagnosis is established, the pregnancy is terminated by suction curettage. Adequate replacement of blood loss is essential and the procedure is accompanied by the infusion of oxytocin to ensure that the uterus remains well contracted. All cases of molar pregnancy should be followed for 1 year and further pregnancy during this time is contraindicated. Serial estimations of subunit hCG are followed; where these remain elevated for more than 1 month after uterine evacuation, or where persistent haemorrhage occurs, repeat curettage should be performed.

If the histological evidence shows malignant change, chemotherapy with methotrexate and actinomycin D is employed and produces good results. In the United Kingdom, management of these cases is concentrated in specialised centres.

It may occasionally be necessary to remove the uterus where haemorrhage becomes life–threatening. It must be remembered that choriocarcinoma sometimes can occur following an abortion or a normal term intra-uterine pregnancy.

Case study
A 27-year-old primigravid woman attended the clinic with a history of 12 weeks' amenorrhoea, complaining of bright vaginal blood loss and lower abdominal discomfort. Abdominal examination revealed that the uterine fundus was 16 weeks in size. There was fresh blood in the vagina and the cervical os was closed. There was a high titre of hCG in the urine and an ultrasound scan showed a ground glass appearance in the uterine cavity with no evidence of fetal parts. Suction evacuation of molar tissue was performed the following day and recovery was uneventful.

Trophoblastic disease

- 1 in 2000 pregnancies in UK
- 16% are invasive mole, 2.5% choriocarcinoma
- Features are large-for-dates uterus, PV bleeding and high hCG
- Curettage should be repeated after one month if bleeding hasn't settled or hCG remains elevated
- Follow-up is by hCG and advise not to get pregnant for 12 months
- Choriocarcinoma blood-borne metastases, treatment with methotrexate

BIBLIOGRAPHY

Fox H, Buckley C H 1982 Pathology of spontaneous abortion. In: Pathology for gynaecologists, p 246. Edward Arnold, London
Fox H, Buckley C H 1982 Trophoblastic disease. In: Pathology for gynaecologists, p 250. Edward Arnold, London

9. Congenital abnormalities and infections in pregnancy

There are a very large number of congenital abnormalities and genetic syndromes documented in the literature, but most clinicians encounter very few of them. Genetic counselling has become an important specialty in its own right. Only those conditions which are encountered relatively commonly will be considered in this section.

CONGENITAL ABNORMALITIES

Incidence

The incidence of serious congenital abnormalities has been estimated at 25–30/1000 births and this figure has remained relatively constant in England and Wales since 1920. Congenital abnormalities account for 25% of all stillbirths and 20% of all deaths in the first week. The commonest five groups of defect include neural tube defects (3–7/1000), congenital heart disease (6), severe mental retardation (4), Down's syndrome (1.5) and hare lip/cleft palate (1.5) (Table 9.1). Whilst the total number of infants born with congenital defects is small, the overall incidence of chromosomal abnormalities is high, as about 30% of early abortions show significant chromosomal abnormalities.

Neural tube defects

The neural tube defects are the commonest of the major congenital abnormalities and include anencephaly, microcephaly, spina bifida with or without meningo-myelocele and encephalocele (Fig. 9.1). The incidence is approximately 1 in 200 and the chance of having an affected child after one previous abnormal child is 1 in 20. Infants with anencephaly or microcephaly do not usually survive. Many die during labour and the remainder within the first week of life. Infants with open neural tube defects often survive — particularly where it is possible to cover the lesion surgically with skin. However, the defect may result in paraplegia and bowel and bladder incontinence. The child often has normal intelligence and becomes aware of the problems posed for the parents.

Table 9.1 Major congenital abnormalities

	Approximate incidence per 1000 births
Neural tube defects	3–7
Congenital heart disease	6
Severe mental retardation	4
Down's syndrome	1.5
Cleft lip/palate	1.5
Talipes	1–2
Cerebral palsy	3
Blindness	0.2
Deafness	0.8
Abnormalities of limbs	1–2
Others including renal tract anomalies	2
Total	15–30

Fig. 9.1 Two common abnormalities of the central nervous system

Anencephaly

Spina bifida

93

Although there is some evidence that multi-vitamin supplementation may reduce the incidence of this condition, the major effort at the present time is directed toward screening techniques (see Chapter 4).

Screening by alphafetoprotein

All women should be offered screening by measurement of serum alphafetoprotein between 16 and 19 weeks gestation. Women who would not accept termination of an abnormal pregnancy should not have the test performed unless it is specifically requested.

An abnormally high value should be investigated by:

1. Repeating the serum measurement on another sample.
2. Checking the gestational age by ultrasound scan.
3. Checking for multiple pregnancy by scan.
4. Screening by scan for neurological abnormality.
5. Performing an amniocentesis and determining the alphafetoprotein content of the amniotic fluid. Acetyl cholinesterase measurement also improves diagnostic precision.

The mother should be advised that there is a risk of abortion which is estimated at about 1%.

Congenital cardiac defects

The next big group is that of congenital cardiac defects. At the present time, prenatal diagnosis is difficult and unreliable. Some of these infants present with intra-uterine growth retardation and oligohydramnios, but in most cases the diagnosis can only be established after delivery. With improvements in real-time ultrasound imaging, recognition of many cardiac defects has become possible but early recognition is essential if any action is to be taken.

Other conditions amenable to diagnosis by amniocentesis

X-linked diseases

This group includes X-linked diseases such as Duchenne's muscular dystrophy and haemophilia. If the mother is a carrier and the karyotype

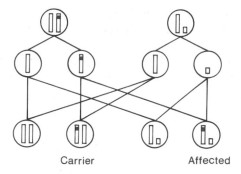

Carrier   Affected

Fig. 9.2   Transmission of recessively inherited X-linked disorder. The abnormal gene is carried on the female X chromosome

demonstrates a male fetus, then the child will have a 50/50 chance of having Duchenne's muscular dystrophy and therefore abortion should be offered (Fig. 9.2).

However, this diagnostic precision can now be improved by fetoscopy and direct samplings from the umbilical and placental blood vessels. Serum creatinine kinase is grossly elevated in the affected infant. Fetoscopy carries a risk of abortion of up to 10%, but this risk is diminishing with the use of finer instruments.

Metabolic disorders

Conditions such as phenylketonuria, which may result in severe mental retardation, are now amenable to prenatal diagnosis by identifying enzyme

Table 9.2   Inherited metabolic disorders most commonly diagnosed antenatally

Sphingolipidoses	
Tay-Sachs disease	Hexoseaminadase-A
Gaucher's disease	Glucocerebrosidase
Metachromatic	Arylsulphatase
Leucodystrophy	
Krabbe's leucodystrophy	Galactocerebroside-B
	Galactosidase
Pompes disease	a-1-4-Glucosidase
(glycogen storage)	
Mucopolysaccharidoses	
Hurler disease	a-L-Iduronidase
Hunter disease	Sulpho-Iduronide Sulphatase
Sanfilippo disease	Heparan Sulphate Sulphatase
Galactosaemia	Galactose-1-Phosphate Uridyl
	Transferase
Homocystinuria	Cystathionine Synthetase
Maple syrup urine disease	Keto Acid Decarboxylase
Methylmalonic acidaemia	Methylmalonic CoA Mutase

deficiencies in cultured fetal cells. The conditions which can be reliably diagnosed in this way are listed in Table 9.2.

Conditions associated with visible abnormalities such as absent eyes, limb deformities, hare lip and encephalocele may also be diagnosed antenatally by fetoscopy.

CHROMOSOMAL ABNORMALITIES

A considerable number of chromosomal abnormalities have been identified from the culture and karyotype of fetal cells in the amniotic fluid and include structural and numerical abnormalities of the karyotype. The commonest abnormality is that associated with trisomy 21 or Down's syndrome.

Down's syndrome

This syndrome is characterised by the typical abnormal facies, mental retardation of varying degrees of severity and congenital heart disease. The karyotype includes an additional chromosome on group 21 and this presents as a trisomy 21, although it sometimes occurs at number 22. The incidence overall is 1.5/1000 births. However, the risk increases with advancing maternal age and over the age of 30 years is 1/300, while over the age of 45 years it is about 1/40. The underlying reason may be related to an increased frequency of non-disjunction at meiosis.

About 6–8% of affected infants have the disease

as a result of a translocation and the extra 21 chromosome is carried on to another chromosome, usually in group 13–15. The mother or the father will usually show evidence of being a translocation carrier. If the mother is a carrier the risk of recurrence is 1/10. Thus, all women over the age of 35 or with a family history of mongolism should be offered amniocentesis with a view to termination of the pregnancy, if the karyotype is abnormal.

Amniocentesis is usually also offered to women who have a previous history of Turner's syndrome (45XO) or Klinefelter's syndrome (47XYY), although the risk of recurrence is low.

Congenital abnormalities

- 25–30/1000 births in England and Wales
- Account for 25% still-births, 20% of neonatal deaths
- Commonest are neural tube defects (7/1000), followed by cardiac defects (6/1000) and chromosomal defects (1.5/1000)
- Incidence of trisomy 21 increases with age
- Amniocentesis can assist in prenatal diagnosis of neural tube defects, chromosome abnormalities, X-linked disorders and some metabolic defects

MATERNAL INFECTIONS WHICH MAY AFFECT FETAL DEVELOPMENT

Rubella

The effect of maternal rubella infection has been discussed in a previous chapter. Congenital malformations include microcephaly, cataracts, deafness,

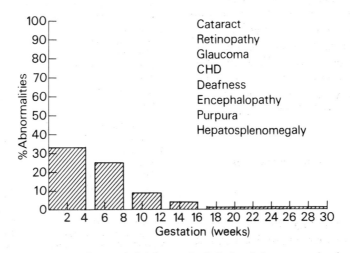

Cataract
Retinopathy
Glaucoma
CHD
Deafness
Encephalopathy
Purpura
Hepatosplenomegaly

Fig. 9.3   Incidence of congenital defects and rubella in relation to gestational age congenital heart disease and osteitis. From 0 to 4 weeks, the risk is 33%, between 5 and 8 weeks 25%, between 9 and 12 weeks 9%, between 13 and 16 weeks 4%, and between 17 and 30 weeks 1% (Fig. 9.3). Injections of gammaglobulin where contact with rubella has occurred may help to prevent infections, but the evidence is equivocal. Diagnosis based on the level of rubella antibodies has been previously discussed.

Hepatitis B

There are two types of viral hepatitis — infective hepatitis (virus A) and serum hepatitis (virus B). Virus A is associated with a short incubation period and virus B with a long incubation time. Hepatitis B surface antigen is known as Australian antigen.

The risk to the fetus of maternal infection appears to be minimal. The infant may become infected by swallowing maternal blood or amniotic fluid during labour and about 25% of these infants subsequently develop hepatitis.

Australia-antigen-positive women are managed with particular precautions as cross-infection may occur from maternal faeces, urine, maternal blood or amniotic fluid. These patients should be managed with barrier nursing, taking especial precautions with the disposal of excreta.

Herpes hominis

Herpes infections are due to two antigenic types, 1 and 2. Type 2 is responsible for 95% of genital tract infections, whereas type 1 occurs in non-genital sites such as the mouth, eyes and central nervous system. Type 2 infections are sexually transmitted.

Genital herpes is associated with a five-fold increase in the incidence of abortion during the first 20 weeks. Genital infection at term results in a 40% incidence of infection in the fetus and this may be manifest in skin vesicles, and in infections involving the brain, liver and adrenals.

At the present time, it is generally considered advisable to deliver the infant by Caesarean section to minimize the risk of infection acquired during vaginal delivery if the culture from the vagina remains positive.

Other infections

Cytomegalovirus

It has been estimated that 4% of women acquire this infection during pregnancy. Both the placenta and fetus may be affected by the viraemia which may result in the development of microcephaly and be the cause of mental retardation of infants in the first 6 years of life. The diagnosis can be established by the presence of a rising antibody titre. Newborn screening is based on raised cord blood IgM levels (>20 mg %).

Pregnancy bacteriuria

Bacteriuria in the mother is associated with an increase in low birth weight infants. Urine specimens yielding more than 10^5 colonies/ml are considered bacteriuric and should be treated with appropriate antibiotic therapy.

Toxoplasmosis

Toxoplasma gondii is a protozoal infection which is found throughout the world. The mode of infection involves the domestic cat. Congenital toxoplasmosis may occur if the mother acquires the infection during pregnancy, and its incidence has been estimated in England at 1 in 20 000 births. In France it may be as high as 1 in 2000 births. Maternal infection may be a cause of recurrent abortion.

HIV infection in pregnancy

Human Immunodeficiency Virus (HIV) is a retrovirus which affects human lymphocytes and other cells in the central nervous system. There are three levels of manifestation of HIV infection:

1. Asymptomatic – a positive test for HIV but no clinical symptoms.
2. AIDS related complex (ARC) – this includes persistent generalised lymphadenopathy, weight loss, lethargy, fever and joint pains.
3. Acquired immune deficiency syndrome – this includes the clinical symptoms plus opportunistic infections and the presence of Kaposi's sarcoma and the presence of Pneumocystis carinii.

Infection is usually asymptomatic and incubation takes 15–58 months. Transmission is sexual or blood-borne and transplacental. There is no evidence to suggest that airborne infection occurs.

Incidence. In the United States AIDS is largely confined to homosexual or bisexual individuals (27%). However, 50% of cases occur in intravenous drugs abusers and following this it is associated with 10% after blood transfusion. Obviously, these clinical incidence figures will continue changing.

In pregnancy, there is no evidence that HIV infection is clinically accelerated. AIDS and ARC depress the T helper cell population. It does not affect fertility.

There is a higher incidence of pre-term labour and low birth weight infants in affected mothers, but there are complicating social factors. There are three routes of infection of the child:

1. Transplacental.
2. At birth.
3. Breast milk.

Incidental perinatal transmission occurs in 30–50% of cases.

Fetal AIDS. This syndrome is manifested by intra-uterine growth retardation, microcephaly, prominent forehead and blue sclerae.

Prognosis. The outlook for survival in infected children is very poor with a high mortality rate. There is some evidence that the extent of maternal illness may determine the risk of infection in the baby.

Maternal infections affecting the fetus

- Incidence of congenital defects in rubella varies in relation to gestational age at time of infection from 33% to 1%
- Hepatitis B transmission is uncommon
- Delivery by Caesarian section is recommended for patients with active herpes (type 2) infection; 40% incidence of neonatal infection
- Cytomegalovirus can cause microcephaly and mental retardation
- Toxoplasmosis affects 1/20 000 births

BIBLIOGRAPHY

Davis P S 1984 Maternal and fetal infection. In: Beard R W, Nathaniels P W (eds) Fetal physiology and medicine. Marcel Dekker, Butterworths, New York
Fitzsimmons J S 1980 A handbook of clinical genetics. William Heinemann Medical Books, London

10. Antenatal disorders

HYPERTENSION IN PREGNANCY

Hypertension is the commonest complication of pregnancy in the United Kingdom and occurs in 10–15% of all pregnancies. In its most severe form, the condition is associated with convulsions, proteinuria and oedema and may lead to fetal and maternal death. In its mildest form, hypertension alone in late pregnancy, it appears to be of minimal risk. The association between pregnancy and convulsions has been described in ancient Egyptian and Greek writings, but that between convulsions and hypertension and proteinuria was first described by Vaquez in 1897.

Classification

Numerous attempts have been made to classify hypertension in pregnancy but the classification should be simple and related to factors which can be clearly defined. Essentially, hypertension may occur as a result of the pregnancy, or it may antedate the pregnancy and be due to underlying renal disease or to essential hypertension. The best classification available at the present time is the one outlined by the American College of Obstetricians and Gynecologists:

Hypertension is defined as a systolic pressure of at least 140 mmHg or a diastolic pressure of at least 90 mmHg on two or more occasions after 20 weeks gestation (Fig. 10.1).

This definition also includes reference to a rise in systolic pressure of at least 30 mmHg or a rise in diastolic pressure of at least 15 mmHg, but it is unlikely that this classification does more than complicate the definition as fetal and maternal risks do not increase if the blood pressure remains less than 140/90 mmHg.

Fig. 10.1 The signs of pre-eclampsia include hypertension, proteinuria and oedema

Proteinuria is defined as the presence of urinary protein in concentrations greater than 0.3 g per litre in a 24-hour collection or in concentrations greater than 1 g per litre on two or more occasions at least 6 hours apart.

Oedema is defined as the development of pitting oedema or a weight gain in excess of 2.3 kg in 1 week. Because oedema of the legs is very common in an otherwise uncomplicated pregnancy, this is the least useful sign and should probably be abandoned in future classifications.

The various types of hypertension are therefore defined as follows:

1. Gestational hypertension.
2. Pre-eclampsia.
3. Eclampsia.

4. Superimposed pre-eclampsia or eclampsia.
5. Chronic hypertensive disease.
6. Unclassified hypertensive disease.

Gestational hypertension is the development of hypertension alone during pregnancy or within the first 24 hours post partum in a previously normotensive woman. The blood pressure returns to normal within 10 days after delivery.

Pre-eclampsia is the development of hypertension and proteinuria and oedema after the 20th week of gestation. It is predominantly a disorder of primigravidae.

Eclampsia is the association of convulsions with pre-eclampsia.

Superimposed pre-eclampsia or eclampsia is the development of pre-eclampsia in a patient with chronic hypertensive disease or renal disease.

Chronic hypertensive disease is the presence of persistent hypertension before pregnancy or before the 20th week of gestation.

Unclassified hypertensive disease includes those cases of hypertension occurring in pregnancy on a random basis, but where there is insufficient information for classification.

Because of the difficulties in classification, hypertension developing during pregnancy is now often classified simply as pregnancy-induced hypertension with or without proteinuria.

Incidence

Approximately 10–15% of all pregnancies are complicated by hypertension, but in the UK only 1 in 10 of these pregnancies is complicated by proteinuria.

Pathogenesis and pathology of pre-eclampsia and eclampsia

The exact nature of the pathogenesis of pre-eclampsia remains uncertain. However, the pathophysiology (Fig. 10.2) is characterized by:

1. Arteriolar vasoconstriction — particularly in the vascular bed of the uterus and the kidney.
2. Disseminated intravascular coagulation.

Blood pressure is determined by cardiac output, blood volume and peripheral vascular resistance. Both cardiac output and blood volume increase substantially in pregnancy, but blood pressure tends to fall in mid-trimester. Thus, the most important regulatory factor is the loss of peripheral vascular resistance that occurs in pregnancy and, as sympathetic tone appears to remain unchanged, the state of peripheral vascular resistance is determined by the balance between humoral vasodilators and vasoconstrictors. There is a specific loss of sensitivity to angiotensin II, which is related to locally active

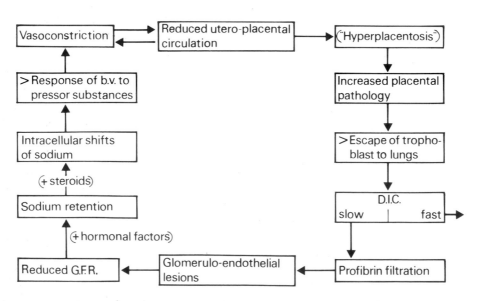

Fig. 10.2   The cycle of pathological changes that occurs in pre-eclampsia

vasodilator prostaglandins. Thus, factors which increase the activity of the renin-angiotensin system or reduce the activity of tissue prostaglandins will result in hypertension. Once vasoconstriction occurs in the utero-placental bed, it results in placental damage and the release of trophoblast into the peripheral circulation. This trophoblast is rich in thromboplastins, which precipitate disseminated intravascular coagulation, giving rise to the pathological lesions in the kidney, liver and placental bed. The renal lesion results in sodium and water retention with most of this fluid accumulating outside the vascular tree. Plasma volume diminishes as the vascular space is reduced. At the same time, increased sodium retention increases vascular sensitivity to angiotensin II and therefore promotes further vasoconstriction and tissue damage in a vicious circle of events which may ultimately result in cerebral haemorrhage, acute cardiac failure with pulmonary oedema, acute renal failure with tubular or cortical necrosis and hepatic failure with periportal necrosis. The placenta becomes grossly infarcted and this results in intra-uterine growth retardation and sometimes fetal death. There are many factors which may trigger this sequence of events, including immunological and dietary factors and the pre-existence of underlying chronic renal disease or essential hypertension.

The renal lesion

The renal lesion is the most specific diagnostic feature of pre-eclampsia (Fig 10.3) and features:

1. Swelling and proliferation of endothelial cells to such a point that the capillary vessels are almost obstructed.
2. Hypertrophy and hyperplasia of the inter-capillary or mesangial cells.
3. Fibrillary material (profibrin) deposited on the basement membrane and between and within the endothelial cells.

The characteristic appearance is therefore one of increased capillary cellularity and reduced vascularity. The lesion is present in 71% of primigravidae, whereas it is found in only 29% of multigravidae. There is a much higher incidence of unsuspected chronic renal disease in multigravidae. The glomerular lesion is always associated with

Fibrin deposition   Swelling of endothelial cells

Fig. 10.3 Renal changes in pre-eclampsia include endothelial swelling and fibrin definition under the basement membrane of the glomerular tuft

proteinuria and with reduced glomerular filtration. Tubular changes result in impaired uric acid secretion leading to hyperuricaemia.

Placental pathology

Placental infarcts occur in normal pregnancy, but are significantly more extensive in pre-eclampsia. The characteristic features in the placenta include:

1. Increased syncytial knots or sprouts.
2. Increased loss of syncytium.
3. Proliferation of cytotrophoblast.
4. Thickening of the trophoblastic basement membrane.
5. Villous necrosis.

In the utero-placental bed, the normal invasion of trophoblastic cells along the luminal surface of the spiral arteries does not occur beyond the deciduo-myometrial junction, and there is apparent constriction of the vessels between the radial artery and the decidual portion (Figs. 10.4, 10.5). These changes may result in reduced uteroplacental blood flow.

Disseminated intravascular coagulation (DIC)

In severe pre-eclampsia and eclampsia, thrombosis occurs in the capillaries. Multiple platelet and fibrin thrombi can be identified in the brain. Similar changes are seen in the periportal areas of the liver

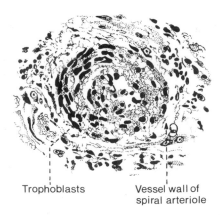

Trophoblasts   Vessel wall of
                      spiral arteriole

Fig. 10.4   Trophoblast invasion of the spiral arterioles is defective in pre-eclampsia

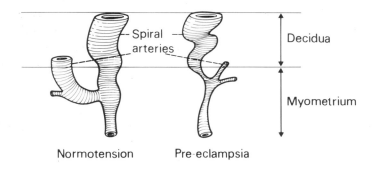

Normotension   Pre-eclampsia

Fig. 10.5   Invasion of the spiral arterioles by trophoblast results
in dilatation of the vessels; this process is defective in pre-eclampsia

and in the adrenal cortex and spleen. In some cases, thrombocytopenia develops and in 10% of eclamptic women the platelet count falls below 100 000/ml. There is an increase in fibrin deposition resulting both from increased fibrin production and from impaired removal of fibrin. There seems little doubt that coagulation changes play a major role in the pathology of eclampsia.

Immunological aspects of pregnancy hypertension

Pre-eclampsia may be due to an abnormality of feto-maternal host response. There is a lower incidence of pre-eclampsia in consanguinous marriages and an increased incidence of hypertension in first pregnancies in second marriages.

Indices of cell-mediated immune response have also been shown to be altered in severe pre-eclampsia. However, the incidence of pre-eclampsia differs markedly in different racial groups and climatic conditions, and it also follows a familial pattern.

Management

Pre-eclampsia and gestational hypertension

The object of management is to prevent the development of eclampsia with its consequent serious sequelae to the mother and to the survival and health of the fetus.

Bed rest. The detection of hypertension is an indication for admission to hospital and bed rest, which results in an improvement in renal and utero-placental blood flow. The improvement in renal blood flow results in a diuresis, loss of weight and a reduction in oedema. In gestational hypertension, there may be a case for home management of hypertension with self-assessment of blood pressure and urine testing for proteinuria. The development of proteinuria is an absolute indication for immediate hospital admission. If the blood pressure returns to normal, the patient can be sent home and observations continued on an out-patient basis.

Sedation. Sedation has little part to play in the management of mild hypertension. In the presence of hyperreflexia and cerebral excitability, diazepam 10–20 mg 6-hourly will reduce the risk of convulsions, but has the disadvantage that prolonged treatment will result in placental transfer of diazepam and its metabolite, desmethyl diazepam, and may lead to hypothermia and hypotonia in the fetus — a condition known as the **floppy baby syndrome** (Fig. 10.6).

Whilst diazepam is particularly useful in the management of the pre-convulsive or convulsive state, longer term prevention of fits may be achieved by the use of sodium phenytoin, intravenously initially and later by the oral route.

Fig. 10.6 The use of diazepam may result in the 'floppy baby' syndrome with hypotonia and hypothermia

Diuretics. Severe pre-eclampsia is associated with hypovolaemia. Further reduction in blood volume with diuretics tends to reduce utero-placental blood flow and renal blood flow. The long-term use of diuretics in pregnancy has been shown to be associated with fetal growth retardation, and has no significant beneficial effect on the development of hypertension or proteinuria. The only positive indications for the use of diuretics are:

1. For the symptomatic relief of oedema.

2. In some cases of essential hypertension in pregnancy.

3. Use of osmotic diuretics such as mannitol in the immediate postpartum period when oliguria develops.

Monitoring of the feto-placental unit

Pre-eclampsia results in impaired placental function and it is, therefore, important to monitor this function and to assess fetal growth and development. Most commonly used techniques now rely on the assessment of biophysical changes and these measurements include:

1. *Oestriol in urine or plasma.* Oestriol reflects in part the function of the fetal adrenal function (see Fig. 6.7) and a fall in oestriol levels may reflect failure of the feto-placental unit. It must be said that the measurement of biochemical parameters is becoming increasingly less common as these measurements have been replaced by the assessment of biophysical changes.

2. *Serial ultrasound measurements.* Assessments of fetal biparietal diameter and abdominal birth are used to examine the role of fetal growth, in association with the assessment of amniotic fluid volume as an index of placental failure.

3. *Doppler flow studies.* The use of pulsed ultrasound enables the measurement of velocity profiles in the fetal and uterine circulation, and from these measurements some estimate can be made of flow rates. A significant reduction in flow in the umbilical arteries or the uteroplacental vessels associated with increased vascular resistance may signify increasing jeopardy to the fetus.

4. *Antenatal cardiotocography.* The antenatal assessment of fetal heart rate and uterine activity provides a useful, but by no means infallible, indication of fetal wellbeing. The presence of episodes of fetal bradycardia, either during the resting phase or during contractions, and the loss of base-line variability of heart rate may indicate fetal hypoxia.

Antihypertensive drug therapy

The role of antihypertensive therapy is currently being explored and re-evaluated. It should be made clear that there is no drug available at the present time that specifically reverses the vascular change of pre-eclampsia. Therefore, the purpose of using antihypertensive therapy is to protect the mother from the effects of the hypertension and to prolong pregnancy to enable greater fetal maturity to be achieved. These objectives can be achieved only if the drug employed has no significant deleterious effects on the mother or infant.

Antihypertensive therapy has its major role in controlling severe hypertension or in treating milder forms of gestational hypertension before 34 weeks gestation.

The drugs most commonly used are:

Methyl dopa.
Hydralazine.
β-blockers such as oxprenolol, atenolol, metoprolol
Combined α- and β-blockers such as labetalol.

The most significant sign in late pregnancy is the development of proteinuria and where this is persistent it is an indication to deliver the patient.

In the milder forms of hypertension, antihypertensive therapy should not be started until the blood pressure has failed to settle after 3 days' bed rest.

An overall profile of the various management strategies in pregnancy hypertension is shown in Figure 10.7. This flow diagram illustrates the various pathways of progression and their management. Mild gestational hypertension may get better after rest, or may progress to proteinuric hypertension with convulsions in the most extreme cases of eclampsia.

Symptoms of pre-eclampsia and eclampsia

Pre-eclampsia is commonly an asymptomatic condition. However, there are symptoms which must **never** be overlooked as they presage the onset of eclampsia and these include frontal headache, blurring of vision and epigastric pain (Fig 10.8). Of these, the most important is the development of epigastric pain — either during the pregnancy or within 24 hours of delivery. It is also extremely

Fig. 10.7 Flow diagram of regression or progression of gestational hypertension and its management.

Frontal headache
Blurred vision

Epigastric pain

Hyperactive
reflexes

Fig. 10.8 Presenting signs of eclampsia

important to remember that the most severe forms of pre-eclampsia and eclampsia may occur in the second trimester, despite the fact that the condition most commonly occurs in the third trimester.

Induction of labour

The decision as to when a pregnancy should be terminated is determined by:

1. The maturity of the fetus.
2. The severity of the pre-eclampsia and, in particular, the development of persistent proteinuria.
3. The presence of additional complications such as placental abruption.

Severe hypertension and proteinuria may sometimes necessitate early induction of labour or Caesarean section to safeguard the health of the mother and because the hazard to the fetus remaining 'in utero' may outweigh the risks of prematurity. No pregnancy should be allowed to proceed past term in the presence of even mild hypertension.

If the cervix is unripe and unsuitable for surgical induction, the cervix can often be ripened by the use of vaginal gel containing prostaglandin E_2. If the cervix is unripe and the condition is severe, it may be necessary to proceed to delivery by Caesarean section, but only after controlling the blood pressure with intravenous hydralazine.

If the cervix is ripe, the labour is induced by:

1. Artificial rupture of the membranes.
2. Oxytocin infusion.
3. A combination of both procedures.

The fetal heart rate should always be monitored as well as the level of uterine activity.

Complications

1. There is an increased incidence of placental abruption in pregnancies complicated by hypertension.
2. Severe pre-eclampsia is associated with reduced glomerular filtration and this may result in severe oliguria. A diuresis can be induced by the administration of mannitol 500 ml of a 20% solution.

Eclampsia

The onset of convulsions in a pregnancy complicated by pre-eclampsia denotes the onset of eclampsia (Fig. 10.9). Eclampsia most commonly occurs in primigravidae, but may occur in women of high parity who have previously had uncomplicated pregnancies. Eclampsia is a preventable condition and denotes a failure to recognize the early worsening signs of pre-eclampsia. It carries serious risks of intra-uterine death for the fetus and of maternal death from cerebral haemorrhage and renal and hepatic failure. All cases must be managed in hospital. Any woman who is admitted to hospital with convulsions during the course of a pregnancy, or who is admitted in a coma associated with hypertension, should be considered to be suffering from eclampsia until proved otherwise.

Fig. 10.9 The differentiating feature of eclampsia is the development of convulsions

Management

The three basic guidelines for management of eclampsia are:

1. Control the fits.
2. Control the blood pressure.
3. Deliver the infant.

Various drugs are used to control the fits but the most widely used regimes include:

1. Intravenous injection of diazepam 20–40 mg followed by intramuscular injection of 10 mg according to the state of sedation.
2. Chlormethiazole by continuous intravenous infusion.
3. Magnesium sulphate by intravenous and intra-muscular administration. This therapy is widely used in the USA but is not commonly employed in the UK. The drug is effective in suppressing convulsions and inhibiting muscle activity. It also reduces platelet aggregation and hence minimizes the effect of disseminated intra-vascular coagulation.

It is important to ensure that a clear airway is maintained and that further fits are prevented and, to this end, patients have traditionally been kept under sedation in a darkened room with minimal noise and light. However, there is now evidence to suggest that they may best be managed in an intensive care unit and managed jointly by the obstetric and ICU staffs.

The best method of controlling blood pressure is the intravenous infusion of hydralazine. In a dosage of 25 mg in 500 ml of 5% dextrose or Hartman's solution, the infusion rate can be regulated according to the blood pressure level. Intravenous infusion of labetalol has also been shown to be effective in regulating blood pressure.

Epidural anaesthesia. Epidural anaesthesia relieves the pain of labour and also lowers blood pressure by causing peripheral vasodilatation in the lower extremities. It will also reduce the tendency to fit by relieving the pain and hence reducing the effect of afferent stimuli from that pain.

Delivery of the infant. Once convulsions have occurred or, indeed, when severe hypertension and proteinuria are present, then the control of blood pressure can usually be sustained only for a short period unless delivery is effected, as the blood pressure will soon rise again. It is therefore necessary to effect delivery and this can be achieved either by forewater rupture and Syntocinon® infusion or by Caesarean section. It is important to remember that delivery should not be attempted until the blood pressure is under control.

Management after delivery

Following delivery, it is important to observe the following points:

1. Maintain the patient in a well-sedated condition in a quiet environment.
2. Special nursing and observation are needed to maintain a clear airway and to avoid further fits.
3. Strict fluid balance charts should be maintained to ensure that fluid overloading does not occur in view of the reduced urinary output.

The risk of fits occurring 24 hours after delivery is minimal. It should also be noted that fits occurring for the first time 24 hours after delivery are rarely due to eclampsia, and are commonly due to epilepsy or superficial cerebral vein thrombosis.

Hypertension in pregnancy

- Occurs in 10–15% pregnancies of which 1 in 10 have proteinuria
- More common in primigravidae, with a new partner, in certain racial groups and where there is a family history
- Defined by hypertension, oedema and proteinuria of > 0.3g/l
- May be associated with chronic hypertensive disease
- Characterised by arteriolar vasoconstriction and DIC
- May lead to cerebral oedema or haemorrhage, cardiac or renal failure, placental infarction and DIC
- Management is to prevent eclampsia, monitor feto-placental unit, control hypertension and deliver the infant
- Important signs to watch for are headache, epigastric pain and hyper-reflexia
- During delivery it is important to control BP, monitor fluid balance and urine output; it may be necessary to sedate

ANAEMIA IN PREGNANCY

Anaemia is a common complication of pregnancy and in some countries may be a major factor in the cause of maternal death.

Maternal difficulties arise in particular where the anaemia is further complicated by antepartum or postpartum haemorrhage.

The fetus tends to withstand maternal anaemia surprisingly well despite the reduced oxygen-carrying capacity in the mother, but is more likely to be damaged if the anaemia is complicated by other conditions such as pre-eclampsia and placental abruption.

Definition

There is no agreed definition of anaemia, but a haemoglobin level of 10 g/100 ml or less is generally accepted as indicating significant anaemia. Normal haemoglobin levels in pregnancy in UK studies have shown first trimester values of 12.0 g/100 ml, 11.9 g in the second trimester, and 11.4 g in the third trimester. There is a fall in haemoglobin in the second trimester associated with a relatively faster expansion of plasma volume than total red cell mass, but this would not account for a significant degree of anaemia.

Nutritional requirements

Anaemia in pregnancy may arise from any recognised cause, but the most important causes are those related to an imbalance between the demands of maternal adaption and the growing fetus, and the actual supply and absorption of essential nutrients (Fig. 10.10). Essential nutrients for haemoglobin synthesis include protein, iron, vitamin B_6 and B_{12}, folic acid, ascorbic acid and numerous trace elements such as copper. The dietary requirement of iron is estimated at 15 mg per day and, unless the dietary intake is above average, this requirement is unlikely to be met.

Fig. 10.10   Basic factors in the aetiology of anaemia in pregnancy

Iron absorption tends to increase in pregnancy and iron is absorbed in the ferrous ionized form. Ascorbic acid may assist in absorption because of its reducing action. Iron absorption may be adversely affected by gastric achlorhydria, protein malnutrition and high carbohydrate diets, chronic diarrhoeal states, and hookworm infestations (Fig. 10.11). Iron

Iron absorption ↑
|
Iron adversely affected by:
  gastric achlorhydria
  protein malnutrition
  high carbohydrate diet
  chronic diarrhoeal state
  hookworm

Fig. 10.11   Factors which influence iron absorption

loss from the body is generally minimal during pregnancy as menstrual loss ceases, although some loss still occurs from hair, nails and sweat. The major reduction in maternal stores is due to the increased demands of pregnancy.

Investigations

Routine management of pregnancy should include measurement of haemoglobin levels at regular intervals during pregnancy. If the haemoglobin falls to less than 11 g/100 ml, then the following investigations should be performed:

1. Complete blood picture — the important measurements are mean corpuscular volume (MCV) and mean corpuscular haemoglobin concentration (MCHC). MCV gives an index of macrocytosis and megaloblastic anaemia, and MCHC gives the best index for iron deficiency anaemia.
2. Serum iron and iron-binding capacity.
3. Serum folate and serum B_{12} levels in all cases of persistent anaemia.
4. Other investigations, including culture of the urine to exclude chronic urinary tract infection and examination of the faeces for ova and parasites.
5. Bone marrow analysis where the diagnosis is in doubt.

Treatment

The management of anaemia in pregnancy depends on the identification of the cause. However, the majority of cases are due to nutritional deficiencies associated with an iron intake inadequate to meet the needs of both mother and fetus.

The use of prophylactic oral iron and folic acid is indicated in nutritional anaemia. Iron should be administered in the form of ferrous sulphate, gluconate, succinate or fumarate. Combined preparations commonly contain 150 mg of ferrous sulphate and 0.5 mg of folic acid and are administered on a once-daily basis.

Where anaemia has become established, oral therapy should always be used first as the response is as rapid as parenteral therapy, excepting when gut absorption is defective.

Parenteral therapy

Parenteral therapy is indicated where iron deficiency anaemia fails to respond to oral therapy. Iron preparations include saccharated iron oxide and an iron-dextran complex such as Imferon®, or an iron-sorbital-citric acid complex such as Jectofer®. All of these compounds may cause severe anaphylactic reactions and a test dose must always be given before a total dose intravenous infusion is given. Intramuscular injections are also sometimes used.

Sickle cell syndrome

These disorders include the heterozygous state for sickle cell haemoglobin (sickle cell trait; HbAS), homozygous sickle cell disease (HbSS), compound heterozygotes for haemoglobin variants such as sickle cell HbC disease and sickle cell thalassaemia.

HbSS. The clinical manifestations of HbSS include chronic anaemia and occasional crises characterised by intravascular sickling leading to vascular occlusion and tissue infarction. Crises are often precipitated by infection and dehydration, and renal complications are common.

Sickle cell HbC disease is a milder variant with near normal haemoglobin levels, but may, on occasions, produce massive sickling crises during pregnancy.

Sickle cell trait (HbAS) rarely causes problems unless there are conditions of extreme anorexia, dehydration and acidosis.

In pregnancy, there are special problems and therefore screening of all potential high risk ethnic groups, such as black people of African origin, Indians, Mediterraneans and Saudi Arabians, is important.

Abortion, pre-term labour and fetal loss are high. These risks can be reduced by regular blood transfusions to maintain a high proportion of HbA.

Adequate hydration, prevention of infection and transfusion during pregnancy are all important management factors in reducing the incidence of crises in pregnancy.

The thalassaemias

These conditions are a genetic disorder associated with a reduced rate of production of one or more of the globulin chains of haemoglobin. They fall into two broad disorders of alpha and beta thalassaemia.

The **beta-thalassaemias** are defined by an inability to synthesise adult beta chains; in the heterozygous state they are symptomless. However, in the homozygous state there is severe and persistent anaemia. These conditions are particularly common in the Mediterranean countries and in India and South-East Asia. The major problems in pregnancy are those related to anaemia and the need for repeated transfusions.

The **alpha thalassaemias** are characterised by an inability to produce the alpha chains common to haemoglobin A. During pregnancy, these women may become very anaemic. Sometimes the fetus may also become anaemic and hydropic and give rise to severe pre-eclampsia.

If routine screening of the parents indicates a risk of carrying a child with alpha thalassaemia, the patient should be referred for prenatal diagnosis. Indeed, this is becoming an increasingly important aspect of management of the homozygous forms of either alpha or beta thalassaemia.

Anaemia in pregnancy

- Commonly dietary but may be due to sickle cell disease or thalassaemia
- Haemoglobin <10 g/l
- Dietary iron requirement is 15 mg/day
- Assessment should include complete blood picture, serum iron and iron binding capacity, serum folate and B$_{12}$ levels.
- Parenteral therapy is indicated only if oral treatment fails, because of risk of reaction

---

DIABETES IN PREGNANCY

Pregnancy affects maternal diabetes and produces

Fig. 10.12 Changes in insulin and glucose levels in normal pregnancy

an increase in insulin requirements; at the same time, diabetes has a significant effect on the pregnancy (Fig. 10.12).

With appropriate management and careful regulation of blood glucose levels, perinatal losses can be minimised and will approach levels in the normal population. This management is best undertaken by a combined team of physicians and obstetricians and delivery should always be effected in a major obstetric hospital which has first class neonatal services.

Nomenclature

All forms of diabetes are associated with increased perinatal loss unless properly managed. The degree of risk is related to the severity of the diabetes. The presentation has been defined by the British Diabetic Association as follows:

1. **Potential diabetes** — patients with no evidence of chemical diabetes but who have a family history of diabetes, a previous history of delivering an infant in excess of 4.0 kg, or a history of an unexplained fetal death. Glycosuria is not a reliable sign, but should be investigated if it is persistent.
2. **Latent or gestational diabetes** — Some women who develop overt diabetes in later life develop chemical or clinical diabetes during pregnancy. This condition is known as gestational diabetes.
3. **Chemical diabetes** — these women have an abnormal glucose tolerance test, but no symptoms of diabetes. Perinatal morbidity is significantly increased.
4. **Clinical diabetes** — insulin dependent diabetes requires careful control throughout pregnancy and should preferably be regulated before pregnancy is commenced.

The American Classification introduced by White in 1965 also linked management and prognosis to further subclassification of the diabetes:

Class A — chemical diabetes only.
Class B — diabetes of adult; onset after 20 years of age.
Class C — diabetes of long duration (between 10 and 19 years) with no evidence of vascular disease.
Class D — diabetes present since before the age of 10 years and present for 20 years or more with vascular disease, calcification of leg vessels or benign retinopathy.
Class E — diabetes associated with calcification of limb vessels.
Class F — diabetes-associated nephropathy.
Class G — the presence of proliferating diabetic retinopathy.

In women with suspected abnormalities of glucose tolerance, a glucose tolerance test should be performed. This test involves the oral administration of 50 g of glucose. An abnormal test is defined by the following criteria:

1. A fasting value of blood glucose in excess of 5.5 mmol/l.
2. A 1-hour value over 9 mmol/l.
3. A 2-hour value over 7 mmol/l.

Maternal complications

1. Pregnancy is diabetogenic and diabetic control therefore becomes difficult. Hyperglycaemia is common and if uncontrolled leads to the development of ketoacidosis with the risk of both fetal and maternal death.

    Hypoglycaemia may result in fetal death only if it is severe and prolonged, and it is more likely to occur in early pregnancy which is complicated by excessive vomiting.
2. Hydramnios is a common complication of the diabetic pregnancy and may result in an unstable lie and premature rupture of the membranes.
3. Pre-eclampsia is common in diabetics and is made worse by poor control of the diabetes. Both fetal and maternal prognosis are significantly worse where the pregnancy is complicated by diabetic nephropathy.
4. Dystocia and operative delivery — the fetus may be abnormally large and an obstructed and difficult labour (dystocia) is a recognized complication. The problem may occur after the head has been delivered because of shoulder obstruction. If there is evidence of potential cephalo-pelvic disproportion, the fetus should be delivered by Caesarean section.

Fetal complication

Babies born to diabetic mothers tend to be larger than normal. There is generalized macrosomia and body fat is commonly increased (Fig. 10.13).

Intra-uterine death tends to occur in the last 3 weeks of pregnancy.

Fig. 10.13   The infant born to the diabetic mother may exhibit macrosomia and abnormal birth weight.

Fetal distress associated with intra-uterine asphyxia and acidosis is a complication of labour.

Neonatal complications

1. *Hypoglycaemia* — there is hyperplasia and hypertrophy of the islets of Langerhans and, as a result, the newborn infant is particularly likely to develop hypoglycaemia. It is therefore important to perform frequent estimations of blood glucose levels in the first 48 hours of life.
2. *Respiratory distress syndrome* — there is higher incidence of respiratory distress syndrome in diabetic infants than in normal infants born at comparable gestational ages.
3. *Congenital abnormalities* — there is a slightly higher incidence of fetal abnormalities in infants born to mothers with diabetes.

Management of diabetes

All grades of diabetes carry a significant risk to the fetus. It may be possible to control gestational diabetes with dietary control, but all other forms of diabetes should be controlled with insulin. In general, the aim should be to keep the blood glucose level below 7 mmol/l at all times by appropriate regulation of diet and insulin administration.

Hospital admission is not essential unless there is an additional complication of the pregnancy or it is not possible to control the diabetes at home. It is the policy in Nottingham to train women to measure their own blood glucose levels and to perform profiles every 2 weeks in the first two trimesters, and weekly in the last 12 weeks. Joint management is undertaken by the physicians and obstetricians and by a diabetic clinic sister who visits patients at home and keeps a close check on the glucose profiles.

The measurement of glycosylated haemoglobin levels (HbA), is a useful method of assessing the longer term stability of the diabetic state; it should normally constitute less than 7% of the total haemoglobin concentration.

Antenatal assessment

Serial measurements of placental function and fetal growth are performed throughout pregnancy.

Placental function tests are of limited value

because oestriol and placental lactogen measurements tend to be abnormally high. However, low values are particularly significant and the tests are therefore worth performing. Cardiotocography is also of value in assessment of feto-placental function.

Serial measurements of fetal growth by ultrasonography and the measurement of biparietal diameter and trunk circumference allow some assessment of fetal size.

Method of delivery

If good diabetic control is achieved and there are no other complications, it should be possible to allow the pregnancy to proceed to full term, although delivery is usually effected between 38 weeks and term. Induction of labour and vaginal delivery can be achieved with careful regulation of blood glucose levels during labour and continuous intrapartum fetal monitoring. If there is any evidence of fetal distress or delay in labour, Caesarean section should be performed.

Amniocentesis performed before induction or elective Caesarean section to measure the lecithin/sphingomyelin ratio or lecithin concentration will enable the prediction of fetal lung maturity.

Neonatal management

The two major hazards that affect the neonate born to a diabetic mother are:

1. Respiratory distress syndrome.
2. Neonatal hypoglycaemia.

These infants should therefore be admitted to the special care neonatal unit to monitor blood glucose levels and to administer oral glucose until feeding is satisfactorily established.

Perinatal mortality

It should be possible to achieve perinatal loss rates that are comparable to the overall perinatal mortality figures. Fetal anomalies occur in 5–6% of cases and are frequently associated with polyhydramnios.

THYROID DISEASE IN PREGNANCY

Thyroid disorders of various types complicate 0.5% of pregnancies.

Hypothyroidism is more common than hyperthyroidism. The most common causes of hypothyroidism which complicates 9 in every 1000 pregnancies are Hashimoto's disease and postablative treatment.

Iodine deficiency is commonest in developing countries and is associated with 30% fetal wastage. The development of cretinism is associated with deafness, mental retardation and spasticity. The diagnosis of hypothyroidism in the mother is made by the presence of low free T_4 and a raised TSH level. Treatment is by thyroid replacement therapy.

Hyperthyroidism occurs in 2 in 1000 pregnancies. Graves' disease or toxic goitre is associated with an increased risk of malformation, low birthweight and premature labour. The condition is diagnosed by the presence of high free T_3 and low TSH, or a flat response to TRH. The condition is treated with carbimazole or propylthiouracial which inhibits iodination of tyrosine. Propylthiouracil does not cross the placenta and does not cause teratogenesis.

Diabetes in pregnancy

- Pregnancy may be associated with changes in pre-existing diabetes, the de novo onset of clinical diabetes or an asymptomatic abnormal glucose tolerance
- A glucose tolerance test should be offered if there is a family history of diabetes, previous baby >4 kg, previous unexplained intra-uterine fetal death or glycosuria
- Maternal complications include poor control, hydramnios, pre-eclampsia and obstructed labour
- Fetal complications include macrosomia, increased risks of; intra-uterine fetal distress after 37 weeks, intra-partum fetal distress and malformation
- Neonatal complications include hypoglycaemia and respiratory distress syndrome
- Management should be to keep blood sugar <7 mmol, monitor fetal growth and placental function
- Delivery should be by Caesarian section if there is evidence of fetal distress or delay

CARDIAC DISEASE IN PREGNANCY

Pregnancy is associated with a 30–50% increase in cardiac output and therefore creates considerable hazards for the mother if there is underlying cardiac disease. The maternal risk varies according to the nature of the cardiac lesion.

Low-risk conditions. These include septal defects, patent ductus arteriosus, pulmonary and tricuspid lesions.

Moderate risk. Mitral stenosis, aortic stenosis,

Marfan's syndrome, previous myocardial infarction and coarctation are associated with significantly greater risk.

High risk. The conditions with maximum risk include Eisenmenger's syndrome, pulmonary hypertension, Marfan's syndrome involving the aorta and cardiomyopathy.

The risks generally are those of cardiac failure and acute pulmonary oedema. Adequate rest and the avoidance of infection are important. The use of antibiotic cover should be routine during labour. Anticoagulant therapy may also be necessary where there has been a valve replacement. It must be remembered that the risk of cardiac decompensation is maximal during labour and in the first 4 days after delivery.

ASTHMA IN PREGNANCY

Asthma complicates 1% of pregnancies. It does not have a consistent relationship with pregnancy as 25% of mothers get better, 25% get worse and the remainder are unaffected by the pregnancy. Severe asthmatic attacks are rare in the last 4 weeks of pregnancy. Sinister signs in the mother include a maternal tachycardia in excess of 120 b.p.m., a respiratory rate in excess of 30/min and a peak flow of less than 120 ml. Management should be maintained with β-agonists, theophylline, steroids and antibiotics.

EPILEPSY IN PREGNANCY

Pregnancy has no consistent effect on maternal epilepsy, with 50% remaining unchanged, 25% becoming worse and 25% improving. Because of a reduction in absorption of anti-epileptic drugs, a reduction in protein-binding, increased liver metabolism and increased plasma volume, serum level of drugs tends to fall and dosage needs to be increased.

Status epilepticus is uncommon in pregnancy.

The effect of epilepsy and its treatment on the fetus

There is an increase in perinatal mortality among epileptic mothers. Ten per cent of infants from mothers taking phenytoin and phenobarbitone have vitamin-K-dependent clotting problems. Also, the incidence of congenital abnormalities in epileptics both on and off therapy is increased, the commonest abnormalities being orofacial, cardiac and limbal.

Management

The first priority is the control of fits using one drug if possible.

Drug levels should be measured every 2–4 weeks. If possible, a pre-conceptual trial of drug withdrawal should be attempted if the woman has been fit-free for a number of years. If possible, treatment changes should be avoided in pregnancy, apart from the regulation of dosage.

INFECTIONS IN PREGNANCY

The effects of rubella in pregnancy are well known, but there are many other infections where the effects are not so well known or are often overlooked. Some of these infections are discussed below.

Listeria monocytogenes

This organism is a Gram-positive cocco-bacillus which is widely distributed in the environment. Some exposure is unavoidable and 1 in 20 people carry the organism in their gut without ill effects. The organism exists in a large number of samples of pre-cooked, ready-to-eat poultry and chilled meats. It is also found in soft, ripened cheeses such as brie, camembert and cheeses of the blue vein type. These cheeses should be avoided by pregnant women, and cook-chilled meals and ready-to-eat poultry should be reheated until they are piping hot.

Clinical manifestations

The mother usually has a short history of a 'flu-like illness' with backache, urinary frequency and fever.

The condition may cause mid-trimester abortion or premature labour, and the infant develops respiratory distress, sepsis, petechial rash and hepatosplenomegaly. There is a high mortality rate. Late onset of the condition may occur 2–5 weeks after delivery, with lethargy, irritability, feeding difficulties and meningitis. Diagnosis is made by culture of the organism from blood or cerebrospinal fluid. The antibiotic treatment of choice consists of ampicillin or amoxycillin in combination with gentamicin.

Mumps

Mumps appears to have no significant adverse effect on the outcome of pregnancy. There is a slight increase in the rate of spontaneous abortions but no increase in the incidence of premature labour. There is an association with the condition of endo-myocardial fibro-elastosis, but basically the condition is benign.

Measles

This infection is a paramyxovirus with droplet transmission. Placental transmission does occur and may result in neonatal death and an increased abortion rate, but the organism is not teratogenic.

Varicella

This is caused by a herpes virus. It may occur in pregnancy and there is evidence of placental transmission. If the infection occurs between 8 and 20 weeks, there is a 5% risk of congenital mal-formations, including muscular atrophy, micro-cephaly, cerebellar or cortical atrophy, cataracts and chorioretinitis.

BIBLIOGRAPHY

Brudenell M, Wilds P L 1984 Medical and surgical problems in obstetrics. Wright, Bristol
Chesley L C 1978 Hypertensive disorders in pregnancy. Appleton-Century-Crofts, New York
de Swiet M 1984 Medical disorders in obstetric practice. Blackwell Scientific Publications, Oxford
MacGillivray J 1983 Pre-eclampsia. The hypertensive disease of pregnancy. W B Saunders, Eastbourne

11. Antepartum haemorrhage

Haemorrhage from the vagina after the 28th week of gestation is classified as antepartum haemorrhage. The factors which cause antepartum haemorrhage may be present before 28 weeks, but the original distinction between a threatened abortion and an antepartum haemorrhage was based on the potential viability of the fetus.

Vaginal bleeding may be due to:

1. Haemorrhage from the placental site and uterine cavity.
2. Lesions of the vagina or cervix.

1. UTEROPLACENTAL HAEMORRHAGE

The major causes of uterine bleeding are:

1. Placenta praevia.
2. Abruptio placentae or accidental haemorrhage.
3. Uterine rupture.
4. Unknown aetiology.

Placenta praevia

The placenta is said to be praevia when all or part of the placenta implants in the lower uterine segment and therefore lies in front of the presenting part (see Fig. 11.1).

Incidence

Approximately 1% of all pregnancies are complicated by clinical evidence of a placenta praevia. Unlike the incidence of placental abruption, which varies according to social and nutritional factors, the incidence of placenta praevia is remarkably constant.

Aetiology

Placenta praevia is due to delay in implantation of the blastocyst so that this occurs in the lower part

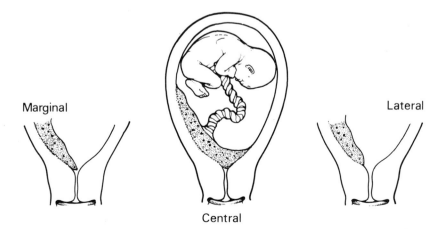

Fig. 11.1 Classification of placenta praevia

of the uterus. It is commoner in high parity, and in conditions where the placental area is large, such as multiple pregnancy or placenta membranacea.

Classification

From the point of view of management, there are three degrees of severity of placenta praevia (Fig. 11.1):

1. Lateral — the placenta encroaches on the lower uterine segment, but does not reach the internal cervical os. This is sometimes known as first degree placentá praevia.
2. Marginal — the placenta encroaches on or covers the internal cervical os before cervical dilatation occurs. This includes both second and third degree placenta praevia.
3. Central — the placenta completely covers the os even with cervical dilatation. This was previously described as fourth degree placenta praevia.

The classification is important in relation to management because spontaneous delivery is extremely rare where there is central placenta praevia, but normal labour and delivery may occur with lateral or marginal implantation.

Bleeding results from separation of the placenta as the formation of the lower segment occurs and the cervix effaces. This blood loss occurs from the venous sinuses in the lower segment. Occasionally, fetal blood loss may occur, particularly where one of the placental vessels lies across the cervical os — a condition known as **vasa praevia**.

Symptoms and signs

The main symptom of placenta praevia is painless vaginal bleeding. There may sometimes be lower abdominal discomfort where there are minor degrees of associated placental abruption.

The signs of placenta praevia are:

1. Vaginal bleeding.
2. Malpresentation of the fetus.
3. Uterine hypotonus.

Development of the lower uterine segment begins at 28 weeks gestation and thus bleeding is likely to occur during the second trimester.

Bleeding is unpredictable and may vary from minor shows to massive and life-endangering haemorrhage.

The presence of the placenta in the lower segment tends to displace the presenting part and when the placenta is posterior the head is pushed forward over the pelvic brim and is easily palpable. When the placenta is anterior, the presenting part is difficult to feel. Lateral placement of the placenta results in contralateral displacement of the presenting part. Where there is a central placenta praevia, the fetal head is held away from the pelvic brim and the lie may be transverse or oblique. If the head does not approach the pelvic brim when the erect posture is adopted, it is strongly suggestive of a placenta praevia.

Case study: placenta praevia

A 29-year-old woman, para 3, was admitted at 32 weeks gestation in her fourth pregnancy with a history of sudden onset of fresh, red vaginal blood loss not associated with pain. On examination the fetal heart beat was present and a breech presentation was diagnosed. Ultrasound scan showed an anterior placenta extending down to, and covering, the internal os. The bleeding settled and the mother was delivered by elective Caesarean section at 37 weeks.

Diagnosis of placenta praevia

1. Clinical findings — painless bleeding occurs suddenly and tends to be recurrent. When labour starts, and the cervix dilates, profuse haemorrhage may occur, although sometimes in a lateral placenta praevia the presenting part compresses the placental site and bleeding is controlled.
2. Abdominal examination —
   a. Displacement of the presenting part — the lie may be oblique or transverse. If the placenta lies on the posterior uterine wall, the presenting part will be easily palpable. If the placenta is anterior, the presenting part is difficult to palpate.
   b. Flaccidity of the uterus — uterine muscle tone is usually low and the fetal parts are easy to palpate.

3. Diagnostic procedures —
    a. Ultrasonic scanning — this is predominantly used to localize the placenta and has largely replaced other techniques. Errors in diagnosis are most likely to occur in posteriorly situated placentae because of difficulties in identifying the lower segment. Anteriorly, the bladder provides an important landmark for the lower segment and diagnosis is more accurate. Localization of the placental site in early pregnancy may result in inaccurate diagnosis as fundal development may lead to an apparent upward displacement of the placenta.
    b. Radiology diagnosis — direct placentography involves localization of the placenta by soft tissue imaging. Indirect placentography involves X-ray in the erect lateral position. The position of the placenta is inferred by displacement of the presenting part.
    c. Magnetic resonance imaging — this is the most accurate method of placental realization, but is not, as yet, widely available.

Management

When antepartum haemorrhage of any type occurs, the diagnosis of placenta praevia should be suspected and hospital admission advised. The diagnosis should be established by ultrasound imaging. Vaginal examination should be performed only in an operating theatre prepared for Caesarean section with blood cross-matched. There are only two indications for performing a vaginal examination:

1. Where there is serious doubt about the diagnosis.
2. Where bleeding occurs in established labour.

It is, in fact, often difficult to establish a diagnosis of placenta praevia by vaginal examination where the placenta is lateral, and there is a serious risk of precipitating massive haemorrhage if the placenta is central. If the placenta is lateral, then it may be possible to rupture the membranes and allow spontaneous vaginal delivery.

Conservative management of placenta praevia involves keeping the mother in hospital with blood cross-matched until fetal maturity is adequate, and then delivering the child by Caesarean section. Providing no active bleeding is occurring, there is no need to keep the mother in bed and she should remain ambulant, as she is as likely to bleed lying supine. Blood loss should be treated by transfusion where necessary, so that an adequate haemoglobin concentration is maintained.

Postpartum haemorrhage is also a hazard of the low-lying placenta.

Placenta praevia

> - Complicates 1% of pregnancies
> - Commoner in multigravidae and multiple pregnancies
> - Painless vaginal bleeding with soft uterus
> - Malpresentation
> - Lateral, marginal or central grades

Abruptio placentae

Abruptio placentae or accidental haemorrhage is defined as haemorrhage resulting from premature separation of the placenta. The term 'accidental' implies separation as the result of trauma, but most cases do not involve trauma and occur spontaneously.

Aetiology

Placental abruption tends to occur more frequently under conditions of social deprivation, in association with dietary deficiencies. Folic acid deficiency, in particular, has been implicated.

The incidence of placental abruption is increased in the presence of pre-eclampsia or essential hypertension. It must be remembered that hypertension and proteinuria may develop as a result of abruption.

Whatever factors predispose to placental abruption, they are well-established before the abruption occurs. The fetus is more likely to be male and the birth weight is often low, indicating pre-existing growth retardation. Trauma is a relatively uncommon cause of abruption and, in the majority of cases, no specific predisposing factor can be identified.

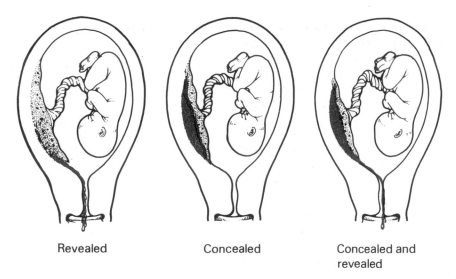

Revealed   Concealed   Concealed and revealed

Fig. 11.2   Types of placental abruption

Case study: abruptio placentae

A 19-year-old primigravida was admitted at 39 weeks with sudden onset of constant abdominal pain. On admission her blood pressure was 160/100 mmHg, pulse 100 b.p.m. and uterine tone increased with marked tenderness to palpation. The fetal heart beat was present, but shortly after admission it fell to 60 b.p.m. and the baby was delivered by emergency Caesarean section. At operation, a large retroplacental blood clot was noted.

Clinical types and presentation

Three types of abruption have been described (Fig. 11.2):

1. Revealed.
2. Concealed.
3. Mixed, or concealed and revealed.

Unlike placenta praevia, placental abruption presents with pain, vaginal bleeding and increased uterine activity.

1. *Revealed haemorrhage* — the major haemorrhage is apparent externally as haemorrhage occurs from the lower part of the placenta and blood escapes through the cervical os. Under these circumstances, the clinical features are less severe.

Abruption tends to occur after 36 weeks gestation with the fetal lie longitudinal and the presenting part sitting well into the pelvic brim. In revealed placental abruption, uterine activity may be increased, but this finding is not consistent.

2. *Concealed haemorrhage* — in this case, the haemorrhage occurs between the placenta and the uterine wall. The uterine content increases in volume and the fundal size appears larger than would be consistent with the estimated date of confinement. Uterine tonus is increased and pain and shock are common features. The uterus may become broad, rigid and tender.

It is important to realize that initially the blood pressure may be raised and the pulse rate slowed but, eventually, the patient becomes shocked, with the development of tachycardia, hypotension and oliguria. The peripheral circulation becomes vasoconstricted and there may be physical signs of this condition even before hypotension develops.

It is most important to remember that initially, even in the presence of substantial intra-uterine haemorrhage where the blood loss is concealed, the blood pressure may remain normal or raised and the pulse rate slow, until collapse suddenly occurs. The estimate of blood loss must therefore be based on uterine size and, in revealed haemorrhage, assessment of external loss. In some severe cases, haemorrhage penetrates through the uterine wall, and the uterus appears bruised. This is described as a **Couvelaire uterus**. On clinical examination, the uterus will be tense and hard and the uterine fundus will be higher than is normal for the gestational age. The patient will often be in labour, and in approximately 30% of cases the fetal heart sounds will be absent and the fetus will be stillborn. The prognosis for the fetus is dependent on the area of placental separation.

3. *Mixed, or concealed and revealed haemorrhage* — in most cases, the haemorrhage is both concealed and revealed. Haemorrhage occurs close to the placental edge and, after an interval when the haemorrhage is concealed, blood loss soon appears vaginally.

Differential diagnosis

The diagnosis is made on the history of vaginal bleeding, abdominal pain, increased uterine tonus, proteinuria and the presence of a longitudinal lie. This must be distinguished from placenta praevia where the haemorrhage is painless, the lie unstable and the uterus hypotonic.

The diagnosis should also be differentiated from other acute emergencies such as acute hydramnios where the uterus is enlarged and tender and tense, but there is no haemorrhage. Concealed placental abruption may simulate other acute abdominal emergencies such as perforated ulcer, volvulus of the bowel and strangulated internal hernia, but these problems are rare during pregnancy.

Management

The patient must be admitted to hospital and the diagnosis established on the basis of the history and examination findings (Fig. 11.3). Mild cases may be treated conservatively and the placental site localized to confirm the diagnosis. If the haemorrhage is severe, resuscitation is the first prerequisite.

It is often difficult to assess the amount of blood loss accurately and intravenous infusion should be started with normal saline, Hartman's solution or blood substitutes until blood is cross-matched and

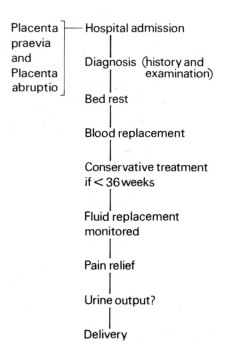

Fig. 11.3   Differential diagnosis and management of antepartum haemorrhage

transfusion can be commenced. Fluid replacement should be monitored by the use of a central venous pressure line. Unlike placenta praevia, any significant abruption should be treated by delivering the fetus as soon as possible.

If the fetus is alive and there are no clinical signs of fetal distress, or if the fetus is dead, surgical induction of labour is performed as soon as possible, and where necessary, uterine activity is stimulated with a dilute Syntocinon® infusion. If the fetus is alive, it should be monitored and Caesarean section should be performed if signs of fetal distress develop. If induction is not possible because the cervix is closed, then delivery should be effected by Caesarean section. Pain relief is achieved by the use of opiates.

Complications (Fig. 11.4)

Afibrinogenaemia. Severe placental abruption results in significant placental damage and the release of thromboplastin into the maternal circulation. This in turn may lead to intravascular coagulation and to defibrination with the development of hypo- or afibrinogenaemia. The con-

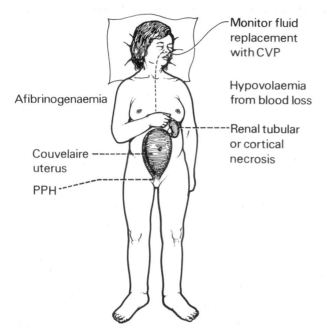

Fig. 11.4 Complications of placental abruption

Fig. 11.5 Non-placental causes of antepartum haemorrhage.

dition may be treated by the infusion of fresh frozen plasma, platelet transfusion and fibrinogen transfusion, but can only be reversed by delivering the fetus. It may lead to abnormal bleeding if operative delivery is attempted, or may result in uncontrollable postpartum haemorrhage.

Renal tubular or cortical necrosis

This is a complication that must always be considered as a possibility, and it is essential to keep careful fluid balance charts and to take particular note of urinary output. It may, on occasion, necessitate haemodialysis or peritoneal dialysis, but this complication is one of increasing rarity.

Abruptio placentae

- Associated with social deprivation, pregnancy-induced hypertension, male fetus, intra-uterine growth retardation
- Pain ± bleeding, ↑ tone
- Revealed, concealed or mixed
- Deranged clotting

Other causes of antepartum haemorrhage
(Fig. 11.5)

Unexplained APH

In many cases, it is not possible to make a definite diagnosis of abruption or placenta praevia. These cases involve a significant increase in perinatal mortality and it is therefore important to monitor placental function and fetal growth. The pregnancy should not be allowed to proceed beyond term.

Vaginal infections

Vaginal moniliasis or trichomaniasis may cause blood-stained discharge and, once the diagnosis is established, should be treated with the appropriate therapy.

CERVICAL LESIONS

Benign lesions of the cervix such as cervical polyps are treated by removal of the polyp. Cervical erosions are best left untreated.

Carcinoma of the cervix is occasionally found in pregnancy. If the pregnancy is early, termination is indicated. If the diagnosis is made late in pregnancy, the diagnosis should be established by biopsy and the lesion treated according to the staging.

12. Multiple pregnancy

Multiple pregnancy presents a series of special problems in obstetric practice. It also has significant implications for the children after birth and during development. The great majority of multiple pregnancies are associated with twins but the increasing use of in-vitro fertilisation has now changed the incidence of higher multiple pregnancies as well as affecting the incidence of twinning. Most of the contents of this chapter will specifically relate to twins.

PREVALENCE OF MULTIPLE PREGNANCY

It is difficult to be precise about the natural prevalence of twins, partly because diagnosis of twins in early pregnancy is often uncertain and partly because the figure varies considerably from one country or race to another. It would be reasonable to assume that the prevalence of twin pregnancies subject to therapeutic abortion would follow the overall incidence, but the prevalence in spontaneous abortion may be higher.

The figures vary from as low as 5.8/1000 pregnancies in Japan to 66.5/1000 in some parts of Nigeria. From 1971–75 the prevalence of twinning in England and Wales was 9.8/1000 pregnancies.

Triplet pregnancy in Japan is 5.6/100 000, in Nigeria up to 177.8/100 000 and in the United Kingdom, 10.2/100 000. Higher multiple births such as quadruplets and quintuplets are commonly associated with the use of fertility drugs, but if one excludes this cause, figures for England and Wales suggest a pregnancy rate of 1.7/million maternities.

The highest naturally occurring multiple pregnancy recorded so far is nontuplets.

TYPES OF TWINNING (Fig. 12.1)

Twins may be monozygotic, derived from one fertilised egg, or dizygotic, derived from two different eggs. With very rare exceptions, all pairs discordant for sex are dizygotic. About one-third of all twin pairs are of unlike sex.

Monochorionic twins are never completely identical but are frequently indistinguishable to the casual observer. Difference in hair and eye colour indicate dizygosity. Thus, it is possible to assign zygosity with reasonable accuracy in most twin pairs by sex, placentation and physical appearance.

The determination of blood group may also help assign zygosity. Discrepant blood groups indicate dizygosity. However, up to 18% of dichorionic twins have similar blood types and therefore concordance of blood group does not determine zygosity.

Monochorionic placentae can be determined by direct examination at the time of delivery or by submitting a sample of the dividing membranes for histological examination. The further approach to confirmation of monochorionicity involves the injection of a contrast liquid into a clamped cord. In monochorionic placentae, positive transfer will occur through the placental circulation, whereas in dichorionic placentae, transfer does not occur. Precise allocation of zygosity can be enhanced by a comparison of blood groups, serum protein and enzyme polymorphism.

THE AETIOLOGY OF TWIN PREGNANCY

Familial factors

Twins tend to occur in families, although there is

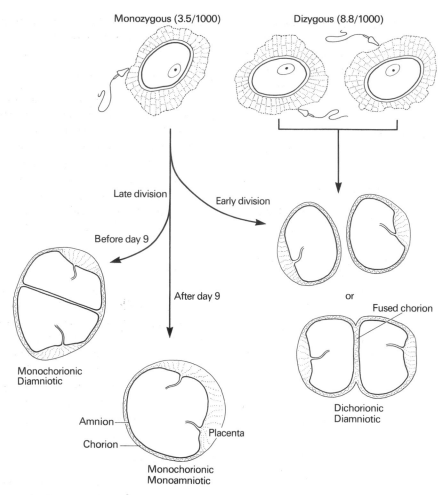

Fig. 12.1 Types of twinning indicating the structure of the membranes and placenta. Note that twins of different sexes are always dizygous and those with a single chorion always monozygous. Dichorionic twins of the same sex can be either monozygous or dizygous.

some debate as to whether this occurs through both female and male partners. The familial tendency is apparent in dizygotic twinning, but this appears to be on the maternal side only. In a study of records at Salt Lake City, the twinning rates of women who were themselves dizygotic twins was 17.1/1000 maternities compared with 11.6/1000 maternities for the general population, but the rate for males who were themselves dizygotic twins was only 7.9/1000 maternities.

A familial tendency to monozygotic twinning is rare but transmission can occur through both maternal and paternal lines.

Parity and maternal age

Twinning rates increase with parity but this increase seems only to apply to dizygotic twinning. Studies in Aberdeen have shown that the rate increases from 10.4/1000 in primigravidae to 15.3/1000 in the para 4+ group.

Dizygotic twinning rates are also age linked, with an increase in twinning in the older mothers.

Ovulation induction

Multiple pregnancy is common following the use of drugs to induce ovulation. It is important to note that the use of gonadotropin therapy commonly results in twin and triplet pregnancy. To some degree this can be avoided by monitoring ovarian follicular development and withholding the injection of human chorionic gonadotropin if excessive numbers of follicles develop.

The use of fertility drugs accounts for 10–15% of all multiple pregnancies and has therefore significantly altered the incidence of multiple pregnancy.

In-vitro fertilization and embryo transfer

The above principles also apply to in-vitro fertilization where the ovaries are hyperstimulated to enable collection of multiple oocytes. Pregnancy rates are enhanced by replacement of a number of embryos, but the risk of this procedure is that it results in a much higher incidence of twin and triplet pregnancy. In ovulation induction and in-vitro fertilisation programmes, twin pregnancies are dizygotic but there are also documented cases of monozygotic twins or of quadruplets where only three embryos were replaced.

COMPLICATIONS OF TWIN PREGNANCY

The normal processes of maternal physiological adaptation are exaggerated in multiple pregnancy. Total weight gain is, on average, 3.5 kg greater than in singleton pregnancy. Plasma volume expansion is significantly greater with twin pregnancy. Between 37 and 40 weeks gestation, the expansion is 17% greater in twin pregnancy. Cardiac output does not seem to be different but there is a greater increase in red cell mass; however, a relative anaemia may develop related to haemodilution in twin pregnancy.

It is thus to be expected that the increased strain put on the system by carrying more than one fetus will result in a higher incidence of complications.

Abortion

Resorption of a fetus in twin pregnancy is a common event in early gestation and on this basis the incidence of 'partial' abortion is high. The incidence of spontaneous abortion is higher in twins and recent evidence from Aberdeen has shown that threatened abortion occurs in 26% of twin pregnancies and 20% of singleton pregnancies.

Antepartum haemorrhage

The incidence of antepartum haemorrhage (APH) has been found by some studies to be 'approximately twice as high in twin pregnancies'. However, not all studies have reported this difference. Despite a general belief that bigger placental size should be associated with a higher incidence of placenta praevia, the differences are marginal. The Aberdeen twin study suggested an overall incidence of 0.70% for twins and 0.42% for singleton pregnancies.

Polyhydramnios

Polyhydramnios is a common finding with multiple pregnancy and complicates 6% of twin pregnancies. Management is difficult and often unsatisfactory. Amniocentesis commonly leads to premature labour and in any case only produces short-term relief of symptoms. Bed rest may help to relieve the physical discomfort, but the condition is often associated with premature rupture of membranes and premature labour.

Pre-eclampsia

There is an increased incidence of both gestational hypertension and pre-eclampsia in twin pregnancies, even allowing for the influence of parity. The incidence of eclampsia is also significantly greater in twin pregnancy. The condition may progress rapidly and is commonly associated with intra-uterine growth retardation (IUGR).

Pre-term labour

The occurrence of premature labour is the most important complication of twin pregnancy. The onset of labour before 37 weeks gestation occurs in 40% of twin pregnancies. The phenomenon appears to be associated with overdistension of the uterus associated with the presence of more than one fetus and the associated increase in amniotic fluid volume. The incidence of pre-term labour is also significantly higher in monozygotic twins than dizygotic twins.

Twin pregnancies

- Incidence in England and Wales 9.8/1000 births, increasing because of IVF (10–15% of twin pregnancies)
- Familial tendency
- Dizygotic twins increase with age and parity
- Increase weight gain, plasma, volume
- Increase risk of spontaneous abortion, APH, polyhydramnios and pregnancy-included hypertension
- IUGR common

MANAGEMENT OF TWIN PREGNANCY

Multiple pregnancies exhibit every type of pregnancy complication at a greater frequency than occurs in singleton pregnancy. Early diagnosis is therefore essential and provides a convincing argument for routine early pregnancy ultrasound scanning. The commonest clinical sign of twin pregnancy is the greater size of the uterus, which is easier to detect in early, rather than late, pregnancy. There are, of course, other reasons why the uterus may be abnormally enlarged, such as hydramnios and uterine fibroids.

Treatment of any antenatal complication is the same as in singleton pregnancies, but remember that the onset of complications tends to be earlier and of greater severity. Routine hospital admission from 28 weeks gestation for bed rest has been advocated in the past, but clinical trials have failed to demonstrate efficacy. However, careful antenatal supervision and more frequent antenatal visits are indicated. It is important that women with multiple pregnancies are booked for confinement in hospitals where there are suitable special care baby units.

Intra-uterine growth retardation is common and therefore serial ultrasound measurements to assess fetal growth are important. If there is evidence of growth retardation in one or both fetuses, then early induction of labour should be considered.

MANAGEMENT OF LABOUR AND DELIVERY

Delivery poses many complexities in twin pregnancy because of the variety and complexity of presentations and because the second twin is at significantly greater risk from asphyxia because of placental separation and cord prolapse.

Presentation at delivery

There are a number of permutations for presentation in twin pregnancy at delivery which are partly influenced by the management of the second twin. Rounded-up figures for these presentations are shown in Figure 12.2. By far the commonest presentation is cephalic/cephalic (50%), followed by cephalic/breech (25%), breech/cephalic (10%) and breech/breech (10%). The remaining 5% consist of cephalic/transverse, transverse/cephalic, breech/transverse, transverse/breech and transverse/transverse.

Method of delivery

A decision about the method of delivery should be made as far as possible before the onset of labour.

Caesarean section

Delivery by elective Caesarean section is indicated for the same indications that exist for singleton pregnancies. However, the threshold to intervene is generally lower. Where an additional complication exists, such as a previous Caesarean scar, a long history of subfertility, severe pre-eclampsia or diabetes mellitus, most obstetricians will opt for elective section. Premature labour between 28 and 34 weeks gestation is an indication for Caesarean delivery, as also is malpresentation of the first twin.

Vaginal delivery

When labour is allowed to proceed normally, it is advisable to establish an intravenous line at an early stage. Labour normally lasts the same time as a singleton labour.

The first twin can be monitored with a scalp electrode or by abdominal ultrasound and, if possible, both infants should be monitored. When the first twin is delivered, the lie and presentation of the second twin must be immediately checked and the fetal heart rate recorded.

For delivery of the second twin, the membranes should be ruptured and cord prolapse excluded. If the uterus does not contract within a few minutes, an oxytocin infusion should be started. If fetal

Cephalic/Cephalic (50%)

Cephalic/Breech (25%)

Breech/Cephalic (10%)

Breech/Breech (10%)

Fig. 12.2 The four major presentations of twin pregnancy. 5% of other variations are not listed in these major groups.

distress occurs, then delivery should be expedited by forceps delivery or breech extraction. Under very exceptional circumstances, it may be necessary to deliver the second twin by Caesarean section. It is important to use oxytocic agents with delivery of the second twin as there is an increased risk of post-partum haemorrhage.

COMPLICATIONS OF LABOUR

There are several complications of labour, some of which are associated with malpresentation. Babies may become obstructed, particularly where there is a transverse lie presenting and that is, in fact, an

indication for delivery by Caesarean section. If Caesarean section is performed in the presence of an obstructed transverse lie, it may be preferable to perform a vertical incision in the lower and upper segment rather than a transverse incision because of the possibility of extension of the lower segment scar into the lower part of the uterus and broad ligaments.

Failed diagnosis

This is now uncommon because of the widespread use of ultrasound imaging in early pregnancy. However, if the diagnosis is made after delivery of the first twin, it is important to withhold syntometrine. If an oxytocin agent is given and the second twin becomes obstructed, delivery must be expedited either by Caesarean section or by reversing the contractions with sympathomimetic agents or deep anaesthesia with delivery of the child by breech extraction or forceps delivery.

Locked twins

This is a very rare complication, where the first twin is a breech presentation and the second is cephalic. Clinically, the twins look chin to chin. The condition is usually not recognised until delivery of part of the first twin has occurred and survival of the first twin is unlikely. It may sometimes be possible to disempact the locked twins, but if this fails a destructive operation may be necessary to the first twin to stand any chance of saving the second child.

Conjoined twins

The union of twins results from the incomplete division of the embryo after formation. It is a rare complication, with a calculated frequency of 1 in 546 twin pregnancies. Union may occur at any site, but commonly is head to head or thorax to thorax.

If the union is recognised by ultrasound or radiology before the onset of labour, then the twins should be delivered by Caesarean section as a significant number of these infants can be surgically separated. If the abnormality is not recognised before the onset of labour, then the labour will usually obstruct.

Perinatal mortality

The perinatal death rate is significantly higher for multiple pregnancies. In general, the mortality rate increases with the number of fetuses. The mortality rate for twins is approximately four times higher than for singleton pregnancies, and the mortality rate for second twins is 50% higher than for the first twin.

The commonest cause of death in both twins is prematurity. Second-born twins are more likely to die from intrapartum asphyxia with separation of the placenta following delivery of the first twin, or where cord prolapse occurs in association with a malpresentation or a high presenting part when the membranes are ruptured.

Twin delivery and labour

- Onset of labour before 37 weeks in 40%
- Second twin at greater risk of asphyxia
- Labour same length as singleton
- Increased risk of PPH and malpresentation
- Mortality rate four times higher than for singleton, and 50% higher for second twin than for first

Twin-to-twin transfusion occurs in 15% of monochorionic twins and two-thirds of the infants die in utero. Death may also occur from lethal congenital malformations, trauma, antepartum haemorrhage and infection.

BIBLIOGRAPHY

MacGillivray I, Campbell D M, Thompson B 1988 Twinning and twins. John Wiley & Sons, London

13. Normal labour

Labour is the process whereby the products of conception are expelled from the uterus after the 24th week of gestation.

Premature labour is defined as labour occurring before the 36th week of gestation.

Prolonged labour is defined as labour lasting in excess of 24 hours in a primigravida and 16 hours in a multigravida.

THE STAGES OF LABOUR

Labour is divided into three stages which are defined as follows:

1. The **first stage** commences with the onset of labour and terminates when the cervix has reached full dilatation.
2. The **second stage,** or stage of expulsion, begins at full cervical dilatation and ends with the expulsion of the fetus.
3. The **third stage,** or placental stage, begins with the delivery of the child and ends with expulsion of the placenta.

THE ONSET OF LABOUR

It is often difficult to be certain of the exact time of onset of labour; however, it is defined as the development of regular, painful uterine contractions producing progressive dilatation of the cervix. There are exceptions to this definition, such as cervical stenosis where labour contractions do not produce dilatation of the cervix. This condition is rare and does not interfere with the general definition. The clinical signs of the onset of labour are:

1. The onset of regular painful contractions.

2. The presence of a 'show' — the passage of blood-stained mucus.
3. Rupture of the membranes.

INITIATION OF LABOUR

The cause of the onset of labour remains uncertain despite extensive research. The subject is of considerable importance particularly in relation to premature labour, which remains the major cause of neonatal death.

Many factors play a part in the initiation of parturition and it is unlikely that any one factor is sufficient to explain the phenomenon. It is more likely that there is a cascade of biochemical events regulated and controlled by the fetus. The fetus increases its production of cortisol towards term and this reduces the production of progesterone by the placenta and increases the production of oestrone and oestradiol. Progesterone inhibits uterine activity and oestradiol increases it. At the same time, these changes lead to an increased production of prostaglandins by the placenta and myometrium, which stimulate increased myometrial activity and also oxytocin release from the posterior lobe of the pituitary gland, which in turn also stimulates myometrial activity. The direct mechanism involved in increasing myometrial contractility is probably related to a release of calcium ions, which increases the activity of the myometrium, and this causes splitting of adenosine triphosphate (ATP) thus stimulating the action of actomyosin.

Uterine activity in labour

The uterus contracts at all times during pregnancy. As full term approaches, the activity increases in

Prelabour   Effacement   Dilatation

Fig. 13.1 Effacement and dilatation of the cervix in labour

frequency and strength. Intra-uterine pressure rises to 20–30 mmHg initially and contractions occur every 10–15 minutes and last approximately 30–40 seconds. Normal resting tonus in labour starts at 10 mmHg and increases slightly during the course of labour. Contractions increase in intensity to reach pressures of 50 mmHg in labour; in the second stage, with voluntary expulsive efforts, they may reach pressures in excess of 100 mmHg. Contractions produce effacement and dilatation of the cervix and shorten myometrial fibres in the upper uterine segment (Fig. 13.1). This process is known as **retraction**. The lower uterine segment becomes elongated and thinned as labour progresses and the conjunction between upper and lower segment rises in the abdomen. Where labour becomes obstructed, the junction between upper and lower segments may become visible near the level of the umbilicus and is known as a **retraction ring**. Contractions are initiated from a pacemaker in the left uterine cornua

and spread downwards through the myometrium. The contractions occur first in the fundus of the uterus where they are stronger and last longer than in the lower segment. The phenomenon is known as **fundal dominance** and is essential to progressive effacement and dilatation of the cervix. As the uterus contracts, its axis appears to straighten and the fundus pushes forward against the anterior abdominal wall (Fig. 13.2). The round ligaments also contract and pull the uterus forward and this brings the uterus into line with the inlet of the pelvis so that the fetus is pushed straight down into the birth canal.

Pain in labour

Contractions in labour are commonly associated with pain, particularly as they increase in strength and frequency (Fig. 13.3). The cause of the pain is uncertain, but may be due to compression of nerve

Resting phase   Contraction phase

Fig. 13.2 Change in direction of the fetal and uterine axis during contractions in labour

Fig. 13.3 Uterine contractions become painful when the intra-amniotic pressure exceeds 25 mmHg

fibres in the cervical area, or to anoxia of compressed muscle cells. Pain is felt as lumbar backache and as pain in the lower abdomen.

The passages

The shape of the bony pelvis has previously been described. Due to softening of pelvic ligaments, some expansion of the pelvic cavity can occur. The soft tissues also become more distensible and substantial distension of the pelvic floor and vaginal orifice occurs during descent and birth of the head. This may result in tearing of the perineum and of the vaginal walls.

The mechanism of labour

The head usually engages in the transverse position and the passage of the head and trunk through the pelvis follow a well-defined pattern. Not all diameters of the fetal head can pass through a normal pelvis. The process of labour therefore involves the adaption of the fetal head to the various segments of the pelvis and the following processes occur (Fig. 13.4):

Fig. 13.4 The mechanism of normal labour involves: (**A**) descent of the presenting part; (**B**) flexion of the head; (**C**) internal rotation; (**D**) distension of the perineum and extension of the fetal head; (**E**) delivery of the head; (**F**) delivery of the shoulders

1. *Descent* — descent occurs throughout labour and is a requisite for the birth of the child. Engagement may not occur until labour is well established, but descent of the head is a measure of progress in labour.
2. *Flexion* — flexion of the head occurs as it descends and meets the pelvic floor bringing the chin into contact with the fetal thorax. Flexion produces a smaller diameter of presentation, changing to the sub-occipito bregmatic diameter from the occipito-frontal diameter.
3. *Internal rotation* — the head rotates as it strikes the pelvic floor and, normally, the occiput gradually moves from its original lateral position towards the pubic symphysis; occasionally it moves posteriorly towards the hollow of the sacrum.
4. *Extension* — the sharply flexed head descends to the vulva and the base of the occiput comes into contact with the inferior rami of the pubis. The head now extends until it is delivered. The maximal distension of the perineum and introitus is followed rapidly by final expulsion of the head, a process that is known as **crowning**. The head now extends again following delivery.
5. *Restitution* — following delivery of the head, it rotates back to its original position in relation to the shoulders.
6. *External rotation* — when the shoulders reach the pelvic floor, they rotate into the anteroposterior diameter. This is followed by rotation of the fetal head so that the face looks laterally at the thigh.
7. *Delivery of the shoulders* — final expulsion of the trunk occurs following delivery of the shoulders. Lateral flexion of the trunk, first posteriorly to deliver the anterior shoulder under the pubic symphysis, and then anteriorly to disengage the posterior shoulder, is followed by rapid expulsion of the remainder of the trunk.

THE THIRD STAGE OF LABOUR

The third stage of labour starts with the completed expulsion of the infant and ends with the delivery of the placenta and membranes (Fig. 13.5). A fourth stage is sometimes described as the time interval following expulsion of the placenta up to 6 hours after delivery. The only implication of this stage is

Fig. 13.5 The normal third stage: (**A**) separation of the placenta from the uterine wall; (**B**) expulsion into the lower uterine segment and upper vagina; (**C**) complete expulsion of the placenta from the genital tract

the possibility of relaxation of the uterus followed by abnormal haemorrhage, which may happen during this time interval.

Once the child is delivered, the uterine muscle contracts, shearing off the placenta and pushing it into the lower uterine segment or upper part of the vagina. The classical signs of placental separation include a show of bright blood, lengthening and descent of the umbilical cord and raising of the uterine fundus. This becomes tent-shaped instead of globular and sits on top of the placenta as it descends into the lower segment. The placenta is accompanied by the fetal membranes, although these often become torn and require additional traction for their removal. The whole process lasts between 5 and 10 minutes. If the placenta is not expelled within 30 minutes the third stage should be considered abnormal. The signs of placental separation may be compressed and obscured by oxytocic drugs administered at the crowning of the head.

Mechanism of labour

> - Initiated by falling progesterone and rising oestradiol, prostaglandins and oxytocin
> - Presenting part undergoes descent, flexion on pelvic floor and rotation
> - Head extends on reaching the vulva then rotates back to original position after delivery
> - Shoulders rotate into antero-posterior diameter and deliver anterior first
> - Uterine muscle contracts and shears off placenta

MANAGEMENT OF NORMAL LABOUR

The management of normal labour begins well before the onset of labour with proper preparation of the mother. This primarily involves education about what actually happens in the various stages of labour. In addition, there are a variety of methods involving controlled respiration, known generally as psychoprophylactic methods, which enable the mother to control pain to some degree and to regulate expulsive efforts during the second stage of labour.

The mother should be advised to come in to hospital when the contractions are at regular 10–15 minute intervals, when there is a show, or if the membranes rupture. If the patient is in early labour, she is given a shower. Shaving of pubic hair is not necessary unless there is likely to be a delivery by Caesarean section. It is also advisable to give a small enema if the bowel is loaded, but this should be left to the discretion of the midwife or doctor attending the patient.

Examination during labour

On admission, the following examinations should be undertaken:

1. *Full general examination* — including temperature, pulse, respiration, blood pressure and state of hydration. The urine should be tested for protein, glucose and ketone bodies.
2. *Obstetrical examination of the abdomen* — inspection, palpation and auscultation to determine fetal lie, and position station of the presenting part.
3. *Vaginal examination* — in labour, vaginal examination should be performed only after cleansing the vulva and introitus and using aseptic technique with sterile gloves and an antiseptic cream.

Once the examination is started, the fingers of the examining hand should not be withdrawn from the vagina until the examination is completed.

The following factors should be noted:

1. The consistency, effacement and dilatation of the cervix.
2. Whether the membranes are intact or ruptured and, if ruptured, the colour of the amniotic fluid.
3. The nature and presentation of the presenting part and the position of the fetal head. The descent or station of the presenting part is also noted in relation to the level of the ischial spines.
4. Assessment of the bony pelvis, particularly of the pelvic outlet.

GENERAL PRINCIPLES OF MANAGEMENT OF THE FIRST STAGE OF LABOUR

The guiding principles of management are:

1. Observation and intervention if the labour becomes abnormal.
2. Pain relief and emotional support for the mother.
3. Adequate hydration throughout labour.

1. Observation — the use of the partogram

The introduction of graphic records has proved to be a major advance in the active management of labour. The partogram is a single sheet of paper which graphically represents progress in labour (Fig. 13.6). The partogram is started as soon as the patient is admitted to the delivery suite and this is recorded as zero time regardless of the time at which the contractions started. The advantage of this record is that it draws attention visually to aberration from normal progress.

Fetal condition

Fetal heart rate is charted as beats per minute, and deceleration in heart rate which occurs during contractions is shown by an arrow down to the lowest heart rate recorded. The type of deceleration is indicated by I (early) or II (late).

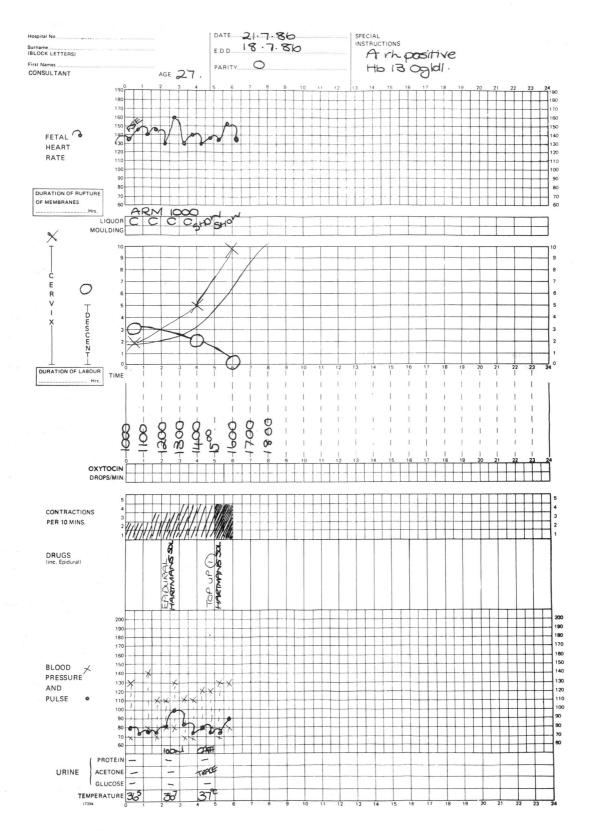

Fig. 13.6   The partogram is a complete visual record of measurements made during delivery

The time of membrane rupture and the nature of the fluid are also noted. Moulding of the fetal head and the presence of caput are also noted.

Progress of labour

Progress in labour is measured by assessing the rate of cervical dilatation and descent of the presenting part. Vaginal examination and assessment of cervical dilatation should be performed on admission to hospital and every 4 hours during the first stage of labour. Cervical dilatation is recorded in centimetres along the 0–10 scale of the cervicograph and a slope of cervical dilatation is constructed. A normal graph is drawn onto the partogram. Dilatation of the cervix occurs in two well-defined phases. The **latent phase** starts at the onset of labour and ends at about 3 cm dilatation. This takes about two-thirds of the time of labour. This is followed by the **active phase,** which extends from the end of the latent phase until delivery. If the dilatation of the cervix lags more than 2 hours behind the expected rate of dilatation, the labour is considered abnormal. The rate of dilatation increases rapidly during this active phase, although it slows down near full dilatation. The head level is also charted on the cervicograph using the following definition (see Fig. 1.22):

1. If the head is high, the level is five-fifths above the pelvic brim.
2. If the head is just descending into the brim, it is four-fifths above the brim.
3. If less than half the head is in the brim, it is three-fifths above the brim.
4. If more than half the head is through the brim, it is two-fifths above the brim.
5. If just the sinciput is palpable, one-fifth is above the brim.

The head level in fifths is plotted on the 0–5 gradations on the cervicograph.

Descent is also assessed in relation to the height of the presenting part above or below the level of the ischial spines. The nature and frequency of the contractions are recorded on the chart by shading in the number of contractions per 10 minutes. Dotted squares indicate contractions of less than 20 duration, cross-hatched squares are contractions between 20 and 40 duration, while contractions lasting longer than 40 are shown by complete shading of the squares.

Management of labour

> - Begins with antenatal education
> - Normally consists of support, pain relief and observation of fetal condition and cervical dilatation
> - Intervention indicated if dilation lags > 2 hours behind expected rate

2. Pain relief in labour

Narcotic analgesia agents

A variety of narcotic agents have been used for pain relief in labour. The most commonly used agents at present include pethidine 50–150 mg, omnopon 10–20 mg, diamorphine 5–10 mg, pentazocine 30–60 mg, phenazocine 1–2 mg or oxymorphone 1–1.5 mg by intra-muscular injection. These drugs are commonly used in conjunction with the phenothiazines or diazepam. The drugs are easy to administer, but have the disadvantage of being relatively ineffective in 30–40% of patients. They also tend to cause nausea and vomiting and may result in respiratory depression of the neonate — particularly if given when they are most needed, i.e. late in the first stage of labour. Despite the tendency to avoid narcotic analgesics in present-day practice, they are still a valuable part of pain relief and are widely used.

Inhalational agents

These are commonly reserved for use in the later part of the first stage and in the second stage of labour. The three agents in common use are nitrous oxide and oxygen 50:50 (Entonox®), trichloroethylene 0.35–0.5% and methoxyflurane 0.35% in air. Nitrous oxide has a low solubility in blood and only about 10% of women obtain complete pain relief. If optimal effects are to be obtained, patients should be trained to self-inhale Entonox® at least 30 seconds before a contraction starts and that is not always easy to judge.

Trichloroethylene and methoxyflurane

These agents have a high degree of solubility in body fat and it therefore takes longer to achieve adequate analgesic concentrations. Inhalation should at first be continuous for 10–15 minutes and thereafter only during contractions. After 30 minutes, inhalation should be necessary only every third or fourth contraction. Nausea and vomiting are common side effects.

Regional analgesia

Epidural analgesia. The most widely used form of regional analgesia is epidural analgesia. The procedure may be instituted at any time during labour. A fine catheter is passed into the lumbar epidural space and local anaesthetic such as Marcain® or bupivacaine injected (Fig. 13.7). This will reduce and usually eliminate the pain of labour but does not affect uterine activity.

The procedure involves the following:

1. Insertion of an intravenous infusion to expand plasma volume, thus reducing hypotensive effects and expanding the vascular tree of the lower third of the body.
2. Insertion of an epidural catheter at L_3L_4 vertebrae. Blood pressure, pulse rate and fetal heart rate should be carefully monitored and the infusion of local anaesthesia should be altered by posture to achieve the desired analgesic effects.

Other forms of vaginal anaesthesia. Spinal anaesthesia is rarely used in the management of normal

Fig. 13.7 Epidural anaesthesis is induced by injection of local anaesthetic agents into the lumbar epidural space

labour because it is not superior to epidural analgesia and it carries greater risk of complications.

Paracervical and pudendal blockade involve infiltration of the paracervical region or infiltration around the pudendal nerve as it leaves the pudendal canal (Fig. 13.8). These procedures are most commonly used for pain relief during operative vaginal delivery and are therefore introduced in the second stage of labour.

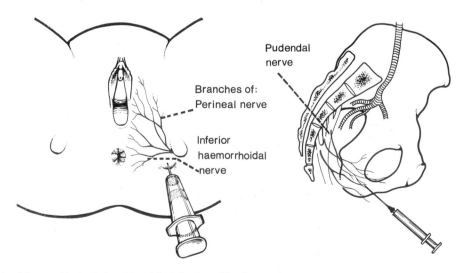

Fig. 13.8 Pudendal nerve blockade is achieved by injection of local anaesthetic around the pudendal nerve at the level of the ischial spine. Additional infiltration is used to block branches of the inferior haemorrhoidal and perineal nerves

Complications of regional analgesia are minimal but include:

1. Toxic symptoms or convulsions with intravenous injection of local anaesthesia.
2. Spinal tap with spinal anaesthesia. Leakage of cerebrospinal fluid (CSF) may result in persistent headache. Total spinal analgesia may result in respiratory paralysis.
3. Hypotension, which is treated by changing the patient to the left lateral position and infusing 500–1000 ml of Hartman's solution.

Regional anaesthesia

> • Epidural catheter inserted at L3/4
> • Need to expand plasma volume
> • Complications are spinal tap, hypotension and intravenous injection of anaesthetic

Posture in labour

Some women prefer to remain ambulant or to sit in a chair during the first stage of labour. However, most women prefer to lie down as labour advances and should be encouraged to lie in the lateral supine position. Women who wish to have epidural analgesia need to remain supine as the procedure inevitably produces some temporary motor impairment of the legs.

3. Nutrition in labour

No patient should be fed by mouth during labour, although occasional small sips of clear fluid are permissible. Delayed gastric emptying may result in vomiting and inhalation of vomitus if general anaesthesia is required. Intravenous therapy should be started where the labour persists for more than 6 hours and delivery is not imminent. The major cause of acidosis in labour is dehydration and not starvation and therefore Hartman's solution and not 5% dextrose should be used at a rate of 1–1.5 litres/8 hours.

Fetal monitoring

Fetal distress (asphyxia) is associated with alterations in fetal heart rate, the passage of meconium-stained liquor and excessive fetal movements. Diminution and cessation of fetal movements may indicate incipient placental failure and fetal demise.

During labour, the fetal heart rate can be monitored every 15 minutes using a Pinard fetal stethoscope and contractions are monitored by manual palpation. However, it is now common practice to use electronic monitors to provide continuous surveillance.

Fetal cardiotocography

The pressure changes in the uterus are recorded by using either internal or external pressure transducers and the resultant pressure wave is recorded on a continuous graphical record (tocograph).

Pressure is recorded either with a pressure sensor applied externally over the anterior abdominal wall

Fig. 13.9 Monitoring during labour—contractions are recorded by intra- and extra-uterine tocography; the fetal heart rate is recorded externally by Doppler ultrasonography or by direct application of an ECG electrode to the presenting part

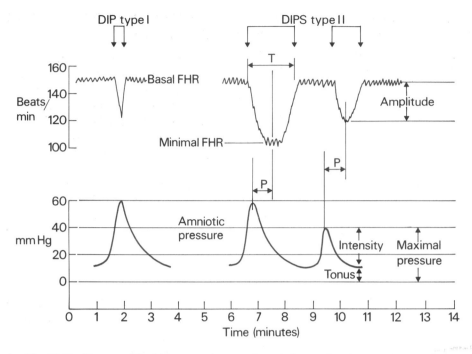

Fig. 13.10 Patterns of fetal heart rate change and amniotic pressure change in labour

and uterus or by inserting a pressure sensitive transducer into the amniotic sac or alternatively a fluid-filled catheter, which is then attached externally to a pressure transducer (Fig. 13.9).

Fetal heart rate is recorded externally by the application of Doppler ultrasound over the fetal heart, or by the direct application of a clip and electrical lead directed to the fetal presenting part, after rupturing the fetal membranes. This has the advantage of giving a much clearer tracing. The heart rate is displayed as a continuous linear trace.

Basal heart rate

The normal fetal heart rate varies between 110 and 160 b.p.m. (Fig. 13.10). It exhibits short-term fluctuations known as beat-to-beat irregularity. The normal heart rate fluctuates between 10 and 25 b.p.m. A 'silent' fetal heart rate of less than 5 b.p.m. indicates fetal distress and jeopardy.

A summary of the definitions of heart rate are shown in Table 13.1.

Table 13.1 Fetal heart rate definitions

Definition	Heart rate (b.p.m.)
Baseline rate	
Normal	120–160
Tachycardia – moderate	160–180
– severe	>180
Bradycardia – moderate	100–120
– severe	<100
Variability	
Normal	>5
Reduced	3–5
Absent	<3

Transient episodes of bradycardia

Three types of fetal bradycardia have been described:

1. *Early decelerations (type I)* – deceleration of the heart rate which commences with the onset of a contraction and returns to normal on completion of the contraction. This is commonly innocuous and indicates head or cord compression.
2. *Late decelerations (type II)* – deceleration occurs well after the contraction has started and does not return to normal until 20 seconds after com-

pletion of the contraction. This is generally considered to be pathological and to indicate fetal asphyxia and placental insufficiency — particularly when it is associated with a resting tachycardia.

3. *Variable deceleration* – this may occur at any time independent of contractions and is sometimes pathological.

The fetal electrocardiogram

The fetal electrocardiogram (FECG) can be recorded from scalp electrodes but the signal is often difficult to interpret because of electrical noise. Techniques are now available using computer technology that allow isolation of the signal from background noise, and continuous real-time monitoring of all changes in time constants and the configuration of the FECG. In the presence of fetal hypoxia, the relationship between the PR interval and heart rate changes from negative to positive, the ST segment becomes depressed and the T wave height increases. This technology is not widely available at the present time, but may prove to have greater specificity than existing methods of monitoring based on heart rate alone.

Fetal acid–base balance

Where abnormalities of fetal heart rate occur in labour, the fetal acid–base status should be examined. Fetal blood can be obtained directly from the scalp through an amnioscope, which is inserted through the cervix and enables direct visualization of the presenting part. A scalp blood pH measurement is made. A pH of less than 7.25 indicates mild acidosis and necessitates repetition of measurement after 1 hour. A value of less than 7.20 indicates a significant degree of asphyxia and the need for delivery.

Fetal monitoring

- Normal basal FHR = 110–160 b.p.m.
- Beat-to-beat variation should be > 5 b.p.m.
- Decelerations are a fall in FHR of > 15 b.p.m. for more than 30 seconds and are described by their relation to contractions
- Significant fetal hypoxia is indicated by a scalp pH of < 7.2
- Significant hypoxia is more likely in the presence of meconium-stained liquor

MANAGEMENT OF THE SECOND STAGE OF LABOUR

The onset of the second stage of labour is indicated by a desire to bear down and, often, to vomit. The diagnosis is confirmed by vaginal examination. This stage occupies less than 2 hours in the primigravida and 1 hour in the multiparous woman. The progress of the second stage is assessed by the degree of distension of the perineum. The desire to bear down may not be present if epidural anaesthesia is effective, and, in this situation, the onset of the second stage can be identified only by the recognition of full cervical dilatation.

Preparation for delivery

The attendant scrubs and puts on gown and gloves. The mother is commonly placed in the left lateral or supine position and may also be placed in the lithotomy position. Some women prefer to deliver in the squatting position. As the head is pushed down with each contraction, it distends the perineum and anus. The anus is covered with a pad and the descent of the occiput controlled with the left hand, the head being kept well flexed until crowned when it is allowed to extend. This process minimises perineal distension. The head then delivers and the eyes and naso-pharynx are cleared.

If the perineum appears to be tearing, an episiotomy is performed, the incision is made in the medio-lateral direction from the midpoint of the posterior margin of the introitus (Fig. 13.11). With the next contraction, the head is gently pulled towards the perineum until the anterior shoulder is delivered under the subpubic angle and then pulled anteriorly to deliver the posterior shoulder and the remainder of the trunk.

The cord is clamped twice and cut between the clamps. The infant will normally cry immediately after birth, but, if the onset of respiration is delayed for more than 1 minute, the naso-pharynx should be aspirated and the baby's lungs inflated with oxygen. If the onset of respiration is further delayed, intubation will be necessary.

The condition of the baby is assessed at 1 minute and 5 minutes using the Apgar scoring system (Table 13.2).

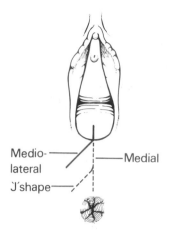

Fig. 13.11 Sites for episiotomy incisions: the object is to avoid extension of the incision or tear into the anal sphincter or rectum

Fig. 13.12 Brandt-Andrews technique for assisted delivery of the placenta: the uterine fundus must be contracted before this technique is attempted

Table 13.2 Evaluation of the Apgar score

	0	1	2
Colour	White	Blue	Pink
Tone	Flaccid	Rigid	Normal
Pulse	Impalpable	< 100 b.p.m.	> 100 b.p.m.
Respiration	Absent	Irregular	Regular
Response	Absent	Poor	Normal

MANAGEMENT OF THE THIRD STAGE

The mother is turned on to her back if she is not already in the supine position. A dish is placed under the cord and beneath the introitus and buttocks to collect any blood loss. The left hand is rested on the abdomen on the uterine fundus. An oxytocic drug such as Syntometrine®, which contains both ergometrine and Syntocinon®, is given by intramuscular injection with crowning of the head, and the uterus should contract firmly shortly after delivery of the fetus.

As soon as the uterus is contracted, cord traction is applied with the right hand whilst monitoring fundal descent with the left hand against the uterine fundus (Fig. 13.12). Assisted delivery of the placenta is usually completed within 5 minutes of delivery.

The placenta and membranes are checked to see if any cotyledons are missing and whether the membranes are complete or incomplete. The blood loss is recorded.

Repair of perineal damage

If there is an episiotomy or tear, this is now repaired (Fig. 13.13). The episiotomy or tear may be first degree, second degree or third degree. First degree tears involve vaginal and perineal skin only. Second degree tears involve the underlying levator ani muscles. Third degree tears involve the anal sphincter and, if gross, the rectal mucosa.

The perineal structures are sutured with size 0 or 1 chromic catgut and the perineal skin may be sutured with non-absorbable or absorbable suture material. The former are removed 5 days later. There are many other satisfactory variants of this procedure. Many practitioners prefer to use absorbable suture materials throughout so that the sutures do not need to be removed. The use of subcuticular sutures results in an excellent scar but demands meticulous haemostasis. The use of synthetic absorbable suture materials which have greater strength and can be used at finer grades are now tending to replace traditional catgut.

Closure of the vaginal wound requires a clear view of the apex of the incision; a 'tagged' pack should be inserted into the vagina to keep the operative field clear of blood. After closure of the vaginal wound, the levator muscle and fascia should be approximated with interrupted sutures and the skin closed with careful haemostasis. If the superficial external sphincter is cut, then the ends should be identified and sutured together.

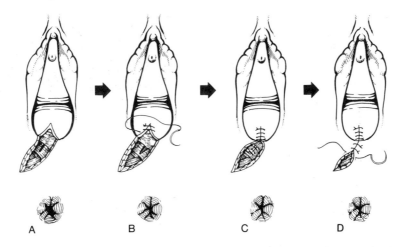

Fig. 13.13 Repair of the episiotomy: the posterior vaginal wall may be closed with continuous or interrupted sutures; apposition of the cut levator muscle ensures haemotasis before skin closure. (A) Episiotomy wound; (B) continuous suture of posterior vaginal wall; (C) interrupted sutures into the cut edges of the levator and; (D) interrupted suture into the perineal skin

On completion of the procedure:

1. Remove the pack.
2. Ensure that the vagina is not constricted and admits two fingers easily.
3. Perform a rectal examination and make sure that none of the sutures have penetrated the rectal mucosa. If this occurs, the sutures must be removed.

BIBLIOGRAPHY

Baylan P 1987 Intrapartum fetal monitoring. In: Fetal monitoring. Baillieres Clinical Obstetrics and Gynecology, Vol. 1, No. 1.
Studd J 1985 The management of labour. Blackwell Scientific Publications, Oxford

14. Abnormal labour

PREMATURE LABOUR

The onset of labour before 36 weeks gestation is described as premature labour. Some 6–10% of all labours are premature. Because uterine contractions may occur at any stage during pregnancy, it is often difficult to identify the onset of labour. However, it must be remembered that the onset of labour is defined as the presence of regular, painful uterine contractions that produce progressive cervical dilatation.

Aetiology

The mechanism of the onset of labour remains uncertain; this also applies to the onset of premature labour. Nevertheless, it is known that there is an association between premature labour and social class, overdistension of the uterus, as with hydramnios and multiple pregnancy, premature rupture of the membranes, antepartum haemorrhage, and uterine abnormalities (Fig. 14.1). A woman has a 30% chance of repeating the situation with her second pregnancy; if she has a second premature labour, there is a 60% chance of a third premature labour.

The danger of premature labour lies mainly in the risk to the fetus and not to the mother. Premature labour remains the most common cause of fetal and neonatal loss.

Management of preterm labour

Once the diagnosis is established, the management of preterm labour is dependent on the stage at which the mother presents and on the quality of available neonatal services. It may, for example, be preferable

Fig. 14.1 Factors predisposing to premature labour

to allow a labour to proceed at 32 weeks gestation if the neonatal unit of a particular service provides a better opportunity of survival than can be achieved by attempting to suppress the labour (Fig. 14.2).

Those factors that indicate impaired prospects of conservative management of preterm labour include:

1. The presence of prematurely ruptured membranes.
2. The occurrence of antepartum haemorrhage.
3. Cervical dilatation in excess of 5 cm at the time of presentation.

Conservative management

If the cervix is less than 5 cm dilated and the membranes are intact, it is reasonable to attempt to

Gestation (weeks)				
20 24 28 32 36				

Half term   Term

Approximate survival rates (%)	0	15	75	97	99.7

Birth weight (g) <500 1000 1500 2500>

Fig. 14.2 Birth weight, gestational age and perinatal outcome

stop labour. This is best effected using intravenous infusion of drugs which are sympathomimetic such as ritodrine, orciprenaline and isoxsuprine. These drugs inhibit uterine contractions when administered by intravenous infusion but they also have significant side effects such as tremor, tachycardia, hypotension, hypokalaemia, nausea and vomiting. Once labour is effectively inhibited, the drug can be administered orally until 36 weeks gestation after which it is doutful that any further advantage is gained by continuing the pregnancy. It is also important to realize that inhibiting labour after 36 weeks gestation will not improve perinatal outcome.

Method of delivery

When labour is established and there is no prospect of effectively inhibiting contractions, the labour should be allowed to proceed with appropriate pain relief. Shortening of the second stage by low forceps delivery and a generous episiotomy will serve to minimize the risk of intracranial haemorrhage.

The chances of survival are substantially enhanced with the availability of high quality neonatal services, and any woman in labour before 34 weeks gestation should be delivered in a hospital with appropriate facilities.

There is evidence that preterm labour with breech presentation is associated with a significant increase in perinatal loss and that survival is improved between 28 and 34 weeks gestation if the child is delivered by Caesarean section.

Perinatal mortality

The survival of infants weighing 1.5 kg or more is now in excess of 95% and this percentage remains remarkably high even for birth weights down to 1 kg.

Premature labour

- Labour occurring before 36 weeks
- 6–10% of labours
- Associated with social class, 'uterine distension', antepartum haemorrhage and premature rupture of the membranes
- Tocolysis indicated if under 32 weeks, intact membranes and < 5 cm dilated

PREMATURE RUPTURE OF THE MEMBRANES

The time of spontaneous rupture of the membranes is determined by:

1. The tensile strength of the fetal membranes.
2. The support of surrounding tissue, i.e. the degree of dilatation of the cervix.
3. Intrauterine pressure.

Premature rupture of the membranes is defined as spontaneous rupture of the membranes before the onset of labour; it occurs in up to 10% of pregnancies.

Aetiology

The membranes may rupture prematurely as the result of:

1. *Weakened membranes.* This is associated with the presence of infection and is the commonest explanation for premature membrane rupture.
2. *Cervical incompetence.* A dilated cervical canal will allow the membranes to bulge through the

Fig. 14.3 Factors which determine the time of rupture of the fetal membranes

cervix and eventually rupture because of poor support.

3. *Abnormally raised intrauterine pressure.* This may be due to hydramnios, distension of the uterus by multiple pregnancy and sometimes abnormal external pressure.

Diagnosis

The mother usually observes that she has had a gush of fluid from the vagina or that she feels constantly wet. It may sometimes be very difficult to be certain whether the symptoms are related to vaginal discharge or to the passage of amniotic fluid. The diagnosis is confirmed by speculum examination and the direct observation of clear fluid in the vagina. The tests for protein in the vaginal discharge are not particularly helpful or reliable, and it can often be difficult to be certain if the membranes have ruptured. Sometimes the drainage of amniotic fluid may cease spontaneously, particularly if there is a high leakage rather than forewater rupture.

Management

It is advisable to admit the mother to hospital for observation.

The risks to the fetus and the mother are those of ascending infection, and in particular infection in the fetal lungs. Furthermore, prolonged drainage of amniotic fluid may lead to oligohydramnios and impaired fetal lung development.

On admission, the diagnosis must be established by direct speculum examination, and a high vaginal swab should be taken for culture. If negative, this should be repeated one week later and weekly thereafter. If the culture is positive or there are clinical signs of infection, then the appropriate antibiotic therapy should be given. After 36 weeks gestation, consideration should be given to the induction, as the risks of prematurity will be minimal, whereas the risk of infection will continue.

If there are maternal signs of infection, such as maternal pyrexia, purulent vaginal discharge and uterine tenderness, then labour should be stimulated. If this is ineffective, as sometimes happens in these circumstances, then the child should be delivered by Caesarean section.

BREECH PRESENTATION

The fetus presents by the breech at delivery in about 3% of all pregnancies at term. The incidence of breech presentation is higher in early pregnancy, but in many cases the presentation spontaneously corrects itself.

Types of breech presentation

The breech may present in one of three ways (Fig. 14.4):

1. Frank breech — the legs lie extended along the body and the buttocks present to the pelvic inlet (see Fig. 14.9).
2. Flexed breech — the legs are flexed and the fetus 'sits' on the legs so that the limbs present to the pelvic inlet.
3. Knee or footling presentation — one thigh is flexed and one is extended so that the foot or knee will descend first through the cervical os into the vagina.

Extended legs   Flexed legs   Footling

Fig. 14.4 Types of breech presentation

The position of the fetus is described by using the sacrum as the denominator, rather than the occiput as with a vertex presentation.

Management

Antenatal

There are various conditions which predispose to breech presentation; these include multiple pregnancy, placenta praevia, congenital abnormalities of the uterus and fetal malformation. Increased muscle tone as found in primigravidae may also be a predisposing factor.

In the presence of any of these factors, it may be necessary to modify management accordingly.

Breech presentation is associated with an increased risk of perinatal loss associated with:

1. Asphyxia from cord compression during delivery.
2. Intracranial haemorrhage and trauma to viscera during delivery.

It is therefore important to be certain that there will be no delay during delivery and that the pelvis is adequate and the fetus is not abnormally large.

External cephalic version

If the breech presentation persists after 34 weeks gestation, it may be appropriate to turn the fetus by manual manipulation to a vertex presentation. This process is known as **external cephalic version**. It is contraindicated if the ultimate intention is to deliver the child by Caesarean section, and if there has been a previous antepartum haemorrhage or placenta praevia.

The procedure is performed by applying pressure to both poles of the fetus after disimpacting the breech from the pelvis and rotating the fetus to a cephalic presentation (Fig. 14.5).

Complications include cord entanglement, fetal distress, premature rupture of the membranes and premature separation of the placenta. It is important to check the fetal heart before and during the procedure. If there are signs of fetal distress it may be necessary to return the fetus to its original presentation. If external cephalic version is not possible, then a decision must be made as to the method of delivery.

Fig. 14.5 External cephalic version: pressure is applied in the opposite direction to the two fetal poles

It may be difficult to define accurately the size of the fetus although modern ultrasound techniques have improved prenatal assessment. It is possible to examine the bony pelvis by clinical pelvimetry and radiological pelvimetry (Fig. 14.6). This should be performed at 36 weeks gestation.

Ilio-pectineal line

Fig. 14.6 Clinical assessment of the pelvis and breech presentation

Method of delivery

Caesarean section

If the pelvis is small or the fetus is large, then delivery should be by elective Caesarean section. A previous Caesarean section, pre-eclampsia or antepartum haemorrhage are also indications for delivery by elective Caesarean section.

Vaginal delivery

If all other factors are normal, vaginal delivery should be planned. The mother should be advised to present as soon as labour starts or the membranes rupture. Vaginal examination must be performed at the time of admission to exclude cord presentation. The length of labour is the same as in a vertex presentation. Analgesia may be provided by epidural anaesthesia.

The presence of meconium-stained liquor carries the same significance of possible fetal hypoxia as with a vertex presentation.

Delivery technique (Fig. 14.7)

When the cervix is fully dilated, the mother is encouraged to bear down until the fetal buttocks and anus come into view (Fig. 14.9). A wide episiotomy is performed and the mother is encouraged to expel the child to the level of the umbilicus. The legs are then lifted out of the vagina and traction is applied to the legs downwards and backwards with the shoulders in the anteroposterior diameter. It should be possible to deliver the anterior arm by sliding the fingers over the shoulder and sweeping the arm downwards. The trunk is then moved laterally until the posterior arm can be delivered. The trunk is then allowed to hang for 30s and this helps to pull the head into the pelvis. The trunk is now swung upwards through 180° until the mouth comes on view. The mouth is cleared of fluid to allow respiration to start and forceps are then applied to the aftercoming head to enable gradual delivery of the head and to protect against sudden expansion and expulsion. Syntometrine® is given by intramuscular injection with delivery of the head. With proper selection and careful management, the perinatal mortality should be no greater than with vertex delivery.

Breech presentation

- 3% of term pregnancies
- Sacrum used as denominator
- Predisposing factors include multiple pregnancy, placenta praevia, and malformation of fetus or uterus
- Associated with increased perinatal morbidity and mortality
- Delivery by section is indicated if previous section, pregnancy-induced hypertension, antepartum haemorrhage or disproportion anticipated
- Length of labour should be normal
- Early deceleration more likely to indicate cord compression or fetal distress than in a vertex delivery
- Delivery of the after-coming head should be assisted

Suction

Fig. 14.7 Technique of breech delivery: initial delivery of the trunk allows descent of the head into the pelvis (left); subsequent anterior rotation of the trunk enables delivery of the fetal head with the application of forceps to safeguard the head from sudden compression and expansion (right)

Left mento-transverse   Right mento-transverse

Fig. 14.8 Position of the face presentation; the denomination is the chin

FACE PRESENTATION (Fig. 14.8).

This occurs in approximately 1 in 600 deliveries. The head is hyperextended so that the occiput rests on the cervical spine. It sometimes occurs as a continuing extension of a deflexed head in the occipito–posterior position. Occasionally the head is pushed back by a cervical tumour. The chin acts as the denominator.

Diagnosis

This can sometimes be made antenatally but it is usually recognized in labour. The head feels large on abdominal palpation and the nuchal groove can often be felt.

On vaginal examination, the fetal nose, eyes, mouth and chin can be felt but are sometimes obscured by considerable facial oedema. The diameter of engagement is the submento-bregmatic diameter, which is the same size as the sub-occipito–bregmatic diameter.

However, in a full-term fetus, delivery can occur vaginally only if the chin lies anteriorly.

Management

Vaginal delivery can be anticipated if the pelvis is normal and the chin rotates anteriorly. If progress is slow, it may be preferable to effect delivery by Caesarean section. The facial bruising and oedema are often gross but usually subside within a few days.

BROW PRESENTATION (Fig. 14.9)

Brow presentation is the cause of obstructed labour and occurs in about 1 in 3000 pregnancies. Unless

Brow presentation   Buttock presentation

Fig. 14.9 Brow and breech presentation at delivery

the head is small or the pelvis very large, vaginal delivery is not possible.

Diagnosis

The head remains high and does not engage and is therefore easily palpable. On vaginal examination, the brow is palpable between the bridge of the nose and supra-orbital ridges and the anterior fontanelle. the management is to deliver the child by Caesarean section.

UNSTABLE LIE, TRANSVERSE LIE AND SHOULDER PRESENTATION

An unstable lie is one which constantly changes. It is commonly associated with multiparity, placenta praevia, uterine abnormalities such as a bicornuate uterus or uterine fibroids. Polyhydramnios may allow undue fetal mobility.

Complications

If the lie is unstable, there is a risk of prolapse of the cord and of obstructed labour from a malpresentation. Provided there is no evidence of placenta praevia, the lie should be corrected and the mother advised to come into hospital immediately labour begins. If the lie is still unstable at 38 weeks, it is safer to arrange hospital admission and await the spontaneous onset of labour. If induction of labour is indicated for other reasons, the lie should be corrected, the membranes, ruptured and labour stimulated with an oxytocin infusion.

TRANSVERSE LIE AND SHOULDER PRESENTATION

If labour starts when the lie is transverse, it is clear that vaginal delivery cannot occur unless the fetus is very small or macerated. The transverse lie may evolve into a shoulder presentation and as the cervix dilates, the arm may prolapse (Fig. 14.10).

Management

If the shoulder is presenting, no attempt should be made to replace or apply traction to the arm. Unless the lie can be corrected before the situation occurs, the only appropriate method of delivery is by Caesarean section. If the lie has been neglected, it may be necessary to perform a classical Caesarean section with a vertical incision in the upper segment.

CORD PRESENTATION AND PROLAPSE

Cord presentation occurs when any part of the cord lies alongside or in front of the presenting part. When the membranes rupture under these circumstances the cord will prolapse (Fig. 14.11).

Shoulder presentation

Anterior arm presentation

Fig. 14.10 Prolapse of the arm into the vagina sometimes results in a shoulder presentation

Fig. 14.11   Cord prolapse (left); pressure on the cord can be minimized by placing the mother in the knee-chest position (right)

Predisposing factors

Any condition that displaces the head or presenting part away from the cervix predisposes to cord prolapse. It is particularly likely to occur in the presence of malpresentations, cephalo-pelvic disproportion and polyhydramnios. If the membranes are ruptured artificially to induce labour the cord may prolapse but it is, in fact, no more likely to occur in this way than spontaneously.

Management

Cord prolapse is an obstetric emergency and delivery must be effected as quickly as possible. This means that unless the cervix is fully dilated and a forceps or ventouse delivery can be effected, Caesarean section is necessary.

As soon as the diagnosis is made, there is no point in trying to replace the cord and indeed it should be handled as little as possible to avoid inducing arterial spasm. Pressure on the cord can be reduced by displacing the presenting part digitally per vaginam or by placing the woman in the knee-chest position (Fig. 14.11).

Despite the acute asphyxial insult inflicted on the fetus under these circumstances, fetal cerebral damage is surprisingly rare — probably because of the short-term nature of the asphyxia.

MALPOSITION OF THE FETAL HEAD

The occipito-posterior position (Fig. 14.12)

This is the commonest malposition of the fetal head and is often associated with prolonged and painful labour with severe backache.

The head normally engages in the transverse diameter and the occiput rotates anteriorly as the head presses onto the pelvic floor. The head occupies the occipito-posterior position in 10% of vertex presentations. The head is deflexed and the presenting diameter — the occipito–frontal — is 11 cm, and therefore produces some degree of cephalo-pelvic disproportion.

Diagnosis

The occipito-posterior position can be diagnosed by both abdominal and vaginal palpation. The anterior abdominal wall looks flattened below the umbilicus as compared with the convexity of the normal presentation and position. The fetal limbs lie anteriorly and are easily palpable. The head engages late and tends to remain high. The occipito-posterior position is the commonest cause of non-engagement of the fetal head in the primigravida at term.

On vaginal examination, the posterior fontanelle lies behind the transverse diameter of the pelvic inlet. During labour, the cervix often dilates

Long anterior rotation-
short posterior rotation

Fig. 14.12   Clinical findings in the occipito-posterior position (left); the head may rotate anteriorly or posteriorly or may arrest in the occipito-posterior position (right)

asymmetrically so that the anterior lip becomes thickened and oedematous whilst the posterior rim dilates normally.

Management

The essential features of management are to ensure that pain relief is adequate and that fluid replacement is maintained to prevent dehydration.

The head may rotate anteriorly and the labour progress normally (see Fig.14.12) or it may rotate posteriorly and adopt a direct occipito-posterior position. The latter is particularly likely to occur in an anthropoid pelvis. It may remain in the occipito-posterior position but, when full cervical dilatation occurs, the head must be rotated either manually or with Kielland's forceps and delivered by forceps extraction.

If the head occupies the occipito-posterior position and is low on the pelvic floor, it may be delivered as a direct occipito-posterior position. This can cause severe damage to the perineum because of the overdistension of the pelvic floor, and may result in a third degree tear.

Deep transverse arrest

Although the head usually engages in the transverse diameter, it normally rotates anteriorly. If this rotation does not occur, the head arrests at the level of the ischial spines. If the pelvis is android in shape, vaginal delivery may be impossible.

If the pelvis is normal, delivery is effected by either manual or forceps rotation. Deep transverse arrest results in a prolonged second stage of labour. This term should not be applied when forceps rotation is required for some other complication before the head has had the chance to rotate normally.

Other presentations

- Face presentation; 1 in 600 births, can be delivered if chin anterior
- Brow; 1 in 3000 births, usually requires Caesarean section
- Unstable lie; associated with multiparity, placenta praevia, polyhydramnios and uterine distortion
- Occipito-posterior position; 10% of births, commonest cause of non-engagement in primigravidae at term

ABNORMALITIES OF UTERINE ACTION

Labour may be prolonged because of abnormalities of uterine action. The degree to which these abnormalities contribute to dystocia has been a subject of considerable debate. Progress in normal labour depends on uterine polarity associated with fundal dominance and the progressive dilatation of the cervix.

Thus, lack of progress may result from either normal polarity and week contractions — **hypotonic uterine inertia** — or abnormal polarity and strong contractions — **hypertonic uterine inertia** (Fig. 14.13). In hypertonic uterine contractions,

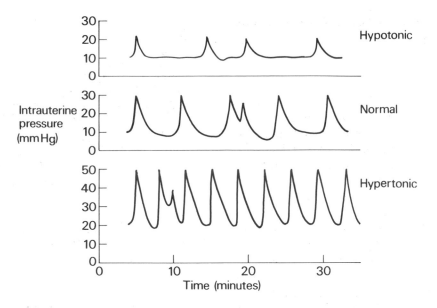

Fig. 14.13 Abnormalities of uterine action which commonly result in prolonged labour

the contraction wave starts in the lower uterine segment and is often prolonged and painful. Contraction waves may also be asymmetrical resulting in a double peak in the uterine contraction wave.

Management

Abnormalities of uterine action are generally recognized by the failure of progress in labour. It is essential to exclude cephalo-pelvic disproportion by careful clinical assessment. Further management should include:

1. Adequate pain relief with epidural anaesthesia.
2. Adequate fluid replacement by intravenous infusion.
3. Stimulation of co-ordinate labour using a dilute solution of oxytocin.

Other disorders of uterine action

Constriction ring dystocia

This is a rare complication of uterine action where one part of the uterus constricts in a ring around the fetus. It commonly results from intra-uterine manipulations such as attempted internal podalic version or from the use of oxytocic agents where there is an abnormal fetal lie.

It is now a rare complication and can generally be reversed only with ether or halothane anaesthesia. It should not be confused with a retraction ring, which occurs as a ridge at the junction of the upper and lower uterine segments and is associated with obstructed labour.

Cervical dystocia

This rare cause of prolonged and obstructed labour is associated with various pathological conditions of the cervix. Factors that cause intensive scarring of the cervix, such as previous cautery or cone biopsy, may lead to a condition where the cervix will not dilate, despite intense uterine activity and, occasionally, this will result in spontaneous annular detachment of the cervix. However, when the condition is recognized, the labour should be terminated by Caesarean section.

TRIAL OF LABOUR AND CEPHALO-PELVIC DISPROPORTION

Every labour in a primigravida is, in a sense, a trial of labour. However, this term is reserved for the conduct of labour where borderline cephalo-pelvic disproportion is suspected. In many women, the only way in which the adequacy of the pelvis can be assessed is to allow the mother to labour and to carefully assess her progress.

Assessment of progress

This is achieved by assessing the rate of progress of cervical dilatation in relation to the normal cervicogram or the nature of the uterine contractions, and the rate of descent of the fetal head. Uterine action is often ineffective in the presence of borderline cephalo-pelvic disproportion and it may be justifiable to employ a dilute oxytocin infusion to stimulate uterine activity.

The mother should be given intravenous fluids and no fluid or food orally. It is also important to ensure that there is adequate pain relief, which is best achieved with epidural anaesthesia. If cervical dilatation remains unchanged over a period of 6 hours, then the trial of labour should be concluded. Likewise, the trial of labour should also be terminated in the presence of fetal or maternal distress.

Causes of failure to progress

- Weak or incoordinate uterine activity
- Cervical dystocia
- Cephalo-pelvic disproportion
- Abnormal lie

ABNORMALITIES OF THE THIRD STAGE OF LABOUR

The third stage of labour starts immediately after the delivery of the infant and ends with expulsion of the placenta. This is normally accomplished within 10–15 minutes and should be complete within 30 minutes.

Postpartum haemorrhage

Primary postpartum haemorrhage consists of blood loss from the vagina in excess of 500 ml and occurring within 24 hours of delivery (Fig. 14.14).

Secondary postpartum haemorrhage

This consists of excessive vaginal blood loss occurring at any subsequent time in the puerperium up

Fig. 14.14 Primary postpartum haemorrhage may occur in the presence of a retained placenta

to 6 weeks after delivery. Haemorrhage may occur from any part of the genital tract, but most commonly from the placental site as a result of (Fig. 14.15):

1. Uterine atony — if the uterus does not contract, then the decussation of myometrial fibres does not exert the usual haemostatic compression of the uterine vessels.
2. Retention of the placenta or placental fragments.

A contracted empty uterus never bleeds.

Fig. 14.15 Causes of postpartum haemorrhage

Case study: primary postpartum haemorrhage

A 37–year–old woman, para 5, was noted to have heavy bleeding following a normal delivery. The uterus was palpable abdominally above the umbilicus and poorly contracted. On vaginal examination, 300 ml of clot was removed from the cervix and vagina, and uterine activity stimulated by rubbing the uterus and starting a Syntocinon® infusion after which the bleeding settled.

Traumatic uterine haemorrhage

This may occur from cervical laceration, which commonly occurs at '3 o'clock' or '9 o'clock' positions, not anteriorly or posteriorly. It may also arise from uterine rupture and in particular, from rupture of a previous Caesarean scar.

Vaginal lacerations

Haemorrhage occurs from vaginal and perineal lacerations and this bleeding may be profuse — particularly when it involves vaginal or vulval varicosities.

Case study: postpartum haemorrhage from vaginal lacerations

A 21–year–old woman delivered by rotational forceps was found to have steady, heavy vaginal bleeding following repair of her episiotomy. The uterus was felt to be well contracted and the bleeding did not respond to intravenous Syntocinon®. Further bleeding required transfusion and the patient was taken to theatre for examination under anaesthesia, when a laceration at the left vaginal fornix was repaired.

Predisposing factors

Various factors predispose to postpartum haemorrhage and these include:

1. Overdistension of the uterus e.g. in multiple pregnancy, hydramnios.
2. Uterine hypotonia associated with prolonged labour.
3. Antepartum haemorrhage — placenta praevia.
4. Multiple fibroids.
5. Grand multiparity.

6. General anaesthesia where agents such as halothane are employed.

Low implantation of the placenta appears to be associated with difficulties in efficient constriction of uterine blood vessels at the site of the implantation. Placental abruption is associated with an increased incidence of postpartum haemorrhage, partly because blood entrapped behind the placenta is expelled during the third stage but also because there may be difficulty with contractility in myometrium damaged by an antepartum haemorrhage. Occasionally haemorrhage may occur because of coagulation disorders.

Management

Postpartum bleeding may be sudden and profound and may rapidly lead to cardiovascular collapse. Treatment is directed towards controlling the bleeding and replacing the blood loss.

Controlling the haemorrhage. A brief visual inspection will suffice to ascertain:

1. The amount of blood loss.
2. Whether the placenta has been expelled.

If the placenta has been expelled, the following actions are taken:

1. Palpate the uterine fundus. If the uterus is soft, then massage of the uterus will immediately stimulate a contraction and expel any retained clot.
2. Inject ergometrine maleate 0.5 mg intravenously and start an oxytocin infusion consisting of 10 units of Syntocinon® in 500 ml of Hartman's solution. Although ergometrine has become less popular because of induced vomiting and raised blood pressure, it is still the most potent oxytocic agent available and should therefore be used as first choice in this situation.
3. Check that the placenta and membranes are complete. If they are not, then manual exploration of the uterine cavity is indicated.
4. If the bleeding continues despite the presence of a well-contracted uterus, the vagina and cervix should be examined with a speculum under good illumination and any laceration sutured to ensure haemostasis.

If the placenta is retained:

1. Massage the uterus to ensure it is well contracted.
2. Apply cord traction and counter pressure against the uterine fundus. The placenta is partially separated and will often deliver with gentle but sustained cord traction as it may be trapped in the cervix.
3. If this manoeuvre fails, then proceed to manual removal of the placenta — with either regional or general anaesthesia.

If bleeding continues after delivery of the placenta and uterine exploration, and the uterus continues to be hypotonic despite physical and pharmacological measures to arrest the bleeding, it may be necessary to apply bimanual compression to the uterus as a first-aid measure. If this fails, it is necessary to proceed to hysterectomy.

There is no place for uterine packing — a technique that has been used in the past but is singularly ineffective.

Recently, the infusion of a solution of prostaglandin E_2 into the uterine cavity has been found to be an effective method of stimulating uterine contractions.

Replacement of blood loss and resuscitation. Although the healthy pregnant woman withstands sudden blood loss remarkably well, adequate replacement by transfusion is essential. Blood substitutes such as Haemacel® can be safely used to replace up to 1500 ml blood loss, but thereafter a blood transfusion should be given.

Vaginal wall haematomas

Profuse haemorrhage does, at times, occur from vaginal and perineal lacerations and it is important to control this bleeding as soon as possible by suturing. Venous bleeding can be controlled by compression but arterial bleeding necessitates ligation of the vessel. If this is not achieved, then formation of haematomas will occur. These may be (Fig. 14.16):

1. Superficial — the perineum will be seen to bulge and distend and will be acutely painful. The sutures must be removed, the haematoma drained and haemostasis secured before closing the wound again with drainage.

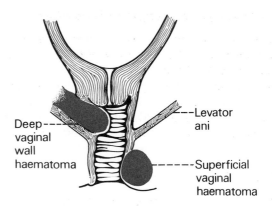

Fig. 14.16 The sites of vaginal wall haematomas

2. Deep — blood loss may occur above the insertion of the levator ani and a large lateral vaginal wall haematoma may develop. This will not be visible externally but presents with continuing pelvic pain, unexplained anaemia and retention of urine. It can be readily recognized by pelvic examination, and must be drained by incision over the haematoma. It is usually very difficult to identify the bleeding point at this stage because extensive tissue damage occurs, but haemostasis should be attempted.

A large corrugated drain is inserted into the cavity and the vagina is packed. A catheter should be left indwelling and adequate blood transfusion and antibiotic therapy instituted.

Bleeding usually arises from a branch of the pudendal artery and may occur spontaneously after a normal vaginal delivery.

Postpartum haemorrhage

- May be primary or secondary
- Common causes are uterine atony, retained products, cervical or vaginal lacerations.
- More likely in multiple gestation, prolonged labour, after antepartum haemorrhage (esp placenta praevia) and in grand multiparity
- Management consists of replacing loss, ensuring an empty well-contracted uterus, repair of lacerations and correction of abnormal clotting

Amniotic fluid embolism

This condition occurs around the time of delivery and results in cardiovascular and respiratory collapse. It is a rare condition occurring about once in 80 000 pregnancies but has a high mortality rate. Amniotic fluid enters the maternal circulation and causes sudden intravascular coagulation resulting in pulmonary insufficiency and a haemorrhage diathesis.

The patient suddenly collapses with dyspnoea, cynanosis and hypotension. Treatment requires immediate oxygenation, monitoring of central venous pressure and adequate restoration of the circulating blood volume. Fresh frozen plasma is given if the fibrinogen level is low.

BIBLIOGRAPHY

Mysercough P R 1982 Munro Kerr's operative obstetrics. Bailliere, London

15. Instrumental and operative delivery

INDUCTION OF LABOUR

Labour is induced when the risk to mother or child of continuing the pregnancy exceeds the risks of inducing labour. The incidence of induction varies widely according to the practice of the obstetrician.

Indications

The major indications for induction of labour are:

1. Pre-eclampsia.
2. Prolonged pregnancy (in excess of 42 weeks gestation).
3. Placental insufficiency and intra-uterine growth retardation.
4. Antepartum haemorrhage — placental abruption and antepartum haemorrhage of uncertain origin.
5. Rhesus isoimmunisation.
6. Diabetes mellitus.
7. Chronic renal disease.

Methods of induction

The commonest method of inducing labour is by surgical rupture of fetal membranes.

Forewater rupture

Rupture of the membranes should be performed under conditions of full asepsis in the delivery suite. Under ideal circumstances, the cervix should be soft, effaced and at least 2 cm dilated. The head should be presenting by the vertex and should be engaged in the pelvis. In practice, these conditions are often not fulfilled and the degree to which they are adhered depends on the urgency of the need to

Forewater rupture

Fig. 15.1 Induction of labour by forewater rupture

start labour. The mother is placed in the lithotomy position and, after swabbing and draping the vulva, a finger is introduced through the cervix and the fetal membranes are separated from the lower segment — a process known as 'stripping the membranes'. The bulging membranes are then ruptured with Kocher's forceps, Gelder forewater amniotomy forceps or an amniotomy hook (Fig. 15.1). The amniotic fluid is released slowly and care is taken to exclude presentation or prolapse of the cord. For purposes of monitoring the uterine activity and fetal heart rate, an intra-uterine catheter is inserted and a scalp electrode is attached.

Hindwater rupture

An alternative method of surgical induction involves rupture of the membranes behind the presenting

Hindwater rupture

Fig. 15.2 Induction of labour by hindwater rupture

part. This is known as hindwater rupture. A sigmoid-shaped metal cannula known as the Drewe-Smythe catheter is introduced through the cervix and penetrates the membranes behind the presenting part (Fig. 15.2). The theoretical advantage of this technique is that it reduces the risk of prolapsed cord. In reality, the risk is even lower with forewater rupture than with spontaneous rupture of the membranes and the technique of hindwater rupture is now rarely used.

Medical induction of labour

Various pharmacological agents can be used to stimulate uterine activity.

Oxytocin infusion. It is common practice to combine surgical induction with a Syntocinon® infusion. A suitable regimen would begin at 1 mU/min and increase 3 mU/min every 15 minutes until adequate contractions become established.

The hazards of induction

The principal hazards of combined surgical and medical induction of labour are:

1. *Hyperstimulation* — excessive and prolonged uterine contractions reduce uterine blood flow and result in fetal asphyxia. Thus, contractions should not occur more frequently than every 2 minutes and should not last in excess of 1 minute. The Syntocinon® infusion should be discontinued if excessive uterine activity occurs or if there are signs of fetal distress.
2. *Prolapse of the cord* — this should be excluded by examination at the time of forewater rupture or subsequently if signs of fetal distress occur.
3. *Infection* — prolonged induction–delivery intervals increase the risk of infection in the amniotic sac with consequent risks to both infant and mother. If the liquor becomes offensive and maternal pyrexia occurs, then the labour should be terminated and the infant delivered.

Medical induction of labour and cervical ripening

Medical induction is indicated where the cervix is unsuitable for surgical induction. The two most commonly used forms of medical induction are:

1. Syntocinon® infusion.
2. Administration of prostaglandins by various routes.

1. *Syntocinon® infusion* — this induces uterine contractions but is a relatively ineffective method of inducing labour unless combined with surgical induction.
2. *Prostaglandins* — the most widely used form is prostaglandin E_2 (Prostin®). This is used to ripen the cervix and may be administered:
   a. orally — tablets of 0.5 mg taken orally are increased to 2 mg/h until contractions are produced.
   b. as an extra-amniotic infusion of PGE_2 — introduced via a catheter into the extra-amniotic space at a dose of 1 mg/min increasing to 4 mg/min until contractions are established. The advantage of this technique is that it produces minimal side effects of vomiting and diarrhoea.
   c. as an intravenous infusion — this is now rarely used because of the severity of side effects and because it often causes thrombophlebitis at the injection site.

Cervical ripening can be achieved using vaginal pessaries of PGE_2 or by a xylose gel suspension in the vagina.

Induction of labour

> - Common indications are pre-eclampsia, post maturity, intra-uterine growth retardation, antepartum haemorrhage, Rhesus disease and diabetes
> - Can be performed by rupture of membranes, oxytocin infusion or vaginal prostaglandins
> - Hazards are hypertonus, cord prolapse and infection

INSTRUMENTAL DELIVERY

Obstetric forceps were first introduced in the 17th century by the Chamberlain family and have been modified and adapted in various forms. Forceps consist of a pair of fenestrated blades with a handle connected to the blades by a shank (Fig. 15.3). The blades normally exhibit both a pelvic and cephalic curve so that they can adapt both to the fetal skull and to the maternal sacral curve. The instruments are designed for application only to the fetal head and not to the buttocks.

Indications

The common indications for forceps delivery are:

1. Delay in the second stage of labour. This occurs most frequently as a result of pelvic floor resistance and a tight perineum. It may, however, also be caused by
   a. poor maternal expulsive efforts;
   b. cephalo-pelvic disproportion;
   c. malposition or malpresentation of the head;
   d. removal of the urge to bear down during epidural anaesthesia.
2. Fetal distress.
3. Maternal distress and maternal conditions necessitating minimal expulsive effort from the mother.
4. Forceps are applied to the after-coming head in a breech presentation and may also be used to extract the fetal head at Caesarean section.

Prerequisites to forceps delivery

When there is an indication for forceps delivery, the mother should be placed in the lithotomy position and the thighs and perineum cleaned and draped. It is then important to check:

1. That the cervix is fully dilated.
2. That the bladder is not overdistended and requiring catheterization.
3. The position, presentation and status of the fetal head; it must be engaged and not palpable in the abdominal cavity.

Anaesthesia

This is commonly achieved with regional anaesthesia — epidural, spinal, sacral block or pudendal

Fig. 15.3 Forceps parts (left); commonly used forceps (right); the absence of the pelvic curve in Kielland's forceps enables rotation of the fetal head

nerve block. On some occasions, general anaesthesia may be indicated.

Method of delivery

Low forceps (outlet forceps)

If the head is direct occipito-anterior in position, below the level of the ischial spine, and resting on the pelvic floor, low forceps delivery is performed (Fig. 15.4).

Low forceps delivery

Fig. 15.4 Low forceps delivery: traction is applied in line with the axis of the pelvis and delivery is effected by lifting the head anteriorly once the occiput has passed beneath the subpubic arch

The forceps used where no rotation of the head is required are:

1. **Neville Barnes forceps** — this has an axis traction handle, which allows considerable force to be applied. This attachment is now rarely used.
2. **Simpson's forceps** — this is similar to Neville Barnes but with no axis traction handle.

Both these forceps have cephalic and pelvic curves.

The two blades of the forceps are designated according to the side of the pelvis to which they are applied. Thus, the left blade is applied to the left side of the pelvis. There is a fixed lock between the blades. Intermittent traction is applied in the direction of the pelvic canal until the occiput is on view and then the head is delivered by anterior extension. An episiotomy is usually, although not invariably, performed.

Mid-cavity forceps

Arrest of the head sometimes occurs in the mid-cavity when the presenting part reaches the level of the ischial spine. At this level, the position of the head is usually transverse or posterior.

The position of the head must first be corrected, by either manual rotation or forceps rotation, to a direct antero-posterior position before application of traction.

Kielland's forceps have a sliding lock and minimal pelvic curve so that rotation of the forceps will not lead to damage by the blades during the process of rotation.

High forceps

This type of delivery, where the head lies well above the level of the ischial spines, is very rarely performed. In fact, if the head can be palpated above the pelvic brim, this is a contraindication to vaginal delivery.

Trial of forceps

Occasionally, a situation arises where there is borderline disproportion and this is an indication for a trial of forceps. This should be attempted only where there is high expectation that vaginal delivery will be achieved without significant trauma to mother or fetus.

Trial of forceps delivery should always be undertaken in an operating theatre with preparation made to proceed to Caesarean section.

Careful assessment of the pelvis and presenting part should be made before proceeding to apply the forceps blades. If firm traction does not produce steady descent of the head, then the blades should be removed and the child delivered by Caesarean section. It may be necessary to disimpact the head vaginally before section.

VACUUM EXTRACTION (**Ventouse**)

An alternative to forceps delivery is the application of a suction cup to the fetal scalp and extraction by traction (Fig. 15.5). The indications for vacuum extraction are the same as those for forceps delivery. The metal suction cups of the vacuum extractor

Ventouse extraction

Fig. 15.5 Ventouse extraction: the suction cup is attached by raising the 'chignon' on the fetal scalp

Lower segment incision

Fig. 15.6 Lower uterine segment Caesarean section: the bladder is reflected and a transverse incision is made in the lower segment

are of three different sizes — 30 mm, 40 mm and 50 mm. The vacuum inside the cup is slowly increased to 0.8 kg/cm^2 and the scalp forms a 'chignon' inside the cup. Traction is applied with the contractions, and rotation of the head will generally occur as the head is pulled on to the pelvic floor.

Laceration of the scalp and caput or haematoma formation may occur with this procedure but the instrument rarely causes any maternal damage. Forceps, if incorrectly applied, may result in considerable maternal laceration, such as uterine rupture and bladder or bowel damage. Fetal damage may involve facial bruising, facial nerve damage, skin abrasions and intracranial haemorrhage.

Instrumental delivery

> - Common indications are delay in second stage, fetal distress, after-coming head in breech
> - Prerequisites are full dilatation, empty bladder, head engaged and occipito-anterior position (for low forceps)
> - Complications include laceration or bruising of scalp, facial nerve palsy and intracranial haemorrhage in fetus and vaginal laceration, fistula formation and uterine rupture in mother

Fig. 15.7 Closure of the uterine wound in layers

Lower segment Caesarean section

The most commonly performed procedure is the **lower segment Caesarean section** where the bladder is reflected from the lower segment and a transverse incision is made (Fig. 15.6). The presenting part is then delivered through the lower segment. The wound is closed in two layers, taking care to exclude the decidua (Fig. 15.7).

The upper segment or classical Caesarean section

In this procedure, a vertical incision is made in the upper segment of the uterus and the child is

CAESAREAN SECTION

This operation is the process whereby the child is removed from the uterus by direct incision through the abdominal wall and the uterus.

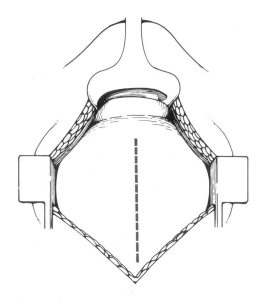

Upper segment incision

Fig. 15.8 'Classical' Caesarean section: a vertical incision is made in the upper uterine segment

delivered through this incision (Fig. 15.8). This is not widely used because it has a much higher morbidity postoperatively, and a much higher incidence of subsequent rupture of the scar.

Caesarean hysterectomy

Caesarean section and hysterectomy are sometimes performed at the same time — where there is uterine rupture, uncontrollable postpartum haemorrhage and, occasionally, cervical malignant disease.

Indications for Caesarean section

It is not particularly helpful to state an incidence figure for Caesarean section because it varies widely from country to country. In the United Kingdom, it is about 10% and the vast majority of the procedures are performed by the lower segment technique. The common indications for Caesarean section are:

1. Obstructed labour.
2. Placenta praevia and antepartum haemorrhage.
3. Fetal distress.

4. Severe pre-eclampsia.
5. Intra-uterine growth retardation and placental failure.
6. Breech presentation and other malpresentations.
7. Failed induction — prolonged labour.
8. Diabetes mellitus.
9. Prolapsed cord.
10. Other rare indications such as cervical dystocia.

The most common indication for Caesarean section is that of a previous section. In some countries, the dictum 'once a section, always a section' is followed.

However, it is reasonable to pursue vaginal delivery following one previous section provided the initial indication is non-recurrent. As a general guideline, one previous Caesarean plus an additional complication indicates a repeat section.

Complications

The immediate complications are those of haemorrhage, shock and the complications of anaesthesia. There may also be damage to the bladder or ureters. Rarely, the fetus may sustain lacerations during the incision of the uterus. Late complications include:

1. Secondary postpartum haemorrhage.
2. Infection — uterine, vesical and wound.
3. Pulmonary embolus.
4. Deep vein thrombosis.

Caesarean section

- 10–15% of deliveries in United Kingdom
- Commonest indication is previous Caesarean section
- Usually transverse lower segment incision
- Complications include secondary postpartum haemorrhage, infection and thrombo-embolism

IMPACTED SHOULDERS

Shoulder impaction occurs where there is a large infant or a small pelvis and particularly where the trunk is large as with diabetic macrosomia. The head is usually delivered without difficulty and, therefore, the condition is one of some urgency as it can only be recognized at this stage. The neck and shoulders do not appear. Unless delivery is

Fig. 15.9 Disimpaction of the anterior shoulder

Fig 15.10 Impacted shoulders: it is sometimes necessary to rotate the fetus to disimpact the posterior shoulder

achieved within 5–7 minutes, the child will die from asphyxia.

Delivery can usually be achieved with firm traction posteriorly to disimpact the anterior shoulder (Fig. 15.9) and then with traction anteriorly to deliver the posterior shoulder (Fig. 15.10). Firm downward pressure should be applied abdominally to the uterine fundus. The danger of this procedure is that excessive traction on the brachial plexus results in Erb's palsy.

Occasionally, the shoulders are disimpacted by rotation through 45° so that either the anterior or posterior shoulder may be disengaged.

BIBLIOGRAPHY

Quillegan E J, Zuspan F P 1982 Douglas-Stromme operative obstetrics. Appleton-Century-Crofts, New York

16. The puerperium

The puerperium is defined as the 6-week period from the completion of the third stage of labour. During this time major physiological changes occur with the adaption of the mother to breast feeding and the return to the non-pregnant state of the various body systems.

PHYSIOLOGICAL CHANGES

Genital tract

The uterus undergoes rapid and massive change by a process of catabolism of muscle fibres. The fibres undergo autolysis and atrophy. Within 10 days, the uterus has involuted from a size where it is palpable at the umbilicus to one where it is no longer palpable as an abdominal organ (Fig. 16.1). By 6 weeks, the uterus has returned to the non-pregnant size. Where breast feeding is established, uterine

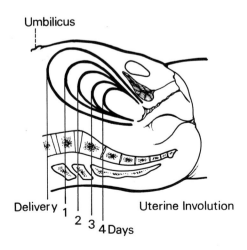

Fig. 16.1 Uterine involution in the puerperium results in a rapid reduction in uterine size

involution may proceed to a level where the size is actually less than the usual non-pregnant state. The endometrium regenerates within 6 weeks and menstruation occurs within this time if lactation has ceased. If lactation continues, the return of menstruation may be deferred for 6 months or more.

Discharge from the uterus is known as **lochia**. At first this consists of blood, either fresh or altered, is called lochia rubra, and lasts from 2 to 14 days. It then changes to a serous discharge, lochia serosa, and finally becomes a slight white discharge, lochia alba. These changes may continue for up to 4–8 weeks after delivery. Abnormal persistence of lochia rubra may indicate retained placental tissue.

Cardiovascular system

Cardiac output and plasma volume return to normal within approximately 1 week. There is a fluid loss of 2 litres during the first week and a further loss of 1.5 litres over the next 5 weeks. This loss is associated with an apparent increase in haematocrit and haemoglobin concentration. There is an increase of serum sodium and plasma bicarbonate as well as plasma osmolality. An increase in clotting factors during the first 10 days after delivery is associated with a higher risk of deep vein thrombosis and pulmonary embolism. There is also a rise in platelet count and greater platelet adhesiveness. Fibrinogen levels decrease during labour, but increase in the puerperium.

LACTATION AND BREAST FEEDING

Breast feeding is the preferred method of infant feeding because, in addition to fulfilling nutritional requirements, it also provides antibodies against infection and protection against various forms of gastro-enteritis associated with unhygienic preparation of artificial feeds. Women tend to avoid breast feeding for social and emotional reasons, and often for reasons of convenience. In a relatively small percentage of cases, there are physical reasons why lactation either is not possible or is inappropriate, such as inverted nipples, previous breast surgery, breast implants or cracked and painful nipples that do not respond to treatment.

Whilst breast feeding is desirable and women should be encouraged, it must be remembered that the majority of infants who are artificially fed also thrive. In other words, the enthusiasm of the attendants should not be allowed to override the mother's wishes. Encouragement and education in antenatal classes are important factors, but many women simply do not like the idea of breast feeding.

Breast preparation

The breasts and nipples should be washed regularly. The breasts should be comfortably supported and the nipples cleared of colostrum. Aqueous-based emollient creams may be used to soften the nipple and thus avoid cracking during suckling. Occasional expression of colostrum in the third trimester helps with subsequent milk secretion. Inverted nipples may present an insuperable barrier to breast feeding and should be treated antenatally by the application of Waller's shields, which apply pressure to the areola and breast tissue surrounding the nipple (Fig. 16.2). These shields are worn inside the breast

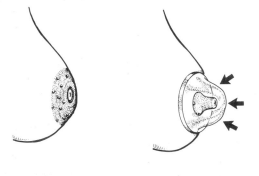

Waller's shield

Fig. 16.2 Inverted or flat nipples (left) may be enhanced by the application of Waller's shields (right)

support for increasing lengths of time during the day.

Breast feeding

The child should be put to the breast as soon after delivery as possible. Suckling is initially limited to 2–3 minutes on each side, but subsequently this period may be increased. Once the mother is comfortably seated, the whole nipple is placed in the infant's mouth, taking care to maintain a clear airway (Fig. 16.3). After suckling, the child is held upright to enable swallowed air to be regurgitated.

Full milk flow supervenes by the third or fourth day after delivery and may be accompanied by painful vascular engorgement.

Fig. 16.3 The mother should be comfortable and the child placed well onto the breast to ensure adequate suckling

Suppression of lactation

Many women elect not to breast feed. Firm support of the breasts, restriction of fluid intake, avoidance of expression of milk and analgesia may be sufficient to suppress lactation. The administration of oestrogens will effectively suppress lactation, but carries some risk of thrombo-embolic disease. It should, however, be noted that the original description of 'risk' was based on observation of doses of oestrogens far in excess of the quantities necessary to suppress lactation. There is, therefore, a case to be made for administering oral oestrogens to suppress lactation. Bromocriptine will inhibit prolactin release and hence suppress lactation, but the dosage necessary to produce this effect tends to create considerable side effects. It should, however, be emphasised that it is preferable to avoid all drug therapy if suppression can be achieved by conservative management.

Physiological changes in the puerperium

- Uterus involutes
- Plasma volume falls
- Increased clotting

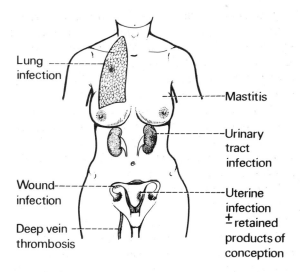

Fig. 16.4 The pathogenesis of puerperal pyrexia

PSYCHOLOGICAL CHANGES AND DISORDERS IN THE PUERPERIUM

Mild degrees of depression and emotional lability are almost the 'norm' in the puerperium, but may become severe in some cases and require psychiatric support. Psychiatric illness may present as severe, incapacitating depression, but the more florid forms of puerperal psychosis involve confusion and delirium with disorientation in time and space, and a complete loss of interest in the child. In some women, frank mania may occur. Early recognition of these symptoms is important if danger to mother and child is to be avoided and early psychiatric support must be sought. These problems are discussed in greater detail in a separate chapter.

COMPLICATIONS OF THE PUERPERIUM

Puerperal pyrexia

The commonest problem of the puerperium is the development of a pyrexia, i.e. a rise of temperature in excess of 38°C.

Aetiology

Puerperal pyrexia must be assumed to be due to infection until proved otherwise. A systematic investigation is undertaken to elucidate the cause and site of the infection (Fig. 16.4).

1. Genital tract infection. The genital tract is particularly vulnerable to infection. The commonest site is within the uterine cavity; infection may be introduced via external sources or arise from contamination from endogenous sources. Infection is particularly common following prolonged labour or prolonged rupture of the membranes.

The clinical signs include subinvolution of the uterus, which remains bulky and larger than would normally be anticipated. The uterus is often tender to palpation. The lochia may be offensive or purulent, but is often normal. Retained products of conception predispose to infection and will also result in excessive and persistent blood-stained lochia. A cervical swab should be taken for culture as a routine procedure in any women with puerperal pyrexia. The common organisms isolated from this site include *E. coli, Staphylococcus pyogenes, Streptococcus faecalis* and *haemolytic streptococcus.*

Infection may also occur in episiotomy wounds of perineal tears, although these infections are relatively uncommon because the vascularity of the perineum provides a higher resistance to infection. The perineum becomes tender and reddened and may be seen to exude purulent discharge. Where genital tract infection is suspected, swabs should be taken for culture and antibiotic therapy started before the culture results are available.

2. Urinary tract infection. The postpartum woman is particularly vulnerable to urinary tract infection.

This is due to a combination of trauma to the bladder, incomplete emptying, particularly related to perineal pain, and the introduction of bacterial organisms by catheterization.

Urinary tract infection is often unaccompanied by any symptoms, with the exception of a low grade pyrexia, but if ascending infection supervenes then acute pyelonephritis may develop. This will produce bilateral loin pain, frequency of micturition and dysuria and lower abdominal pain after voiding. In cases of puerperal pyrexia, a midstream specimen of urine should be sent for culture.

3. Breast infection. Mastitis most often occurs in the second week after delivery and, therefore, may develop after discharge from hospital. Infection may be introduced through a cracked nipple and often originates from the mother's skin or nasopharynx or from the infant's nasopharynx.

4. Other sites of infection. Following Caesarean section, infection may occur in the skin wound or in the peritoneal cavity. Where general anaesthesia is used, lung infection may occur although, with modern anaesthesia, this is an uncommon complication.

Signs and symptoms

The development of pyrexia is accompanied by pain and local tenderness. The breast develops a reddened, tender area and, if abscess formation occurs, the skin becomes oedematous and develops the classical 'peau d'orange' appearance.

Early recognition of infection enables early introduction of antibiotic therapy. If abscess formation occurs, then surgical drainage is necessary.

If the mother is still lactating, feeding is discontinued from the affected breast. In most cases, lactation should be suppressed unless there is strong motivation to continue.

Thrombo-embolic disease

Thrombophlebitis

This is the commonest form of thrombo-embolic disease and tends to arise within the first 3 or 4 days after delivery. Localized inflammation, tenderness and thickening occur in the superficial leg veins. Although the condition is painful and may spread along the leg veins, it rarely leads to serious embolic disease and does not require anticoagulant treatment. Anti-inflammatory drugs and local applications of glycerine and icthyol should be used.

Phlebothrombosis

Deep vein thrombosis is a much more serious complication which tends to arise 7–10 days after delivery, and is particularly likely to occur after operative delivery or prolonged immobilization. Clotting occurring in deep veins may be silent and presents only when the clot breaks loose and lodges in the lung as a pulmonary embolus, with consequent chest pain and haemoptysis. Massive pulmonary embolus results in sudden death unless treated by prompt surgical management.

Deep vein thrombosis may also present as pain in the leg associated with swelling and tenderness and impaired peripheral circulation.

Management of phlebothrombosis. As soon as the diagnosis is established, anticoagulant treatment should be started with intravenous heparin. The limb should be rested until the anticoagulant therapy produces pain relief; then gradual mobilization may be introduced. When the acute process has been controlled, the anticoagulant therapy can be changed to warfarin and should be continued for 3 months. Specialized leg supports such as TED stockings are used to provide support for the affected leg.

Other complications of the puerperium

Urinary retention is a common problem in the immediate puerperium and may result in overflow incontinence. The major cause of retention is pain from the perineum. Traditional methods of encouraging micturition include hot baths, relief of perineal pain by a nalgesic drugs and local applications of ice-packs. If these procedures fail, then the bladder should be catheterized on an intermittent basis until the residual urine is less than 50 ml.

True incontinence is a rare complication and is usually associated with a vesico-vaginal fistula resulting from pressure necrosis during obstructed labour, or following direct injury to the bladder. Injection of a coloured dye into the bladder will establish the diagnosis. A catheter is left indwelling until there is evidence of closure of the fistula or surgical repair is undertaken.

Faecal incontinence may occur following a third degree tear where a recto-vaginal fistula is present. Correct repair of the original tear with proper separation of tissue layers should avoid this complication. Surgical closure is necessary, but repair is delayed until the wound area is clear. Some faecal incontinence may occur where the external anal sphincter is damaged.

Complications of the puerperium

- Genital tract infections
- Urinary infection
- Wound infection
- Mastitis
- Thrombo-embolism
- Incontinence/urinary retention

BIBLIOGRAPHY

Briggs G G, Bodendorfer T W, Freeman R K, Yaffe S J 1983 Drugs in pregnancy and lactation. Williams and Wilkins, Baltimore
Ledward R S, Hawkins D F 1983 Drugs and breast feeding. In: Ledward R S, Hawkins D F (eds) Drug treatment in obstetrics. Chapman and Hall, London

17. Psychiatric disorders of pregnancy and the puerperium

Dr M. Oates

MENTAL ILLNESS IN PREGNANCY

Incidence

At least 15% of all women can be identified as having an episode of mental illness during the first trimester of pregnancy. Many general practice surveys have shown the same prevalence of mental disorder in women of reproductive age, so it could be thought that pregnancy does not involve an increased risk of becoming mentally ill. However, 10% of all pregnant women can be identified as suffering from a new episode of mental illness, having been mentally quite well for at least 3 months before conception, and only 5% of all pregnant women can be identified retrospectively as having suffered from a mental illness before conception. It would therefore seem that the first trimester of pregnancy does constitute an increased risk of mental illness. The incidence of new episodes of mental illness in the second and third trimester is about 5% and does not represent an increased risk of becoming mentally ill.

Minor mental illness

The majority of new episodes of mental illness identified during pregnancy are minor mental illnesses, or neuroses. The depressive neurosis with anxiety is the commonest diagnosis; phobic anxiety states and obsessional compulsive disorders are less common. Eighty per cent of these neurotic mental illnesses resolve by the second trimester and do not predispose the woman to developing postnatal depression. However, a woman who begins her pregnancy with a chronic neurotic condition is likely to continue with her illness throughout the pregnancy (Table 17.1).

Table 17.1 Risk factors – mental illness in pregnancy

Before pregnancy	FH
	Severe mental illness
	PH
	Postnatal mental illness
	Maternal deprivation
	Single
	Young mother/early baby
	Older mother/late baby
	Marital/family discord
	Loss of last baby
During pregnancy	Question of termination of pregnancy
	Concern over fetus
	Anxiety
	3rd trimester
	Depression
	Antenatal admission
	Life events
After pregnancy	CS
	Neonatal illness
	Maternal illness
	Life events
	Loss of self-esteem
	Unrealistic expectation
	Social isolation

NB Risk factors cluster
    Risk factors can be reduced
    Risk factors do not respect social class

FH = Family history; PH = past history

These few women are predisposed to developing an exacerbation of their condition in the puerperium. It would appear that a past history of neurotic disorder occurring earlier in a woman's life, a consideration of terminating this pregnancy, marital tension, a previous abortion, and marked neurotic traits in the premorbid personality predispose to the development of a neurosis in the first trimester of pregnancy. Although less common, the occurrence of a neurotic mental illness towards the end of pregnancy does predispose to the development of postnatal depression, which suggests that it is important to detect such conditions and to treat with psychosocial as well as with medical strategies so that the woman has recovered from her illness before the baby is born. Third trimester mental illness appears to be more common, again, in those women who have marital tension and who have considered termination of pregnancy, but it also seems to be more common in women over the age of 30 and in those women who have had difficulty in conceiving and who have had infertility investigations. Third trimester illness is not related to a previous psychiatric history nor to having been depressed earlier on in pregnancy.

Management of minor mental illness

Neurotic depression is fairly common in pregnancy and will affect about 15% of women in the first trimester. Prescribing psychotropic medication should not be the first line of treatment. The majority of these illnesses will spontaneously resolve by the second trimester and, if help is required, such illnesses will usually respond to non- medical forms of treatment. Adequate information and reassurance, particularly if the anxiety and depression are centred upon the pregnancy, may be sufficient. Sources of distress from marital, family and social problems should be tackled appropriately by a social worker. Midwives, physiotherapists and psychologists can help with relaxation and anxiety management training, and such techniques may well be as effective as tranquillizers. As a general rule, benzodiazepines should be avoided in the first and third trimesters of pregnancy. The neonate may not be able to metabolize them adequately and may experience excessive sedation or withdrawal symptoms if the mother has been taking benzodiazepines regularly in the last 2 weeks before delivery. If absolutely necessary in the midtrimester and up to 2 weeks before delivery, a benzodiazepine such as diazepam can be given during the day in a dosage of up to 15 mg daily, but should be gradually withdrawn as delivery approaches. If night sedation is required towards the end of pregnancy, then the use of a shorter-acting benzodiazepine is indicated, such as lorazepam or temazepam, in order to avoid the risk of sedating the new-born baby.

Major mental illness

New episodes of major mental illness (manic depressive illness, severe depressive illness and schizophrenia) are relatively uncommon during pregnancy. The risk of developing such conditions is lower than at other times during a woman's life. Presentation to the psychiatric services and, in particular, admission to a mental hospital, is much less common amongst pregnant women than amongst other women of reproductive age, and is in marked contrast to the increase in the incidence of major mental illness in the first 3 months following delivery. Provided they are well stabilized and their illness is in remission, women with a past history of major mental illness are at no particular risk of relapse in pregnancy.

Management of major mental illness

Women who have had single episodes of manic depressive illness, or schizophrenia or a schizophrenia-like illness and who have been well for some time, should be advised to withdraw their medication before conception and to continue with their pregnancies without medication. There is no substantial risk of relapse during pregnancy. However, there is a marked increase in their risk of developing a puerperal psychosis in the first 3 months after delivery, and the obstetrician should therefore liaise with the patient's psychiatrist. If the patient has had multiple episodes of major mental illness and her psychiatrist feels that the risk of relapse is substantial if the medication were to be withdrawn, then the obstetrician, psychiatrist and patient must weigh the risks to the fetus from the continuation of psychotropic medication against the risk to the fetus and its mother from the consequences of maternal mental illness.

Schizophrenia and schizophrenia-like conditions

These patients may be maintained on either oral phenothiazines, e.g. chlorpromazine, trifluoperazine, or depot long-acting phenothiazines, e.g. fluphenazine decanoate. These drugs are frequently administered together with antiparkinsonian agents, e.g. benzhexol. The well-stabilized patient whose symptoms are in remission will probably be receiving these substances at the lower end of the dosage range. If the risk of relapse is substantial, then it is probably safe to continue this medication at the minimal level throughout pregnancy. The evidence for teratogenesis in the first trimester being inconclusive in human beings, providing that severe extrapyramidal side effects have not been experienced in the recent past, it is sensible to withdraw the antiparkinsonian agent for the first 12–16 weeks of pregnancy and only re-institute it thereafter if it should prove necessary. Occasionally, a patient becomes pregnant whilst still actively psychotic and still in receipt of dosage in the higher range. Such a patient's mental state may deteriorate with the stress of pregnancy and she may incorporate the pregnancy into her delusional system. In these patients, the possible hazard to the developing fetus from giving higher dosages of phenothiazines will be outweighed by the risks of a deterioration in maternal mental health and consequent non-compliance with antenatal care. In these cases, and in the rare cases of a new episode of schizophrenia occurring in pregnancy, the rapid control of the mental state will be the clinician's first priority, but the dosage of the phenothiazines should be reduced as soon as possible.

Affective illnesses

These include manic depressive illness, mania and severe depressive illness. Again, if the patient has had a single episode of this illness and has been well for some time, she should be advised, under the supervision of her psychiatrist, to withdraw her medication before conception. She will not be exposed to a substantially increased risk of relapse during pregnancy; however, she will be at a greatly increased risk of developing such an illness in the puerperium. Again, liaison between the obstetrician and psychiatrist is advisable. If her illness has been predominantly manic, and the risk of relapse on withdrawal of medication is thought to be substantial, the patient may be taking either an oral phenothiazine as described above, or a butyrophenone, usually haloperidol. Again, this medication is often taken with an antiparkinsonian agent. She may also be taking lithium, which is frequently used in manic depressive illness as a mood stabilizer and prophylactic against a recurrence of the illness.

Lithium is probably teratogenic in the first trimester and may be hazardous in the last trimester of pregnancy when it can affect the infant's thyroid, produce infantile diabetes insipidus and produce hypotonia and cyanosis at birth. It is therefore contraindicated in pregnancy and should be withdrawn at least 1 month before conception, or immediately if the patient is found to be pregnant. However, phenothiazines and butyrophenones can probably safely be continued throughout pregnancy, but again in the minimum dosage, with the withdrawal of antiparkinsonian agents during the first trimester.

Major depressive illness

A woman who has had a single severe depressive episode and is symptom-free but still on tricyclic antidepressants should be advised to withdraw these before conception. However, if there is a substantial risk of relapse, conventional antidepressants such as amitryptyline, imipramine and dothiepin can probably be safely continued throughout pregnancy. There is little information about the effects of the newer antidepressants such as mianserin, maprotilene and nomifensine on the developing fetus and they should not be used in preference to conventional tricyclic antidepressants unless there are specific indications for their use, for example if a patient is epileptic (mianserin) or has cardiac problems. After delivery, tricyclic antidepressants are very slowly metabolized by the neonate, who no longer has the assistance of the maternal circulation. Some adverse effects have been reported in recently delivered babies whose mothers have been receiving tricyclic antidepressants in full therapeutic dosage (150 mg a day), including irritability, jitteriness and neonatal fits. It is therefore sensible to reduce the tricyclic antidepressants to a minimum maintenance dosage in the third trimester of pregnancy, and to gradually withdraw them before delivery, even if they are restarted immediately following the delivery of the infant. Most depressive illnesses that occur during pregnancy, particularly in the first trimester, will be minor depressive illnesses and will not require antidepressant medication. It is particularly important therefore that depressive illness is accurately diagnosed during pregnancy and that major depressive illness requiring a tricyclic antidepressant is distinguished from cases of neurotic depression or situational unhappiness, which will rarely require such help. Such a distinction may require the help of a psychiatrist. The indication for the use of tricyclic antidepressants at any time, but in particular during pregnancy, should be the presence of the so-called biological symptoms of depression — early morning wakening, a diurnal variation of mood, impaired concentration, interest and ability, and a marked slowing of psychomotor function, together with morbid and guilty ideation. If new episodes of major depressive illness do occur during pregnancy, particularly in the second and third trimesters, they should be treated with tricyclic antidepressants to effect resolution of the depressive illness before the birth of the baby, as there is a correlation between depressive illness in the last trimester and postnatal depressive illness.

Major mental illness in pregnancy

- Increased in first trimester
- Mostly neuroses
- Do not predispose to postnatal illness
- New major illness rare
- Consider withdrawal of medication prior to conception in patients with only one previous episode

MENTAL ILLNESS IN THE PUERPERIUM

Incidence (Fig. 17.1)

Sixteen per cent of all women delivered will develop an episode of mental illness during the first 3 months after childbirth. The majority of these illnesses will be new episodes — that is to say the women will have been mentally well before delivery. The risk of becoming mentally ill during the puerperium is therefore increased from other times in a woman's reproductive life. However, the most dramatic increase in risk is that of suffering from a major mental illness. The risk of developing such an illness in the first 3 months after delivery is 16 times as great as in nonpuerperal women. Two out of every thousand women delivered will require admission to a psychiatric unit with a puerperal psychosis, but the incidence of puerperal psychosis in the community is probably double this, if not higher. About 5% of women delivered will suffer from a major but nonpsychotic depressive illness, and about 10% will be suffering from neurotic or minor mental illnesses. This latter group rarely comes into contact with psychiatrists or obstetricians and, uncommonly, even with their own general practitioners.

PSYCHIATRIC MORBIDITY AFTER CHILDBIRTH

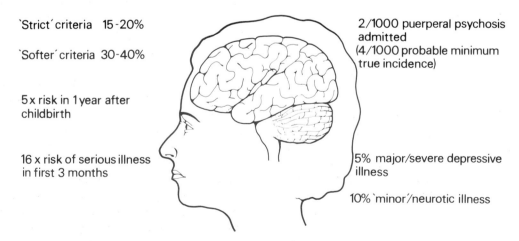

'Strict' criteria   15-20%

'Softer' criteria   30-40%

5 x risk in 1 year after childbirth

16 x risk of serious illness in first 3 months

2/1000 puerperal psychosis admitted
(4/1000 probable minimum true incidence)

5% major/severe depressive illness

10% 'minor'/neurotic illness

Fig. 17.1   The incidence of psychiatric morbidity after childbirth

Using less strict criteria, between 30 and 40% of all women are depressed in the puerperium. Despite the fact that unhappiness, mental illness and, in particular, severe mental illness are so common in relation to childbirth, affecting at least a fifth of all women, very little of this morbidity is presented for medical help. Community surveys have suggested that less than 1% of women suffering from postnatal illness are known to their doctors, and even in areas such as Nottingham which have a psychiatric service for postnatal mental illness only 2% of the recently delivered population presents to psychiatric services. Hopefully, the majority of the remainder will spontaneously recover, but a significant minority of both major and minor illnesses do not, and their illnesses become chronic, persisting well into the second year of their child's life.

General aetiology

Over the past century, there have been marked changes in attitudes towards childbearing, family and social structures, obstetric practice, and maternal and perinatal mortality. Marked differences also exist in these areas between our society and other cultures. Despite this, there has been little change in the incidence of major mental illness related to childbirth over the past century, and in minor mental illness over the past 20 years. Similar rates, for both major and minor mental illness, have been observed in a variety of other cultures. It would seem, therefore, unlikely that a single aetiological factor such as the 'medicalization' of childbirth, or the decline in the extended family, can be implicated in the development of these conditions, or in the increased risk that women are exposed to after delivery. It is probable that there is a multifactorial aetiology for a heterogeneous group of illnesses, and that other factors are required before women develop mental illness. Current evidence suggests that for major mental illness the most important factor is the family history, or personal history, of major mental illness. Other factors include obstetric difficulties and major life events, and for minor mental illness chronic personal and social difficulties.

Implications for maternal and child welfare

Postnatal mental illness in Western society is the greatest cause of avoidable morbidity in the puerperium. More effective prevention, detection and earlier treatment of such illness will have a major impact on maternal and child health. Longstanding untreated depressive illness has been implicated by many authorities in many parameters of childhood ill heath, whether physical, emotional or psychiatric. Its swift resolution is, therefore, important for the child as well as the mother.

Puerperal psychosis

Definition

This is a clinical, descriptive term used to describe a group of illnesses which occur in a close temporal relationship with childbirth, and which are hallmarked by delusions, hallucinations and impaired perception of reality. The majority of puerperal psychoses are affective — manic or depressive psychoses. A minority are schizophrenia-like conditions. True chronic schizophrenia arising for the first time in the puerperium is very uncommon.

Clinical presentation (Fig. 17.2)

The majority of the manic and schizophrenia-like illnesses and a third of the depressive psychoses will present very abruptly between day 3 and day 14 of the puerperium. Women may become psychotic whilst still on the postnatal ward and frequently do so whilst the community midwife is still visiting. These illnesses are some of the most severe that occur in psychiatry. In the first few days the clinical picture is one of perplexity, confusion, fear and distress, restlessness and insomnia. The patient often looks physically unwell and, unusually for functional mental illness, may be disorientated for time and for place. In the last century, French psychiatrists described this initial phase of the puerperal psychosis as the 'delire triste'. At this stage it is difficult to make a specific psychiatric diagnosis. The mental state then changes rapidly with prominent delusions, hallucinations, and disturbance of behaviour. Within a few days of the onset of the condition, the symptoms usually settle enough for a more recognizable depressive, manic or schizophrenia-like psychosis to emerge. Apart from the classical delire triste, the clinical features

PUERPERAL PSYCHOSIS

Risk factors:
    family/personal history
    caesarean section

Abrupt onset 80% 3-14 days

Rapidly changing clinical picture

Delire triste

99% manic depressive/
    schizo-affective

Treatment:
    admission/alternatives
    with baby

breast feeding

prognosis

next baby

N.B. Schizophrenia very rare

Fig. 17.2 Risk factors, presentation and treatment in puerperal psychosis

of puerperal psychosis are not unique, merely distinctive. The illnesses of these patients are more severe than in an age-matched control group of nonpuerperal psychiatric patients. They are more hallucinated, more deluded, more behaviourally disturbed and, if depressed, more likely to become grossly retarded or even stuporose. Another distinctive feature of puerperal psychosis is that patients suffering from this condition are much more likely to be manic than other patients with manic depressive illness. Even those patients with schizophrenia-like conditions are likely to have marked affective features, usually of mania, but sometimes of depression as well. Although the form of puerperal psychoses has much in common with psychoses occurring at other times in life, the content will frequently reflect upon the presence of the baby and of the recent delivery as well as the mood state of the patient. Delusions that the baby has died or has been substituted for another, and marked perceptual distortions of time and bodily function relating to pregnancy and delivery, are very common, as well as a fearful delusional preoccupation that something dreadful is about to happen to either mother or baby.

Aetiology

It is fashionable, particularly amongst the lay public,

to implicate hormonal abnormalities in the aetiology of puerperal psychosis. There is strong evidence to suggest that the dramatic alteration in hormonal status that occurs between 3 and 5 days postpartum is associated with the normal postnatal 'blues'. However, there is no evidence to suggest that the hormonal status of women suffering from puerperal psychosis is different from other puerperal women not so afflicted. There is an increase in family history of manic depressive illness in women who suffer from puerperal psychosis, as compared with the rest of the psychiatric population. Thirty per cent of such patients have a family history of either manic depressive illness or schizophrenia, as opposed to only 5% of a nonpuerperal schizophrenic population, and 15% of a manic depressive population. Although uncommon, a personal prepregnant history of major mental illness would also seem to increase the risk of developing puerperal psychosis. Women who suffer from a puerperal psychosis after the birth of their first child are more likely to have had a Caesarean section, or major obstetric difficulties, than the rest of the puerperal population. There is a tendency also for them to be of higher social class, to be of older age at the birth of their first child, to be married, to have had a longer interval from marriage to the birth of their child, and to have had a major life event shortly before or after the birth of their child, as compared with the rest of the puerperal population. These differences are even more marked when women suffering from puerperal psychosis are compared with the non-puerperal psychiatric population. The most striking finding in studying women with puerperal psychosis is how ordinary and well adjusted they are before the birth of their first child.

Management (Fig. 17.2)

Because these women are so profoundly disturbed, they usually require both skilled psychiatric nursing and in-patient care and should always be admitted with their babies. Few women will be prepared to accept voluntary admission to a psychiatric unit without their baby and to do so almost inevitably causes an increase in the intensity of the disturbance and, in particular, delusions that harm is to come to their child. There is evidence that admitting mother and baby together both facilitates the treatment of the mother and shortens her stay in hospital, as well as improving the mother/baby relationship when she is well. However, safe management of a disturbed mother and a new-born baby requires specialist skills and, fortunately, many psychiatric units now have specialized mother and baby facilities.

When puerperal psychosis first presents, the immediate priority is to sedate the patient to a level that makes them safely containable within their environment and allows for adequate hydration and nutrition. This is usually done with either phenothiazines or butyrophenones, e.g. haloperidol. Such medication will also reduce the perplexity and fear, and over a period of 48 hours should begin to make some impact upon the hallucinations and delusions. If the patient can be safely managed on a postnatal ward or at home, it is often worthwhile trying such treatment 48 hours before transfer to the psychiatric unit, because in a significant minority of cases the illness will resolve quickly and obviate the necessity of a psychiatric admission. This is particularly likely if a psychotic episode arises within a few days of a Caesarean section. A suggested initial regimen would be 50 mg of chlorpromazine three times daily, together with 75 or 100 mg at night as the mental state is frequently at its worst at this time. This dose can then be titrated up or down; a single bolus of up to 150 mg of chlorpromazine can be given if necessary. After a few days, when the clinical picture becomes clearer, the appropriate treatment for the underlying diagnosis can be instigated.

Both **mania** and **schizophrenia-like conditions** will respond to either a phenothiazine or a haloperidol. If the patient is not responding within 3–7 days of a regimen of regular medication for mania and for schizophrenia-like conditions because of a strong affective component, then ECT may be the treatment of choice.

For the early onset **depressive psychoses**, electroconvulsive therapy (ECT) is usually the treatment of choice from the initial diagnosis. Tricyclic antidepressants take between 10 and 14 days to begin their effect, and are rarely appropriate as a first line treatment for a severely disturbed, depressive psychosis. These patients may also require phenothiazines in the early stages of their illness before they begin to recover. The presence of a life-threatening condition in depressive psychosis, such as not eating or drinking, or a state of extreme depressive retardation known as **depressive stupor**, constitutes a primary indication for the use of ECT.

Prophylactic medication. There is no evidence that in those women who are well and symptom free, but who are at high risk of developing puerperal psychosis because of a previous history of puerperal or non-puerperal psychosis, that prophylactic medication after delivery prevents the occurrence of puerperal psychosis. However, it is sensible to monitor them closely in the early weeks, and start treatment early if symptoms emerge. In the small number of women who have well-established recurring mental illness, and who have been on maintenance medication, for example lithium, before pregnancy the psychiatrist may wish to start maintenance treatment after the birth of the baby. In such cases, the woman should be advised not to breast feed.

Immediate prognosis

Despite the fact that this illness is often very frightening, in both its intensity and severity, the short- and long-term prognosis is very good. Manic patients will usually respond quickly to treatment within 2 weeks, often within a matter of days. Most of the severe depressive puerperal psychoses will resolve between 4 and 6 weeks, and the schizophrenia-like conditions between 6 and 8 weeks. Although the majority of women with puerperal psychosis will have fully recovered and be back to their normal functioning by 6 months, a significant minority pursue a more protracted recovery.

Risk of relapse

Many early onset puerperal psychoses, although initially responding to treatment very well, relapse, particularly in the early weeks after recovery. Therefore, continuation of the phenothiazines, albeit at a reduced dosage, is important for a number of weeks, or at least until the baby is 3 months old. A patient who has presented with a manic psychosis may relapse with a depressive psychosis or a further episode of mania. If this happens on at least one occasion, the clinician may well think of using lithium in an attempt to stabilize the mood over the period of a few months after delivery. This mode of treatment would also be indicated if the patient has a past history of manic depressive illness or has previously been stabilized on lithium. For a patient who has had only one episode of relapsing manic depressive illness in association with the puerperium, prophylactic lithium therapy would not normally be continued beyond the first year. However, for a patient who has a previous history, lithium prophylaxis may be continued for longer.

Next birth prognosis

One in five of the women who have had a puerperal psychosis will be at risk of developing a further illness following the birth of their next child. For those women with a previous history of major psychiatric illness, be it puerperal or nonpuerperal, or who have a strong family history of mental illness, the risk will remain constant for all births at one in three. For those women who developed a puerperal psychosis following the birth of their first child by Caesarean section, or associated with major life events, the risk of a further puerperal psychosis will be lower. If it does occur, it is likely to have the same diagnosis, the same duration, and occur at the same time in relation to delivery. It will also have the same prognosis. Given adequate information about the likelihood of their becoming mentally ill following the birth of the second baby, women will be able to make up their own minds as to whether they are prepared to take these risks in order to complete their family. Should they decide to embark upon a further pregnancy, it is important for the obstetrician and psychiatrist to liaise and to monitor the woman closely following delivery, as prompt and effective treatment will minimize disability and distress (Table 17.2).

Table 17.2 Prevention of mental illness in pregnancy — what can we do?

Prediction/risk reduction
Early detection
Early treatment
Minimize disability
Primary and secondary prevention
Modify (antenatal classes)
(postnatal check)

Lifetime prognosis

Thirty per cent of all women who suffer from puerperal psychosis will at some later stage in their life develop a manic depressive illness which is not related to the process of childbearing. It is because of this latter point and the strong evidence of a family history of manic depressive illness that the current psychiatric thinking has developed that puerperal psychosis is not a unique diagnostic entity, but represents rather the increased vulnerability to manic depressive illness of women in the puerperium.

Major depressive illness

Definition

This is a term used to describe women suffering from an illness which involves not only a profound and consistent lowering of mood, but also depressive ideation, biological symptoms of depression and slowing of psychomotor functioning. They do not have hallucinations and delusions and, to some extent, remain in touch with reality. None the less, they are profoundly ill and disabled, and such illnesses do not commonly occur in people of this age group outside the puerperium. About 5% of all recently delivered women will suffer from such an illness in the first 3 months.

MAJOR DEPRESSIVE ILLNESS

Risk factors:

Onset in 1st two weeks
    more gradual

2 peaks presentation:
    2-4 weeks
    10-14 weeks

Early presentation:
    profound verging psychotic

Later presentation:
    often missed because atypical

Atypical-covert classical symptoms:
    EMW
    DVM
    SLOWING

Overt-guilt/worthlessness
    anomie
    ruminative worry
    anxiety

Treatment:
    medical/psychotherapeutic

    prognosis

    self-help groups

    next baby

Fig. 17.3   Risk factors, presentation and management of major depressive illness in the puerperium

Clinical features (Fig. 17.3)

This illness too begins in the first 2 weeks after delivery, but develops gradually. One-third of these women will have presented by 4 weeks post-partum, but two-thirds present between 10 and 14 weeks. Those who present early have very profound illnesses, are often severely retarded, and their mental states verge on the psychotic. However, those who present later are often sadly missed because their symptoms appear 'atypical'. This is partly because the stereotype of depressive illness is that of depression in a middle-aged person, and partly because many of the classical symptoms of early morning wakening, psychomotor slowing, and feeling much worse in the morning (diurnal variation of mood) are present but can easily be attributed by the uninformed observer to the presence of the baby interfering with sleep, or a difficulty in adjusting to motherhood. There are usually prominent feelings of guilt and worthlessness, openly expressed doubts about their fitness for motherhood, and fears for the health and safety of the baby. Anxiety and a ruminative worry are much more conspicuous in puerperal depressive illness than they are in depressive illnesses in an older age group.

One of the most distressing and misleading symptoms of severe postnatal depression is the symptom of 'anomie'. This is a painful feeling of an inability to experience love or pleasure, and is often expressed as 'I can't or 'don't' love my baby. As this is often in marked contrast to the obvious loving and concerned handling of the baby on the part of the mother, it should be an important diagnostic point. However, all too commonly, the woman is taken at her word and the dissonance between her expressed comments and behaviour is not noticed. Postnatal depression of this severity may be life threatening, not least because of prominent suicidal ideation — the women believing that their babies and their husbands would be better off without them, and that they will never recover, but also because of the dangers of depressive stupor and death through dehydration, inanition and physical complications.

If untreated, most severe puerperal depressive illness will resolve spontaneously within 6 months, but one-third of these patients will continue to suffer from depression into the second year of their child's life. For many reasons, therefore, it is very important to detect and to treat swiftly severe post-natal depression. The postnatal examination at

6 weeks postpartum would seem to be an ideal opportunity for both obstetricians and general practitioners to enquire routinely for depressive symptoms of their patients.

Aetiology

The risk factors for postnatal depressive illness are broadly similar to those for puerperal psychosis. Major life events in the third and fourth trimesters, and major health problems with the baby, are also important.

Management (Fig. 17.3)

Women suffering from major depressive illness, with active suicidal ruminations, or with marked retardation and difficulties in eating and drinking, should be admitted with their babies to a psychiatric unit. However, many less severely disturbed patients can be effectively managed at home, providing they are closely supervised. The early presenting depressive illnesses, particularly with life-threatening features, will respond swiftly to ECT, whilst at the same time patients should be started on antidepressants which should be continued for at least 6 months postpartum. The later presentations should respond satisfactorily to a therapeutic dose of a tricyclic antidepressant within 2 weeks, and achieve a recovery by 6 weeks, although again the antidepressant will need to be continued for at least 6 months. Delusional ideas of unworthiness and guilt, marked suicidal ideation and states of hopeless despair are indications for ECT as a first line treatment.

Further pregnancies

There is an increased risk of suffering from a severe depressive illness following the birth of the next baby, probably to the order of one in five. Again, if this illness is associated with an operative delivery and recent life events, the risk may be lower than if it is associated with a family history or personal history of major depressive illness. Women suffering from severe postnatal depression gain a tremendous amount of help, both in the recovery from their illness and in the longer term with the recovery of self-esteem and self-confidence, from self-help

groups where they can talk about their experiences with fellow sufferers. There are many such organizations both locally and nationally, the most famous of which is the national Association for Post-Natal Depression, and it may help if a patient suffering from such a condition is put in touch with one of these organizations.

Minor mental illness

Definition

The term minor mental illness, or neurosis, is used to describe a very common group of conditions where the symptoms and signs vary only in quantity from those which are part of the normal human reaction to stress. Both the timing of the illnesses and the symptoms are usually understandable as the result of the interaction of the personality with stress. None the less, the symptoms may be very distressing and disabling, but there is not usually any impairment in the patient's perception of reality. Symptoms of emotional turbulence and unhappiness and anxiety tend to predominate. The commonest neurosis is that of the depressive neurosis, sometimes known as **reactive depression**. Anxiety states, panic disorder and phobic anxiety states are also quite common. Obsessional compulsive illness is much rarer.

Aetiology

Such illnesses are very common in the general population and may not, in fact, be much commoner in the puerperium than at other times. Some women are more vulnerable to developing puerperal neuroses than others by virtue of personality problems, on-going social and family problems, or recent major stresses or life events. The young, unmarried, socio-economically deprived with unhappy marriages and poor family relationships are more likely to suffer from these conditions than other people.

Clinical features (Fig. 17.4)

Although these illnesses often have an insidious onset within the first few weeks after delivery, they rarely present until 3 months or later after delivery

Fig. 17.4 Risk factors, presentation and management of minor puerperal neurosis

of the child. Content of the neurotic illness is frequently concerned with the baby and problems with mothering and child care. However, the form of the illness, most commonly a depressive neurosis or anxiety state, is not different from that occurring at other times. Because of its late presentation, it is most usually first noticed by the health visitor, and not infrequently presents through the well baby clinic, with manifest problems with the child.

Management (Fig. 17.4)

Psychotropic medication is very rarely the first line of treatment in such cases. Combating social isolation, reducing overly high expectations of motherhood and babies, and introducing women to other mothers in the same situation through mother and toddler groups etc. will do much to reduce the guilt and feeling of alienation that such patients have. Benzodiazepines are very commonly prescribed for such states of minor depression and anxiety. They are probably best avoided in women who present with predominant feelings of irritability and difficulty in controlling their tempers because they can disinhibit them and make their behaviour and 'depression' worse. The opportunity to ventilate their feelings, self-help groups, and anxiety management techniques, social work and other forms of non-medical intervention will often prove to be just as effective as medication.

Breast feeding and psychotropic medication (Fig. 17.5)

Many women who present with mental illness early in the puerperium are breast feeding and its continuation is usually very important to them. Stopping breast feeding because of a mental illness will add to the burden of guilt they feel once they recover. Continuing with it will help the recovery of their self-esteem and their relationship with their baby once their mental state improves. Continuing breast feeding requires a great deal of skill on the part of the psychiatric nurse when women are so very disturbed. Totally breast feeding the infant may not be possible in the first few days of a severe puerperal psychosis. None the less, it should be possible to maintain lactation with a combination of expressing the milk and frequent suckling of the infant. When it is clearly important to continue breast feeding, the choice of psychotropic medication becomes very important. Lithium should probably not be given to breastfeeding women. The available evidence suggests that tricyclic antidepressants in full dosage are safe for breast feeding. They are present in only very small amounts in breast milk and significant quantities are not detectable in the infant's serum. Phenothiazines such as chlorpromazine (in single dosage of 100 mg and not more than 300 mg a day) and trifluoperazine (in a single dosage of 5 mg and not more than 20 mg a

DRUGS AND BREAST FEEDING

1. Tricyclic antidepressants safe in full dosage

2. Chlorpromazine
   Trifluoperazine } safe in moderate dosage
   Haloperidol

3. Benzodiazepines/ alcohol best avoided

4. Lithium dangerous

Fig. 17.5   Drug secretion in breast milk

day) are also probably safe for breast-feeding mothers. The infant should be closely monitored and the breast feeding suspended if the baby is drowsy, does not wake and cry for its feeds, or does not suckle strongly. If the severity of the mental state requires the use of parenteral medication, or a single dosage of more than the equivalent of 100 mg of chlorpromazine, it is probably safer to suspend breast feeding for a period of 12–24 hours and express the milk. Paediatric advice should be sought if the baby is premature, of low birth weight or jaundiced.

Summary

Although few psychotropic drugs are known to be teratogenic or to have adverse effects on the developing fetus or neonate, no psychotropic drug is of proven safety. It is therefore very important that psychotropic medication should not be prescribed lightly during pregnancy or lactation and that such drugs should be prescribed only where there are positive indications for their use. Close collaboration between obstetrician and psychiatrist is rec-

ommended before treatment of a mental illness with psychotropic medication. Breast feeding should not routinely be suspended in mothers who require psychotropic medication. There is an adequate range of psychotropic drugs available to treat safely the pregnant or lactating woman who is mentally ill.

Mental illness in the puerperium

- Affects 16% of women in first 3 months
- 2 in 1000 require hospital admission
- Highest risk time of woman's life
- Major illness incidence constant
- Family or personal-history of mental illness most important risk factor
- $\frac{1}{5}$ risk of recurrence

BIBLIOGRAPHY

Brockington I F, Kumar R (eds) 1982 Motherhood and mental illness. Academic Press, London
Tyrer P J 1983 Drugs in psychiatric practice. Butterworths, London

18. Perinatal mortality

DEFINITIONS

The definition of perinatal death is linked to the concept of viability and, as the likelihood of survival of a low birth weight infant has increased progressively over the last 20 years, current British definitions are not satisfactory. These definitions are:

- Stillbirth — the term stillborn is used when there are no signs of life in a child born after the 28th week of gestation. The stillbirth rate is the number of stillbirths per 1000 total births per year.
- Neonatal death — this is defined as death of a liveborn infant within 28 days of birth. Neonatal death rate is the number of infants dying within 28 days after birth per 1000 live births per year.
- Perinatal death rate — this is the total number of stillbirths and first-week deaths per 1000 total births per year.

INCIDENCE

Perinatal mortality rates vary widely — both between different countries and within different regions of the same country. For example in 1980 the highest rate occurred in Mexico and the lowest in Sweden. In Western European countries, perinatal mortality has fallen markedly over the last 20 years; these trends are clearly demonstrated in the figures for England and Wales (Fig. 18.1). The causes for this improvement include:

1. Improved antenatal and intrapartum care.
2. Improved socio-economic conditions.
3. Reduction in parity.
4. An active screening programme for common congenital abnormalities such as Down's syndrome and abnormalities of the central nervous system such as anencephaly and spina bifida.

Factors which are known to affect perinatal mortality in England and Wales include social class, country of birth of the mother, maternal age and parity and marital status. Smoking also has a significant adverse effect on birth weight and perinatal mortality.

Many third world countries in Africa and Asia do not collect routine statistics and the data available are collected by governmental and other agents. In the poorest countries, such as Bangladesh and the Central African Republic, the perinatal mortality rate appears to be in the order of 50 per 1000 total births. A comparison of the role of obstetric care in perinatal mortality must take account of the incidence of congenital abnormalities and low birth weight.

Table 18.1 International comparisons, perinatal mortality rates 1980 (per 1000 total births)

Country	Rate/1000 births
Mexico	23.8
Kuwait	21.3
Chile	18.8
Italy	17.4
East Germany	13.6
USA	13.6
England & Wales	13.4
France	13.0
West Germany	11.6
Netherlands	11.1
Canada	10.9
Switzerland	9.5
Denmark	9.0
Sweden	8.7

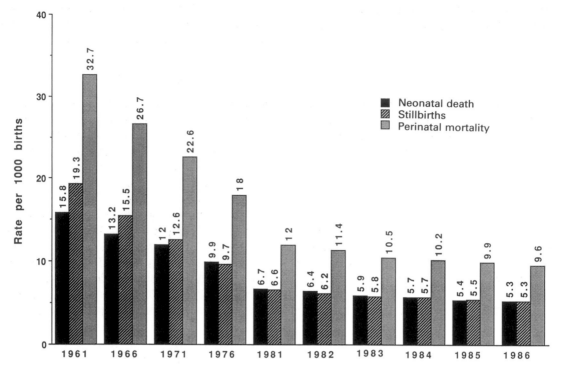

Fig. 18.1 Perinatal mortality in England and Wales.

AETIOLOGY

The commonest causes of stillbirth are those related to:

1. Major congenital abnormalities incompatible with life, such as heart disease and abnormalities of the central nervous system and renal agenesis.
2. Asphyxia — a final diagnosis of intra-uterine asphyxia may represent the end product of a variety of different pathological processes including:
   a. placental abruption;
   b. pre-eclampsia and eclampsia;
   c. placental dysfunction associated with intra-uterine growth retardation;
   d. cord entanglement or prolapse;
   e. abnormal uterine activity and cephalo-pelvic disproportion.
3. Traumatic cerebral haemorrhage and intra-cranial damage from difficult labour and delivery.
4. Blood group incompatibility — this is now a rare cause of intra-uterine death associated with

severe rhesus iso-immunization and hydrops fetalis.

The common causes of neonatal death are those related to:

1. Major congenital abnormalities incompatible with life.
2. Prematurity — the most important single factor in causing neonatal death associated with:
   a. respiratory distress syndrome and hyaline membrane disease;
   b. pneumonia;
   c. intracranial haemorrhage and cerebral damage sustained either during labour and delivery or in the early neonatal period;
   d. necrotizing enterocolitis.

SOCIAL FACTORS AND PERINATAL MORTALITY

1. Maternal age

Maternal age at both extremes is associated with

an increase in perinatal mortality. The death rate in the under 16 age group is twice as high as at any other age.

2. Parity

There seems to be little doubt that the introduction of the 1967 Abortion Act has been a major factor in the reduction of perinatal mortality. High parity is associated with high fetal and neonatal loss.

3. Social class

Each country tends to exhibit in microcosm the international differences that are dependent on economic status. The impact of socio-economic class on perinatal mortality means that women of social classes 4 and 5 have a higher perinatal mortality rate.

Many countries do not collect annual routine statistics and in those countries where figures are published, there are often difficulties in interpreting the data because of inaccuraies in the data collection. However, the more gross discrepancies generally do say something about social indices in a country and the quality of medical care.

The figures published for 1980 in World Health Statistics (1983) show a threefold difference between Mexico and Sweden (see Table 18.1). Although all of these figures have fallen, there are still marked differences in mortality rates which are tending, if anything, to become more marked.

Perinatal mortality

- Major causes are congenital abnormalities, asphyxia and prematurity
- Predisposing factors are maternal age, high parity, low social class

---

THE IMPACT OF LOW BIRTH WEIGHT ON NEONATAL MORTALITY

Low birth weight is defined as a live birth of less than 2500 g. The rate varies from 4% in Sweden to an estimated 25% in Bangladesh. The overall figure in Britain is 6.7% of all live births. The mortality rate in relation to birth weight is shown in

Figure 14.2. The figures shown are national figures and tend to vary substantially in relation to the quality of special intensive care units.

MATERNAL MORTALITY

Maternal mortality rate is the number of maternal deaths per 100 000 maternities in 1 year. A maternal death is defined as death occurring within 1 year of delivery. Death may be directly due to pregnancy and childbirth including abortion, or may simply occur within a year of childbirth, but be unrelated to the process.

The statistics in Figures 18.2 and 18.3 are based on the triennial reports from the DHSS in England and Wales. The most recent report for 1982–84 showed a direct death rate of 5.5/100 000 maternities (Fig. 18.2) and an 'indirect' death rate of 5.57/100 000 (Fig. 18.3). The rates in Britain vary according to the region — as with perinatal mortality rate.

The major causes of maternal death in order of importance are as follows:

1. Pulmonary embolism.
2. Anaesthesia, including deaths associated with abortion and ectopic pregnancy.
3. Hypertensive diseases of pregnancy.
4. Uterine haemorrhage.
5. Ectopic pregnancy.

Fig. 18.2 Deaths due to direct maternal causes per million maternities.

Fig. 18.3   Maternal deaths associated with pregnancy.

reports of all those staff involved in management of the pregnant woman, together with the results of the postmortem are passed to regional obstetric assessors and finally to central assessors who are the DHSS advisers in obstetrics and gynaecology. Strict confidentiality is maintained throughout this procedure and the name of the patient is removed from the public record. An attempt is made to classify deaths into avoidable and unavoidable groups.

Maternal mortality

- Deaths within 1 year post-partum
- 11/100 000
- Major causes include pulmonary embolism, pregnancy-induced hypertension, anaesthetic, haemorrhage

6. Sepsis excluding abortion.
7. Abortion.
8. Ruptured uterus.
9. Amniotic fluid embolism.

The system of confidential enquiries into maternal death

The system of confidential enquiry was introduced in England and Wales in 1952 and triennial reports have been published since that time. Ninety-nine per cent of all deaths have been documented in the most recent report. Information gathered by the area or, now, district medical officers, based on

BIBLIOGRAPHY

Antonov A 1947 Children born during the siege of Leningrad in 1942. J. Paediatrics 30: 250–259
Brit. Med. J. 1980 Quality, not quantity, in babies. 1:347–348
Field D J, Hopkin I, Milner A D, Madeley R J 1985 Changing overall workload in neonatal units. Brit. Med. J. 290: 1539–1542
OPCS Monitors Series DH3
Pharoah P O D, Alberman E D 1981 Mortality of low birthweight infants in England and Wales 1953 to 1979. Arch. Dis. Childh. 56: 86–89
Report on confidential enquiries into maternal deaths in England and Wales 1976–1978. DHSS, HMSO
WHO 1980 The incidence of low birthweight — a critical review of available information. World Health Statistics Quarterly 33(3)

19. Imaging techniques in obstetrics and gynaecology

The major techniques used in imaging the fetus and the pelvic organs are:

1. Radiological imaging.
2. Ultrasonography.
3. Magnetic resonance imaging.
4. Immunoscintigraphy.

The latter two new methods are beginning to assume importance but are not yet widely used.

X-RAYS IN OBSTETRICS AND GYNAECOLOGY (Figs 19.1–19.7)

Radiological imaging in pregnancy has now largely been replaced by ultrasound imaging because of risk factors. Nevertheless, there are specific examples where it is still used, although replacement by magnetic resonance imaging may happen in the near future.

Indications for X-rays in pregnancy

X-ray pelvimetry

Assessment of the bony pelvis remains the commonest indication for the use of X-rays in pregnancy. The erect lateral views of the pelvis are the most valuable because they enable assessment of the true conjugate diameter and the shape of the sacrum. Pelvic inlet views are used for assessment of the transverse diameter of the inlet and also for measurement of the narrowest diameter of the pelvic cavity — the interspinous diameter. Outlet views are less important because the pelvic outlet is amenable to clinical assessment.

Gestational age

Ultrasound measurement of biparietal diameter and abdominal circumference have largely replaced radiological assessment. Nevertheless, these measurements are not particularly useful if first undertaken in late pregnancy as single measurements can be misleading. The presence of ossification in the lower femoral epiphysis indicates a maturity of 36 weeks, although this is determined to some degree by race and sex. The proximal tibial epiphysis undergoes ossification at term. The order of appearance of the centres of ossification is:

1. Calcaneus.
2. Talus.
3. Distal epiphysis of the femur.
4. Proximal epiphysis of the tibia, cuboid bone, head of the humerus, capitate, hamate, third cuneiform and head of the femur.

Intra-uterine death (Fig. 19.1)

As the diagnosis can be established with pulsed ultrasound, radiological diagnosis of intra-uterine death is now rarely employed. There are three commonly recognized signs:

1. Spaldings sign — liquefaction of the brain results in collapse and overlap of the skull bones (Fig. 19.2). This becomes apparent within 2–3 days.
2. Gas in the blood vessels.
3. Exaggerated spinal curvature.

Fig. 19.1   X-ray of intra-uterine death: note the exaggerated curvature of the spine

Fig. 19.2   X-ray of Spalding's sign: intra-uterine death is associated with collapse of the cranial vault and overlap of the skull bones

Fig. 19.3   X-ray of an anencephalic fetus: the absence of cranial vault bones makes the diagnosis readily apparent

Fig. 19.4   X-ray of twin pregnancy associated with hydramnios with a characteristic ground glass appearance

Fig. 19.5   X-ray of multiple pregnancy and hydramnios

Fig. 19.6   X-ray of the defeated Lippes loop: a mature fetus in the presence of an intra-uterine contraceptive device

Fig. 19.7   X-ray of head engaged in the pelvis in advanced labour; a scalp electrode can be seen

Other diagnoses

X-ray can be used to diagnose skeletal abnormalities such as anencephaly (Fig. 19.3), achondroplasia and intra-uterine fractures associated with osteogenesis imperfecta. It may also be used to diagnose multiple pregnancy or conjoined twins (Figs 19.4, 19.5), and pregnancy in the presence of an intra-uterine device (Fig. 19.6), and to look at head engagement in labour (Fig. 19.7). Most functions related to fetal imaging have now been taken over by ultrasound techniques. It must be remembered that there is an association between X-ray exposure and childhood leukaemia and lymphoma. The risk is low but it is sufficient to reduce the use of X-rays in pregnancy and to shield the fetus where X-ray pelvimetry is performed. Localization of the placenta by radiological techniques is now rarely used. It was never a precise method and its only use in this context would arise if no ultrasound equipment was available.

Radiological diagnosis in gynaecology

Plain X-ray of the abdomen has a role to play in the diagnosis of pelvic tumours. Dermoid cysts often contain radio-opaque material such as teeth and bone, which can be seen in the pelvis. Uterine fibroids are not visible radiologically but can be detected if there is calcification in the fibroid.

Hysterosalpingography (Fig. 19.8)

The injection of a radio-opaque water soluble dye through the cervix into the uterine cavity is used to visualize the cavity of the uterus, the cervical canal and the Fallopian tubes. This procedure is performed by injecting the dye through a Leech–Wilkinson or Ruben's cannula, having first filled the instrument with dye to exclude air bubbles. The cavity of the uterus is filled with 2–3 ml of dye and the presence of filling defects caused by polyps or submucous fibroids can be demonstrated. These defects usually show a rounded margin. Intra-uterine synechiae have a sharp demarcation but an irregular edge. Abnormalities of the uterine cavity such as uterus bicornis bicollis and septate uteri can also be demonstrated (Fig. 19.9).

Fig. 19.8 Hysterosalpingogram of a subseptate uterus; the fallopian tubes can also be clearly defined

Tubal obstruction associated with fimbrial confluence shows up as a retort-shaped structure. If dye leaks through the tube, it can be seen smeared over the surface of the bowel. If it becomes loculated around the end of the tube, it may indicate the presence of peritubal adhesions.

The site of tubal obstruction can also be demonstrated. It is important to be gentle in performing the procedure. Rough manipulation of the uterus may result in utero-tubal spasms and thereby give a false indication of organic tubal obstruction.

X-rays

- Obstetrics – assessment of bony pelvis, gestational age, skeletal malformations, multiple pregnancy
- Risk of leukaemia in child
- Gynaecology — dermoids, hysterosalpingography and lost IUCD

ULTRASONOGRAPHY IN OBSTETRICS AND GYNAECOLOGY (Figs 19.9–19.15)

The principle of ultrasound usage in medical diagnosis is based on the direction of sound frequencies in the order of 2–20 MHz into human tissues and the subsequent measurement of returning echoes from interfaces of differing densities. Ultrasound will not penetrate a gaseous medium and has therefore not been particularly useful in the diagnosis of disorders of the bowel and lung.

Ultrasound is produced by excitation of a piezo-electric crystal, which vibrates at a predetermined frequency. The transmitting phase is short and the crystal reverts to a receiving phase. Scanners are divided into static and real-time machines.

Static scanners

The ultrasound probe is moved manually over the patient's skin and a two-dimensional 'slice' of information is obtained. This is known as a B-scan image. The technique enables accurate fetal measurement.

Fig. 19.9 (**A**) Crown-rump length in an 8-week fetus;
(**B**) the measurement of femur lenght may enhance the accuracy
of the assessment of gestational age and fetal growth

Fig. 19.10 (**A**) Biparietal diameter as measured by ultrasound; the midline
shadow of the falx cerebri can be clearly identified;
(**B**) abdominal circumference measured at the level of the umbilical
vessels

Real-time scanners

There are three forms of real-time scanners: linear array, mechanical array and phased array. These techniques enable positive identification of moving or pulsating parts, particularly fetal movements and fetal heart beats. Modern machines produce images of comparable quality to those obtained by static scans.

Estimation of gestational age

In the first 90 days of pregnancy, the most accurate measurement for estimation of gestational age is the measurement of crown-rump length (Fig. 19.9). This is best performed with real-time apparatus as it is possible to measure the maximum longitudinal axis.

In the second trimester, gestational-age can be estimated by measurement of biparietal diameter (Fig. 19.10). The scatter around the mean increases with gestational age and the most accurate estimate of gestational age can be obtained between 16 and 20 weeks gestation.

Images of the normal fetus

Modern ultrasound real-time techniques have increasingly high resolution and enable high quality images of the general structures of the fetus to be obtained. Figure 19.11 for example shows a saggital view of the face and brain in a normal fetus in a low power section (A) and in a high power section (B).

Ultrasound assessment of blood velocity profiles in the fetus

The assessment of the velocity of blood flow in blood vessels can be calculated using the principle of Doppler shift. Ultrasound waves reflected from a moving target such as red blood cells in a vessel produce a frequency change which is proportional to the velocity of the target. The y-axis records the height of the Doppler shift and the x-axis reflects the time (Fig. 19.12). A typical waveform in the fetal umbilical artery is shown in Figure 19.12A. This shows a cross-sectional image of the umbilical vessels. It also shows a profile of the waveform. All profiles in this section should be considered to provide an index of blood velocity. The peak of the waveform is known as the A wave and the trough of the wave is known as the B wave. The AB ratio therefore represents the ratio of peak systole to end diastole.

The resistance index is the ratio of peak systole minus end diastole over peak systole. In general terms, fetal growth retardation is associated with an increase in the AB ratio, suggesting an increase in resistance to flow in the placenta. An increase in the resistance index also suggests a deterioration in the condition of the placenta. These tests are being used increasingly in the assessment of placental function.

A

B

Fig. 19.11 (**A**) Ultrasound image of the fetal face and brain. (**B**) The same view with greater magnification.

Fig. 19.12 (**A**) The velocity profile of the umbilical artery measured from insonation of the fetal umbilical artery. (**B**) shows the vessels.

Abnormalities in early pregnancy

Ectopic pregnancy

Direct identification of an ectopic pregnancy by ultrasound is difficult. Indirect evidence can be obtained from recognition of free fluid in the Pouch of Douglas and the absence of an intra-uterine pregnancy. However, echography is of limited value in the diagnosis of tubal pregnancy.

Missed abortion

In this condition, the fetus can be clearly ident-ified and usually grows at a normal rate until death occurs, and the fetal heartbeat can no longer be seen. One of the difficulties created by routine scans in early pregnancy is that the diagnosis of missed abortion may be established before there is any indication that the pregnancy is abnormal. It is sometimes preferable to repeat the scan a week later rather than proceed to immediate uterine evacuation, to enable the mother to come to terms with the diagnosis.

Blighted ovum

The absence of fetal development results in the presence of a gestational sac which does not contain a fetus. This can be readily identified but, as with missed abortion, it is advisable to repeat the scan after at least one week.

Hydatidiform mole

The classic appearance of a molar pregnancy makes this condition easy to recognize. The uterus is filled with echoes which give it a snowstorm appearance. There is usually no evidence of a fetus but this is not invariably the case. The presence of haemorrhage within the molar tissue may lead to some confusion with the possibility of a missed abortion and fetal resorption.

Detection of fetal malformations

Ultrasound is widely used for the diagnosis of congenital abnormalities. Real-time scanning enables imaging in both longitudinal and transverse sections and is particularly useful in the diagnosis of abnormalities of the central nervous system.

Spina bifida

The entire length of the fetal spine can be demon-strated by real-time imaging with both longitudinal and transverse scans (Fig. 19.13). The normal spine appears as a complete bony ring, but with spina bifida the posterior aspect of the ring is open, with a bulging meningo-myelocoele, and the neural elements can be seen outside the spinal canal. The most difficult area to visualize is the lower lumbar and sacral spine.

Fig. 19.13 (**A**) Ultrasound image of the fetal spine; (**B**) a fetal hand can be seen to the right of the clear space of amniotic fluid

Anencephaly

Ultrasound diagnosis of anencephaly is relatively easy but also less important than the diagnosis of spina bifida, because the anencephalic fetus does not survive.

Hydrocephaly can be diagnosed by the abnormal enlargement of the biparietal diameter and lateral ventricles. In the detection of microcephaly, the head circumference must be compared with trunk measurements in order to obtain a sure diagnosis.

Renal tract anomalies

The bladder can be visualized after 14 weeks gestation but may vary considerably in size according to the voiding cycle of the fetus. Renal agenesis can be recognized by the absence of kidneys and of urine in the bladder. Other anomalies that can be diagnosed by ultrasound include isolated renal cysts, multicystic dysplasia, infantile polycystic kidneys and obstructive uropathy.

Abnormalities of the gastrointestinal tract

Oesophageal atresia can be identified by the absence of a stomach bubble and the presence of poly-hydramnios. Duodenal atresia is associated with a double bubble, and diaphragmatic hernia is suggested by deviation of the heart and a fluid-filled space in the chest. It is also feasible to establish a diagnosis of omphalocoele and gastroschisis. Foreign bodies can also be identified in the uterus (Fig. 19.14).

Fig. 19.14 Ultrasound diagnosis of a plastic intra-uterine contraceptive device

Ultrasound imaging of the placenta

The placenta can be easily identified on ultrasound scan but is often difficult to localize in relation to the lower uterine segment and the cervix. The reflection of the bladder from the uterus facilitates the demarcation of the lower uterine segment anteriorly, but it is difficult to identify the cervix with ultrasound and localization of the posterior placenta with any great degree of accuracy is not possible. Apparent placental migration is due to the changing shape of the uterine musculature with advancing gestational age.

The role of ultrasound in the diagnosis of placental abruption is limited because it is difficult to differentiate between normal intravascular blood and retroplacental clot. A diagnosis of abruption should be made only where the state of the blood collection is non-physiological.

Assessment of fetal growth

The assessment of fetal growth is dependent on serial measurement of various parts of the fetus and no valid estimate can be obtained from an isolated measurement. **Cephalometry** involves the measurement of the fetal biparietal diameter. These measurements can be misleading in breech presentation because of the dolico-cephalic shape of the head; in this instance it is necessary to measure the occipito-frontal diameter as well, to establish a ratio between the two measurements.

Abdominal measurements

The size of the fetal abdomen provides a sensitive indication of fetal growth. Measurements are aimed at the lower edge of the liver and are expressed in terms of either abdominal circumference or abdominal area. Abdominal size in relation to head size gives a sensitive indication of intrauterine growth retardation. Late onset of placental insufficiency gives rise to a 'head-sparing' effect and asymmetrical growth retardation. Symmetrical growth retardation may be associated with fetal abnormality or infection, and intra-uterine growth retardation of early onset. Various nomograms have been devised for growth of the long bones of the limbs. In particular, measurements of the femur in relation to abdominal girth are useful in the assessment of fetal growth.

Detection of pelvic pathology

Ultrasound is now used extensively for the detection of pelvic pathology. It can be used to measure the size of various pelvic tumours such as ovarian cysts, be they benign or malignant, and the presence of minor cysts in the ovary as with polycystic ovarian syndrome (Fig. 19.15).

Ultrasound

- Uses frequencies of 2–20 MHz
- Static and real time
- Most valuable in estimation of gestational age, missed abortion, mole, fetal CNS and renal tract malformations, fetal growth, anterior placenta praevia
- Less useful in ectopics, posterior placenta praevia, abruption

Fig. 19.15 Bilateral polycystic ovarian disease showing the mottled appearance in both ovaries characteristic of multiple small cysts.

Fig. 19.16 Magnetic resonance imaging; a sagittal section of a mature fetus:
A: cerebral cortex, B: cerebellum, C: umbilical cord vessels,
D: spinal cord, E: anterior placement of the placenta, F: bladder

MAGNETIC RESONANCE IMAGING (MRI)
(Figs 19.16–19.18)

Magnetic resonance tomography is a new technique of imaging. Soft tissue definition is at a premium with this method and it has the advantage that images can be obtained in any plane. Furthermore, the technique is not dependent on ionizing radiation and at the present time does not appear to be associated with any hazard. The nucleus of the hydrogen atom contains a single spinning proton which generates a small magnetic field. The application of a powerful external magnetic field polarizes the hydrogen-ion-containing sample and aligns the hydrogen ions. When radio-waves of the appropriate frequency are passed through the tissue, the protons are displaced and, in returning to their basal state, energy is emitted as a radio frequency. Images are created from a series of measurements in the time domain. The use of this technique in obstetrics is now under investigation. It enables very accurate localization of the placental site because the cervix can be identified with considerable clarity. The fetal brain can also be imaged in late pregnancy (Fig. 19.16), but it is difficult to image the fetus in early pregnancy using existing techniques because of fetal movement.

MRI is particularly useful in the diagnosis of pelvic tumours (Fig. 19.18). Endometrial carcinoma can be clearly identified and the depth of invasion into the myometrium accurately measured. Tumour invasion for cervical, uterine and ovarian carci-

Fig. 19.17 Sagittal section of the normal non-pregnant female pelvis with magnetic resonance imaging: A: outer layers of the myometrium, B: endometrium, C: low resonance band of the myometrium, D: bladder, E: pubic symphysis, F: vagina

Fig. 19.18   Magnetic resonance imaging of a large ovarian cyst; the tumour can be seen indenting the bladder

nomas can be seen in transverse, sagittal and coronal sections.

The technique promises considerable advances in morphological and biochemical imaging.

IMMUNOSCINTIGRAPHY

This technique involves the injection of specific monoclonal antibodies to tumours into the circulation for the purpose of targeting radioactivity isotopes on to tumour deposits. Remote metastases can be identified and so far the technique has been principally used in studies in ovarian tumours to identify recurrent disease. Perhaps its greatest potential use lies in the prospect of using the target antibody to carry cell toxins to the tumour cells.

BIBLIOGRAPHY

Bennett M J 1984 Ultrasound in perinatal care. John Wiley & Sons, Chichester
Campbell S, Bennett M J 1980 Real time ultrasound in obstetrics. Blackwell, Oxford

20. Contraception and sterilization

The ability to control fertility by reliable artifical methods has transformed both social and epidemiological aspects of human reproduction. Family size is determined by a number of factors including social and religous customs, economic aspirations, knowledge of contraception and the availability of reliable methods to regulate fertility.

The most fertile phase of the menstrual cycle occurs at the time of ovulation. In a 28-day cycle, this occurs between day 12 and day 14 of the cycle. Thus natural methods of family planning include:

1. The **rhythm method** — avoiding intercourse midcycle and for 3–4 days either side of midcycle. The efficacy of this method depends on the ability to predict the time of ovulation.
2. **Coitus interruptus** — a traditional and still widely used method of contraception which relies on penile withdrawal before ejaculation. It is not a particularly reliable method of contraception.

Artificial methods of contraception act by the following pathways:

1. Inhibition of ovulation.
2. Prevention of implantation of the fertilized ovum.
3. Barrier methods of contraception whereby the spermatozoa are physically prevented from gaining access to the cervix.

Efficacy. The effectiveness of any method of contraception is measured by the number of unwanted pregnancies that occur during 100 women years of exposure, i.e. during 1 year of 100 women who are normally fertile and having regular coitus. This is known as the **'Pearl Index'**.

BARRIER METHODS OF CONTRACEPTION

These techniques involve a physical barrier which prevents spermatozoa from reaching the female upper genital tract.

Condoms

The basic condom consists of a thin, stretchable latex film which is moulded into a sheath, lubricated and packed in a foil wrapper. The sheath has a teat end to collect the ejaculate. The disadvantages of sheaths are that they need to be applied before intercourse and that they reduce the level of sensation for the male partner. The advantages are that they are readily available, that they are without side effects for the female partner, and that they provide a degree of protection against infection. The failure rate is variable, but averages around 3.9 pregnancies per 100 women years.

Diaphragms

The female equivalent of the sheath is the diaphragm. The modern diaphragm consists of a thin latex rubber dome attached to a circular metal spring. These diaphragms vary in size from 45–100 mm in diameter. The size of the diaphragm required is ascertained by examination of the woman. The size and position of the uterus are determined by vaginal examination and the distance from the posterior vaginal examination and the distance from the posterior vaginal fornix to the pubic symphysis is noted. The appropriate measuring ring is inserted. This usually varies between 70 and 80 mm and,

Fig. 20.1   Insertion of the vaginal diaphragm to cover the cervix and anterior vaginal wall

when correctly in position, the anterior edge of the ring or diaphragm should lie behind the pubic symphysis and the lower posterior edge should lie comfortably in the posterior fornix (Fig. 20.1).

The woman should be advised to insert the diaphragm either in the dorsal position or in the kneeling position whilst bending forwards. The diaphragm can be removed by simply hooking an index finger under the diaphragm rim from below and pulling it out. The diaphragm should be smeared on both sides with a contraceptive cream, and it is usually advised that the diaphragm be inserted dome down. However, some women prefer to insert the diaphragm with the dome upwards.

The diaphragm must be inserted prior to intercourse and should not be removed until at least 6 hours later. The main advantage of this technique is that it is free of side effects to the woman, apart from occasional reaction to the contraceptive cream. The main disadvantages are that the diaphragm must be inserted before intercourse and that there is a failure rate of 7.2 per 100 women years. There are a variety of vault and cervical caps which are of much smaller diameter than the diaphragm. These are suitable for women with a long cervix or with some degree of prolapse, but otherwise have no particular advantage over the diaphragm.

Spermicides

Spermicides in general are only effective if used in conjunction with a mechanical barrier.

Pessaries or suppositories have a water-soluble or wax base and contain a spermicide. They must be inserted approximately 15 minutes before intercourse. Common spermicides are nonoxynol-9 and benzalkonium.

Creams consist of an emulsified fat base and tend not to spread. Care in insertion is essential so that the cervix is covered.

Jellies or pastes have a water-soluble base which spreads rapidly at body temperature. They therefore have an advantage over creams as they spread throughout the vagina.

Foam tablets and foam aerosols contain bicarbonate of soda so that carbon dioxide is released on contact with water. The foam spreads the spermicide throughout the vagina. Pregnancy rates vary with different agents, but average around 9–10 per 100 women years.

Sponges consist of polyurethane foam impregnated with nonoxynol-9. The failure rate is between 10 and 25% and is not recommended as an isolated method.

Barrier contraception

- Condom: 3.9 pregnancies/100 women years but also some protection against infection
- Diaphragm: 7.2/100
- Spermicides: 10/100 (need to be used with other barrier)

INTRA-UTERINE CONTRACEPTIVE DEVICES (IUDs)

A wide variety of devices have been designed for

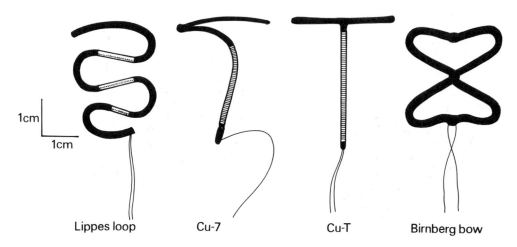

Fig. 20.2 Some intra-uterine contraceptive devices

insertion into the uterine cavity (Fig. 20.2). These devices have the advantage that, once inserted, they are retained without the need to take alternative contraceptive precautions. It seems likely that they act by preventing implantation of the fertilized oocyte, although some produce changes in cervical mucus which interfere with the ability of spermatozoa to penetrate into the uterine cavity.

The first device to be widely used was the Grafenberg ring and was made of a silver–copper alloy. Introduced in the 1930s, it ran into considerable difficulties with haemorrhage, infection, abortions and uterine perforations. With the development of plastic devices in the 1960s, intrauterine devices entered a new phase of acceptance and are now in common usage.

Types of device

The devices are either inert or pharmacologically active.

Inert devices

Lippes loops, Saf-T-coils and Margulis spirals are plastic or plastic-coated devices. They have a thread attached which protrudes through the cervix and allows the woman to check that the device is still in place. Inert devices tend to be relatively large.

Pharmacologically active devices

The addition of copper to contraceptive devices produces a direct effect on the endometrium by interfering with endometrial oestrogen-binding sites and depressing uptake of thymidine into DNA. It also impairs glycogen storage in the endometrium. Examples of such devices are Copper-T or Copper-7 or combined Multiload Copper-250. Copper has both bactericidal and spermicidal properties.

Devices containing progesterone

Some devices such as the Progestosert® contain 38 mg of progesterone, which is released at 65 μg per day. These devices, like those containing copper, need to be changed on a regular basis as elution of the pharmacological agent occurs.

Progesterone-containing devices have been associated with a high incidence of ectopic pregnancy and menstrual distrubances.

Selection of patients

Intra-uterine devices are best reserved for older parous women where there are difficulties with other methods of contraception, or where the motivation to remember to use methods which involve action before intercourse is deficient. These devices are not really suitable for nulliparous women under the age of 20, as the infection rate can be up to 18%. There are often difficulties with insertion of the device and expulsion rates are high. Menorrhagia, dysmenorrhoea and dyspareunia are common.

Insertion of devices

The optimal time for insertion of the device is in the first half of the menstrual cycle. With postpartum women, the optimal time is 4–6 weeks after delivery. Insertion at the time of therapeutic abortion is safe and can be performed when motivation is strong. It is unwise to insert intrauterine devices following spontaneous abortion because of the risk of infection. Devices may be inserted within a few days of delivery, but there is a high expulsion rate. Ideally, the woman should be placed in the lithotomy position. A cervical smear should be taken and a swab taken for culture if there is any sign of infection. The uterus is examined bimanually and the size, shape and position ascertained. The cervix is swabbed with an antiseptic solution and a vulsellum can be applied to the anterior lip of the cervix, although this is not essential and may cause discomfort. The passage of a uterine sound will indicate the depth and direction of the uterine cavity, and the dimensions of the cavity may be assessed by devices known as cavimeters, which measure its length and breadth. Many IUDs are available in different sizes, and cavimeters help to choose the appropriate IUD. Insertions vary in construction, but generally consist of a stoppered plastic tube containing a plunger to extrude the device, which may be linear or folded (Fig 20.3). The device is inserted in the plane of the uterine lumen and care is taken not to push it through the uterine fundus.

Attempts at insertion of a device where the cervical canal is tight may result in vagal syncope.

Acute pain following insertion may indicate perforation of the uterus.

The woman should be instructed to check the loop strings regularly and to notify her doctor immediately if the strings are not palpable. Copper devices generally require replacement every 3–5 years, but other devices may be left in situ for longer periods.

Complications (Fig. 20.4)

Pregnancy rates

Unwanted pregnancies occur at a rate of 2–3 per 100 women years. If the device or its strings are easily grasped, it is sensible to remove it to reduce the incidence of a septic abortion, there being a high incidence of spontaneous abortion in such pregnancies. If it is not accessible, it should be left and removed at the time of delivery. The risk of failure of the IUD diminishes with each year after insertion.

Perforation of the uterus

About 0.1–1% of devices perforate the uterus. In many cases, partial perforation occurs at the time of insertion and later migration completes the perforation. If the woman notices that the tail of the device is missing, then it must be assumed that one of the following has occurred:

1. The device has been expelled.
2. The device has turned in the uterine cavity and drawn up the strings.

Fig. 20.3 Insertion of the intra-uterine decide

COMPLICATIONS OF IUCD

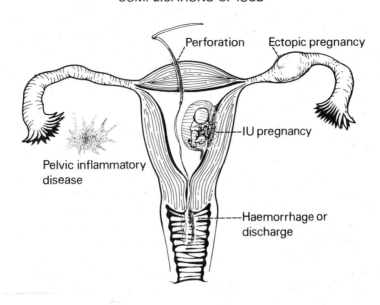

Fig. 20.4 Complications of intra-uterine devices

3. The device has perforated the uterus and lies either partly or completely in the peritoneal cavity.

If there is no evidence of pregnancy, an ultrasound examination of the uterus should be performed. If the device is located within the uterine cavity, then it is removed and, unless part of the loop or strings is visible, it will generally be necessary to remove the device with formal dilatation of the cervix under general or local anaesthesia. If the device is not found in the uterus, an X-ray of the abdomen will reveal the site in the peritoneal cavity. It is advisable to remove all extra-uterine devices by either laparoscopy or laparotomy. Inert devices can probably be left with impunity, but copper devices promote considerable peritoneal irritation and should certainly be removed.

Pelvic inflammatory disease

Acute pelvic inflammatory disease occurs in 1–2% of high income patients and 8–10% of indigent populations. Pre-existent pelvic inflammatory disease is a contraindication to this method of contraception.

If pelvic inflammatory disease does occur, then the device should be removed immediately and antibiotic therapy commenced. If the infection is severe, it is preferable to complete 24 hours antibiotic therapy before removing the device.

Abnormal uterine bleeding

Increased menstrual loss occurs in most women with an intra-uterine device, but can be tolerated by the majority. However, in 15% of such women it is sufficiently severe to necessitate removal of the device. It can be controlled by drugs such as dicynene, amino-caproic acid, or danazol. Intermenstrual bleeding may also occur, but if the loss is slight it does not constitute a reason for removal.

Pelvic pain

Pain occurs either in a chronic low grade form or as severe dysmenorrhoea. The incidence is widely variable with up to 50% of women suffering some pain. However, the pain may be acceptable if it is not severe, and this is a decision that has to be made by the patient in relation to the convenience of the method.

Vaginal discharge

Vaginal discharge may be due to infection, but most women with an intra-uterine device develop a slight watery or mucoid discharge.

Ectopic gestation

There is an increased incidence of ectopic pregnancy with a rate of 0.6 per 100 women years. It is therefore essential to think of this diagnosis in any woman presenting with abdominal pain and irregular vaginal bleeding and who has an intrauterine device in situ.

IUDs

- Prevent implantation
- Inert or pharmacologically active
- Best for older multiparous women
- Can be inserted at TOP
- Replace after 3–5 years
- 2 failures per 100 women years
- Complications: perforation, pelvic inflammatory disease, abnormal bleeding, ectopic pregnancy

HORMONAL CONTRACEPTION

Oral contraception is given as a combination of oestrogen or progestogen, either as a combined pill or triphasic pill, or as progesterone only.

Combined pill

These preparations contain oestrogen and a progestogen in a variety of combinations. The oestrogen used is either oestradiol or mestranol, and is given in a dosage between 20 and 50 μg daily. The progestogens used are derived from 17-hydroxyprogesterone or 19-norsteroids.

The only derivative of 17-hydroxyprogesterone commonly used is medroxyprogesterone acetate in the form of Depo-provera®. The 19-norsteroids used include:

1. Norethisterone.
2. Ethynodiol.
3. Norgestrel.
4. Laevonorgestrel.
5. Norethisterone acetate.
6. Lynestrenol.

Triphasic pill

These pills have a variable dose of progestogen and oestrogen components and are used to reduce the side effects from the progestogen.

Progesterone-only pill

Progesterone-only pills contain either norethisterone or ethynodiol diacetate and are taken continuously on the basis of one tablet daily. Because of the low dose, they should be taken at the same time every day.

Injectable compounds

Medroxyprogesterone acetate is administered as a depot preparation given in a single injection which lasts for 3 months. This compound has been criticized because of its side effects, which include irregular vaginal bleeding, loss of hair and skin eruptions.

Norplant® contains 36 mg of levonorgestrel, impregnated into a silicone rubber rod, and implanted subcutaneously in the arm. The effects last from 3 to 5 years and it requires surgical removal.

Mode of action

Combined and triphasic pills act by suppressing gonadotrophin secretion and, in particular, the LH peak. The endometrium becomes unsuitable for nidation and the cervical mucus becomes hostile. Progesterone-only pills alter the endometrial maturation and affect cervical mucus. Ovulation is suppressed in only 40% of women.

Contraindications

There are various contraindications to the pill, some being more absolute than others.

The absolute contraindications include pregnancy, pulmonary embolism, deep vein thrombosis, sickle cell disease, porphyria, liver disease and jaundice — particularly where it is associated with a previous pregnancy or carcinoma of the breast. It is necessary to maintain a high level of vigilance in women with varicose veins, diabetes, hypertension, renal disease, chronic heart failure and oligomenorrhoea but none of these conditions constitutes an absolute contraindication, and, in some cases, the adverse effects of a pregnancy may substantially outweigh any hazard from the pill. Women who smoke and those over the age of 35 have a significantly increased risk of thrombo-embolic disease.

The occurrence of migraine for the first time, severe headaches or visual disturbances, or transient neurological changes are indications for immediate cessation of the pill. There are a series of minor side effects which may sometimes be used to advantage or may be offset by using a pill with a different combination of steroids.

Oestrogenic effects
Fluid retention and oedema
Premenstrual tension, and irritability
Increase in weight
Nausea and vomiting
Headache
Mucorrhoea, cervical erosion
Menorrhagia
Excessive tiredness
Vein complaints
Breakthrough bleeding

Progestogenic effects
Premenstrual depression
Dry vagina
Acne, greasy hair
Increased appetite with weight gain
Breast discomfort
Cramps of the legs and abdomen
Decreased libido

Therapeutic uses other than contraception include the treatment of menorrhagia, premenstrual syndrome, endometriosis and dysmenorrhoea.

Major side effects

The mortality rate from thrombo-embolic disease is 1.3 per 100 000 below 34 years of age and 3.4 per 100 000 above 35 years. Cardiovascular problems are increased and this appears to be associated with increased levels of low density lipoproteins or reduced levels of high density lipoproteins. Prolonged amenorrhoea may occur in women coming off the pill, but the direct relationship remains unclear. Smoking increases the risks of thrombo-embolic disease two- to three-fold.

Counselling

It is important to obtain a complete general history and examination before presenting the pill, and also to perform annual check-ups and cervical cytology. There are a large number of compounds commercially available, and some pills marketed by different companies contain the same compounds at the same concentrations.

Interaction between drugs and contraceptive steroids

Many drugs affect the contraceptive efficacy of the pill and therefore additional precautions should be taken (Table 20.1). Vomiting and diarrhoea also result in loss of the pill and hence the return of fertility — particularly with the low-dose pills now widely in use. Progesterone-only pills must be taken every day if they are to be effective.

Failure rates

The failure rate of combined pills is 0.5 per 100 women years. The failure rate for progesterone-only preparations is higher and varies between 0.9 and 4.3 per 100 women years.

The pill and surgery

The pill increases the risk of deep vein thrombosis and should therefore be stopped at least 6 weeks before surgery. It should not be stopped before minor procedures — particularly before laparoscopic sterilization procedures. The risk of an unwanted pregnancy occurring before admission is substantially greater than the risk of thrombo-embolism.

The pill and lactation

Combined preparations tend to inhibit lactation and are therefore best avoided. The pill of choice at this time is the progesterone-only pill as it has minimal effect on lactation and may, indeed, promote it.

Post-coital pill

Following unanticipated intercourse around mid-cycle, there is sometimes a need for emergency measures to prevent conception.

Table 20.1 Interactions of various drugs with oral contraceptives

Interacting drug	Effects of interaction
Analgesics Amidopyrine Phenazone Phenacetin Pethidine	Breakthrough bleeding Possible decrease in contraceptive reliability Possible increased sensitivity to pethidine
Anti-inflammatory agents Phenylbutazone Oxyphenbutazone	Possible decrease in contraceptive reliability
Anticoagulants Dicoumarol	Possible reduction of effect of anticoagulant. An increased dosage of anticoagulant may be necessary

Anticonvulsants
Hydantoins
  ethotoin
  methoin
  phenytoin
Methylphenobarbitone
Phenobarbitone
Primidone
Ethosuximide
Carbamazepine
	Possible decrease in contraceptive reliability
	Careful observation is necessary for signs of fluid retention

Tricyclic antidepressants Imipramine Clomipramine Amitriptyline	Reduced antidepressant response; increase in antidepressant toxicity
Antihistamines Antihistamines	Possible decrease in contraceptive reliability
Anti-infective agents Ampicillin Chloramphenicol Neomycin Nitrofurantoin Penicillin V Rifampicin Sulphamethoxypyridazine	Possible decrease in contraceptive reliability Possibility of breakthrough bleeding This is most likely with rifampicin
Antimigraine agents Dihydroergotamine	Possible decrease in contraceptive reliability
Barbiturates Phenobarbitone Methylphenobarbitone	Probable decrease in contraceptive reliability
Hypoglycaemic agents Insulin Oral hypoglycaemics	Control of diabetes may be reduced
Anti-asthmatics Anti-asthmatics	Asthmatic condition may be exacerbated by concomitant oral contraceptive ingestion
Sedatives and tranquillizers Chlordiazepoxide Chlorpromazine Diazepam Meprobamate	Possible decrease in contraceptive reliability Possibility of breakthrough bleeding
Systemic corticosteroids Systemic corticosteroids	Increased dosage of steroids may be necessary as plasma corticoid-binding protein increases

The regime recommended by the Committee of Safety in Medicines as an emergency measure is that of a combined oestrogen-progestogen pill. The preparation of choice should contain 50 μg of ethinyloestradial and 250 μg of levonorgestrel. Two pills of this combination should be given with 72 hours of exposure and then repeated 12 hours later. If one dose is lost through vomiting the complete course should be repeated.

Combined oral contraceptive pill

- Suppress gonadotrophins
- Oestradiol and progestogen
- Pregnancy, thrombo-embolism and liver disease contraindicate
- 1.3/100 000 mortality
- 0.5/100 women years failure rate

STERILIZATION

Contraceptive techniques have the major advantage that they are easily reversible and provide a high level of protection against pregnancy. They have the disadvantage that they require a conscious act on behalf of the individual before intercourse. When family size is complete or there is a specific medical contraindication to continuing fertility, then sterilization becomes the contraceptive method of choice.

Counselling

It is essential to counsel both partners about the nature of the procedures and their implications and to discuss whether it is better for the male or female partner to be sterilized. In many cases, only one partner will be seeking sterilization, in which case only one point of view needs to be considered.

Counselling should include reference to the failure rates and to the question of reversibility. With the improvements brought about by micro-surgery, it is no longer acceptable to say that sterilization is irreversible and the patient should be counselled according to the technique to be used. The partner to be sterilized will be a matter of choice and motivation. If one partner has a reduced life expectancy from chronic illness, then that partner should be sterilized.

Timing of sterilization

The operation is best performed in the first half of the menstrual cycle. If this is not possible, then it is important to ascertain that the woman is not pregnant. Sterilization at the time of abortion or delivery is generally unwise because of the high failure rate and relatively high 'regret' rate. It is preferable to perform sterilization as an 'interval' procedure some 3 months after delivery.

Techniques

Female sterilization

The majority of procedures involve interruption of the fallopian tubes, but may vary from the application of clips on the tubes to total hysterectomy. In general terms, the more radical the procedure, the less likely there is to be a failure. However, very low failure rates can now be achieved using methods with high reversibility prospects and these should be the methods of choice.

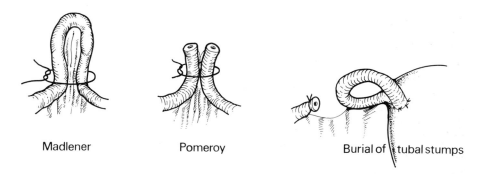

Madlener   Pomeroy   Burial of tubal stumps

Fig. 20.5 Sterilization by tubal ligation and excision

Tubal ligation (Fig. 20.5). The common technique involves simple ligation of a loop of tube using a 'mini' laparotomy procedure. This is known as the **Madlener procedure**.

The **Pomeroy technique** is the same, but the loop of tube is excised and absorbable suture material used for the ligation. There are several variations to this technique, including the separation of the cut ends of the tubes on contralateral sides of the broad ligament.

Failure rates vary with the technique but may be as high as 3.7% with the Madlener operation, and as low as 0.6% for the Pomeroy technique. This type of procedure may also be performed by the vaginal route, either through the Pouch of Douglas or through the utero-vesical fold of peritoneum. The failure rates tend to be higher than those achieved via abdominal incision.

Laparoscopic sterilization. The use of the laparoscope for sterilization procedures has substantially reduced the duration of hospital stay.

1. Tubal coagulation and division — Sterilization is effected by either unipolar or bipolar diathermy of the tubes in two sites 1–2 cm from the utero-tubal junction. A considerable amount of tube can be destroyed with this technique. Division of the diathermied tube is said to reduce the risk of ectopic pregnancy. The failure rate with this procedure is about 0.7%. The major complication of the procedure is the danger of burning bowel with subsequent leakage and faeculent peritonitis.

2. Tubal clips — The application of clips or rings through the laparoscope has become popular because it avoids the risk of diathermy damage. The clips are made of plastic and inert metals and are locked on to the tube (Fig. 20.6). They have the advantage of causing minimal damage to the tube, but their disadvantage is a higher failure rate.

   The **Hulka-Clemens clip** has been reported as having a failure rate of up to 2.6%. Failures may be due to application on the wrong structure or extrusion of the tube from the clip, recanalization, or fracture of the clip so that it falls off the tube.

   The **Filshie clip**, which has a titanium frame lined by silicone rubber, has a lower failure rate (0.2%) and is easier to apply.

   Yoon rings are applied over a loop of tube and

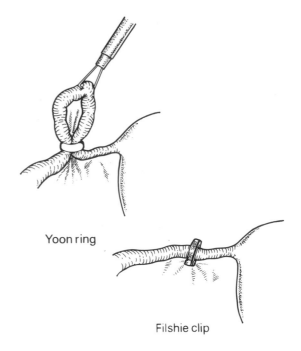

Yoon ring

Filshie clip

Fig. 20.6 Sterilization by clip occlusion

are similar to a Madlener procedure. This technique is associated with considerably greater abdominal pain postoperatively and the failure rates vary between 0.3 and 4%. The rings are not suitable for application to the tubes in the puerperium where the tube is swollen and oedematous.

Complications. Apart from the complications of laparoscopy, the longer term complications are those of tubal recanalization and pregnancy, ectopic pregnancy, menstrual irregularity and loss of libido.

Table 20.2 Comparative failure rates

Method	Pregnancies (per 100 wy)
Sheath	3.9
Diaphragm	7.2
Spermicides	10
Combined pill	0.5
Progesterone-only pill	0.9–4.3
IUCD	2–3
Clip sterilization	0.2 (%)
Vasectomy	1–2/1000

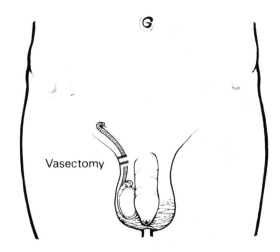

Fig. 20.7 Vasectomy involves excision of a segment of the vas deferens

Vasectomy

This procedure is generally performed under local anaesthesia. Two small incisions are made over the spermatic cord and 3–4 cm of the vas deferens are excised (Fig. 20.7).

The advantage of the technique is its simplicity. The disadvantages are that sterility is not immediate, and should not be assumed until all spermatozoa have disappeared from the ejaculate. On average, this takes about 14 ejaculations. The procedure is more difficult to reverse and, even when satisfactory re-anastomosis is achieved, only about 50% of patients will sire children, because of the production of sperm-immobilizing and sperm-agglutinating antibodies. Failures may follow spontaneous re-canalization and excision of an inadequate length of vas deferens. The excised segments should always be examined histologically to confirm that the vas has been excised. Complications of the operation include haematoma formation, wound infection and epididymitis. Also a painful granuloma may form at the cut end of the vas due to a foreign body reaction induced by spermatozoa.

Sterilization

- Counsel re irreversibility, failure rate and risks
- Laparoscopy/mini-laparotomy
- 0.2–4% failure rate
- Complications: laparoscopic, ectopic pregnancy, menstrual irregularity

BIBLIOGRAPHY

Department of Health 1990 Handbook of contraceptive practice. HMSO
Loudon N 1991 Handbook of family planning, 2nd edn. Churchill Livingstone, Edinburgh

21. The changes of the menstrual cycle

The nature of the menstrual cycle has been described in a previous chapter. Menstruation is the periodic change occurring in primates which results in the flow of blood and endometrium from the uterine cavity, and which may be associated with various constitutional disturbances.

Fig. 21.1 Development of the female breast during the thelarche

PUBERTY AND MENARCHE

Puberty is the process of sexual maturation beginning with the maturation of the hypothalamus. This results in an increased release of pituitary gonadotrophins and, hence, stimulation of the ovary with the production of sex hormones. Other trophic hormones such as ACTH, thyroid-stimulating hormone (TSH) and growth hormone also gradually increase over a period of 3–4 years. The sexual changes of puberty can be divided into three phases.

Thelarche

The first of the sexual changes to occur is the development of the breast (Fig. 21.1). Nipple enlargement begins between 9 and 11 years of age with thickening

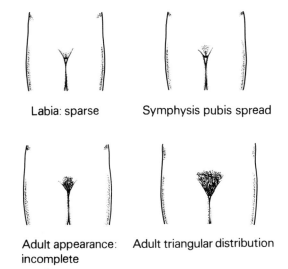

Fig. 21.2 Pubic hair distribution leading up to full sexual maturation during the adrenarche

209

of the duct system as a result of increasing oestrogen production. At the same time, the vaginal epithelium increases in thickness and vaginal pH decreases.

Adrenarche

The growth of pubic hair occurs at about 11–12 years of age and is followed by the development of axillary hair (Fig. 21.2). Both phenomena are dependent on adrenal development.

Menarche

The final manifestation of sexual maturity in the female is the onset of mestruation. The average age of the menarche in the United Kingdom is 13 years and occurs in 95% of girls between the ages of 11 and 15 years. There has been a lowering of the age of the menarche in Western Europe and there is some variation between different ethnic groups.

The menstrual cycle is often irregular in the first 2 years and may show intervals of 4–6 months between periods. The cycles are frequently anovulatory and prolonged bleeding may occur.

The growth spurt

Throughout the period of sexual maturation, marked changes occur in growth (Fig. 21.3). A rapid increase in growth occurs between 11 and 14 years. The legs lengthen first and this is followed by increases in shoulder breadth and in trunk length. The pelvis enlarges and changes in shape. Maximal height occurs between 17 and 18 years and growth is terminated by the fusion of femoral epiphyses.

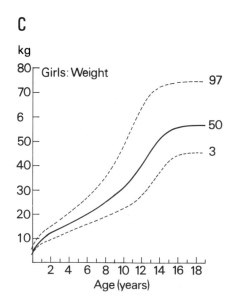

Fig. 21.3 (**A**) Centile change for height in the female; (**B**) height velocity indicates the slowing down of the rate of growth with a secondary acceleration around the time of puberty; (**C**) Changes in weight show a wider scatter than with height

Puberty/Menarche

- Hypothalamic maturation
- Breast enlargement 9–11 years
- Pubic hair 11–12 years
- Menarche 11–15 years
- Growth spurt 11–14 years

Precocious puberty

The development of physical signs of sexual maturation before the age of 8 years and the onset of menstruation before the age of 10 years are indications of precocious puberty. The majority of cases carry no pathological connotation.

Aetiology

Precocious puberty may occur at any point in the hypothalamic/pituitary/ovarian axis or as a result of abnormalities in the adrenal or thyroid glands. Causes may be (Fig. 21.4):

- Constitutional.
- Neurological — meningitis, encephalitis, polyostotic fibrosis, dysplasia, neurofibromatosis, cerebral tumours, hydrocephalus, cysts.
- Ovarian tumours.
- Adrenal tumours.
- Gonadotrophin-secreting tumours — chorioepithelioma, hepatoblastoma.
- Others — hypothyroidism, exogenous oestrogens.

Constitutional

Neurological

Ovarian tumours

Adrenal tumours

Gonadotrophin secretory tumours

Others: hypothyroidism, exogenous oestrogens

Fig. 21.4 The aetiology of precocious puberty

The majority of cases of precocious puberty are constitutional in origin. It is, however, important to exclude other organic causes before classifying the problem as constitutional. There are a group of cases where activity of the hypothalamic/pituitary axis is stimulated by intracranial lesions such as meningitis, encephalitis, ventricular hamatoma and pineal tumours. The **McCune-Albright syndrome** is a disorder of bone involving widespread polyostotic fibrous dysplasia with disturbed function of the hypothalamus and pituitary resulting in premature menstruation. There is also a skin disorder manifested by the development of skin pigmentation and cafe-au-lait spots. Of the ovarian lesions, the commonest are the granulosa cell tumours. These must be differentiated from follicular cysts, which may be associated with hypothalamic causes.

Investigation

All children exhibiting precocious sexual development must be investigated to exclude any underlying pathology. General and pelvic examination may reveal evidence of ovarian lesions. A skeletal survey should be undertaken for any bony abnormalities. Skull X-ray and computerized axial tomography (CAT) scanning may reveal the presence of abnormalities of the sella turcica, suprasella calcification and lesions involving the floor of the fourth ventricle.

Ultrasound scanning of the pelvis should reveal any ovarian tumours.

Management

In children where there is a specific lesion causing precocious sexual maturation, the management depends on the treatment of the condition. In constitutional precocious puberty, management is concerned with the abnormal bone growth and the emotional and psychological problems contingent on early sexual maturation. Advanced bone growth results in the girl initially being much taller than her classmates but the early fusion of epiphysis means that her ultimate stature is smaller than normal. It is sometimes possible to inhibit hypothalamic activity by the administration of medroxyprogesterone acetate 100–200 mg i.m. every 2–4 weeks or by

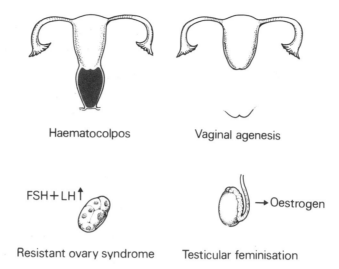

Haematocolpos   Vaginal agenesis

FSH+LH↑   →Oestrogen

Resistant ovary syndrome   Testicular feminisation

Fig. 21.5   The aetiology of primary amenorrhea

giving the anti-androgenic agent, cyproterone acetate, by the oral route.

These children may need protection from sexual assault as they may conceive if coitus occurs. The youngest recorded pregnancy and confinement occurred in a 6-year-old child with precocious sexual development.

Precocious puberty

- Menarche before 10 years of age
- Usually constitutional
- Exclude intracranial/ovarian lesions
- Investigations, ultrasound scanning of pelvis, X-ray pituitary fossa, skeletal survey

Delayed puberty

Delayed puberty commonly presents as primary amenorrhoea. This is defined as the failure to menstruate by the age of 16 years. However, delayed puberty is also revealed by failure in development of secondary sexual characteristics.

If the secondary sexual characteristics are normal apart from amenorrhoea, the diagnosis is likely to be (Fig. 21.5):

1. Hematocolpos — the retention of menstrual fluid because of an imperforate hymen.

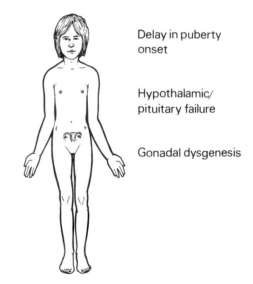

Delay in puberty onset

Hypothalamic/ pituitary failure

Gonadal dysgenesis

Fig. 21.6   Aetiology of delayed puberty with poor secondary sexual characteristics

2. Vaginal agenesis — congenital absence of the vagina.
3. Resistant ovary syndrome (see below).
4. Testicular feminization or other chromosomal abnormalities.

If the secondary sexual characteristics are poor, then the amenorrhoea may be due to (Fig. 21.6):

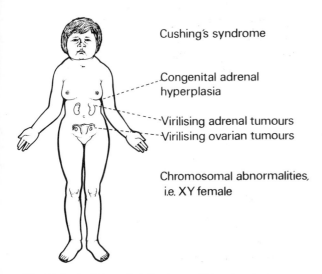

Cushing's syndrome

Congenital adrenal hyperplasia

Virilising adrenal tumours

Virilising ovarian tumours

Chromosomal abnormalities, i.e. XY female

Fig. 21.7 Aetiology of virilization and hirsutism in the female

1. Constitutional delay in puberty.
2. Gonadal dysgenesis — primitive streak ovaries or the congenital absence of ovarian tissue.
3. Hypothalamic/pituitary failure.

If there are signs of virilization in the female, then the following diagnosis should be considered (Fig. 21.7):

1. Congenital adrenal hyperplasia.
2. Virilizing adrenal tumours.
3. Virilizing ovarian tumours.
4. Cushing's syndrome.
5. Chromosomal abnormalities such as the XY female.

General examination should take account of the age, height, weight and arm span of the individual and also features of abnormal somatic structures such as neck webbing and short metatarsal bones. Pelvic examination will reveal whether there are any abnormalities of the genital tract.

The resistant ovary syndrome

This is a rare but important cause of primary amenorrhoea. Secondary sexual characteristics are usually normal. FSH and LH levels are raised to the menopausal range but, unlike true ovarian failure, the ovaries contain numerous ova. Stimulation with human menopausal gonadotrophin or with human chorionic gonadotrophin meets with little success. It must be remembered that these women are able to conceive and may sometimes ovulate spontaneously. Prognosis for childbearing must be guarded, but, unlike true ovarian failure, ovulation and spontaneous menstruation may occur.

Intersexuality

Ambiguous genital development is a rare but disturbing problem and successful management at a physical and psychological level should be started as soon after birth as possible.

Causes of ambiguous genitalia may be:

1. Where the fetus has a Y chromosome and so is karyotypically male, the testes may not form, or they may function abnormally and produce oestrogens as in testicular feminization. The failure of androgen production or androgen insensitivity at the target organ site will result in development of female external genitalia.
2. Virilization may occur in a karyotypic female with androgens being produced from some outside source such as in congenital adrenal hyperplasia.
3. Mosaicism — on occasions, true hermaphroditism does occur and testicular and ovarian tissues form in the same fetus.

The appearance of the hermaphrodite, the undermasculinized male and the masculinized female are all similar. Differential diagnosis is dependent on establishing the karyotype, and measuring 17-oxosteroids and the intermediate products of cortisol metabolism as well as electrolyte levels.

Congenital adrenal hyperplasia needs early recognition if fetal and neonatal survival are to occur. Salt loss may be a major factor in this condition and the infant should be treated with cortisone acetate and prednisone or bromohydrocortisone.

Sexual assignment is particularly important in all intersex cases and should be allocated on the basis of phenotypic sex.

Delayed puberty

- Primary amenorrhoea
- Poor secondary sex characteristics
- Consider chromosome disorders and adrenal tumours

THE MENOPAUSE

At the other end of the spectrum, the termination of menstrual life occurs and is accompanied by a variety of different manifestations.

The **climacteric** is that part of the ageing process which embraces the transition from the reproductive to the non-reproductive phase of life. It is divided into the **premenopause, menopause** and **postmenopause**. The menopause marks the end of menstruation but, as with the menarche in relation to puberty, it reflects only one manifestation of a series of changes. The age of the physiological menopause varies with race and socio-economic conditions, but in Western Europe and the USA the average age of onset is between 49 and 50 years.

Spontaneous cessation of the periods before the age of 40 years is defined as premature menopause. The menopause may be physiological or artificial, when it is associated with removal of the ovaries or the uterus.

Hormonal and menstrual changes in the premenopause

The menstrual cycle shortens in women over the age of 40 years and the change in the cycle length is related to shortening of the follicular phase. FSH levels are higher at all stages of the cycle than levels seen in younger women, whilst oestradiol levels are lower.

The transition from menstruation to amenorrhoea is often characterised by menstrual irregularity. Prolonged episodes of bleeding following a period of amenorrhoea may be associated with anovulatory cycles and with hyperplastic endometrium. Persistent irregular bleeding in the premenopausal phase should never be considered normal, because it may be associated with uterine neoplasms.

Vaginal bleeding which occurs more than 1 year after the menopause is known as postmenopausal bleeding. The possibility of carcinoma of the body of the uterus should be considered and diagnostic curettage performed in all cases (Fig. 21.8).

Hormone changes in the menopause

There is a marked reduction in ovarian production of oestrogen and, in particular, of oestradiol. Some oestrogen production occurs in the adrenal gland, but the major source of oestradiol appears to be the 'fat' organ with peripheral conversion of both oestrone and testosterone. Thus heavy women have higher circulating oestradiol levels than slender women. There is considerable variation in the circulating levels of oestradiol in the menopause and this may account for the variation in severity of menopausal symptoms. The absence of any significant oestrogen production results in excessive release of FSH and LH, with the major increases occurring in FSH. The levels of gonadotrophins continue to show random oscillations similar to the pattern seen in the premenopausal phase. Androgens produced in the ovary and adrenal gland are mainly androstenedione and testosterone and these levels fall in menopausal women. There is also a

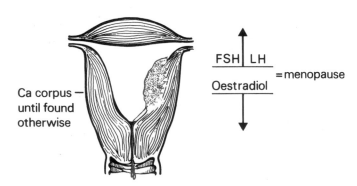

Fig. 21.8 Postmenopausal bleeding must always be assumed to result from corpus carcinoma until the diagnosis is excluded. The menopause can be confirmed by the presence of high FSH/LH levels and low oestradiol levels in the plasma

reduction in adrenal androgen secretion, including that of dehydroepiandrosterone (DHEA) and DHEA sulphate. Oestrogen production by the ovary is reduced, but the production of testosterone persists.

Symptoms and signs of the menopause

Vascular distrubances

The commonest symptom of the menopause is the development of hot flushes. These episodes consist of flushes and perspiration, occur in about 80% of the female population and may persist for up to 5 years after the menopause. The flushes are associated with an increase in skin temperature and conductance. They are also associated in some way with high gonadotrophin levels, but this relationship is not as clear as might at first appear. There are other women where oestrogen levels are low and gonadotrophin levels are high, but who do not develop hot flushes. There is no doubt that the administration of oestrogens relieves these symptoms, but they return when the oestrogen therapy is discontinued.

Changes in target organ response

The reduction in ovarian oestrogen production results in involution and regression of target organs (Fig. 21.9).

The most obvious response is the cessation of menstruation. Periods generally exhibit a gradual reduction in both amount and duration with occasional delays in menstruation. The vaginal walls lose their rugosity and become smooth and atrophic. In severe cases, this may also be associated with chornic infection and atrophic vaginitis. The cervix diminishes in size and there is a reduction in cervical mucus production. The uterus also shrinks in size and the endometrium becomes atrophic.

The breasts exhibit parallel changes with involution of breast structure and the disappearance of cyclical breast changes, which may bring considerable relief to some women.

Although it is not in any proper sense an endocrine target organ, the bladder epithelium may also become atrophic with the development of frequency, dysuria and urge incontinence in the absence of any overt urinary tract infection. It is important to recognize these symptoms because they can be relieved by oestrogen replacement therapy.

Epidermal appendages

The skin tends to become thinned and wrinkled after the menopause as a result of oestrogen deprivation; these changes can be reversed by the use of local oestrogen creams or by hormone replacement therapy. There is loss of scalp hair and of pubic and axillary hair. There is an androgen-based increase in growth of coarse terminal hair so that a slight moustache may develop and loss of scalp hair sometimes results in partial or complete baldness, but this is uncommon.

Involution of breast structure   Cervix diminished in size   Vaginal rugosity lost

Fig. 21.9 Characteristic changes in the breasts and genitalia following the menopause

Bone changes

Osteoporosis is an important health hazard in the menopausal woman. The loss of trabecular bone is the major disorder. Bone loss occurs at a rate of about 2.5% per year for the first 4 years after the menopause so that fractures become a major source of morbidity in the menopausal female. Thus, by the age of 65 years, vertebral fractures occur in 25% of all women.

Bone loss is most severe in women who have an artificial menopause. Hip fractures increase in incidence from 0.3/1000 at an age of 45 years to 20/1000 at age 85 years, and there is also a 10-fold increase in Colles' fractures.

Osteoporosis is associated with increased bony resorption with normal bone formation. There is no doubt that there is a net loss of calcium. These changes are associated with oestrogen deficiency and there is little doubt that prolonged and early hormone replacement therapy can prevent the development of osteoporosis. The means by which these effects are achieved remains uncertain. Fractures late in life carry serious implications in relation to life expectation because of the immobilization of the elderly woman.

Cardiovascular complications

There is evidence of an increase in coronary heart disease following the menopause which is not simply an age-related phenomenon. However, hormone replacement therapy with oestrogens does not reduce the incidence of coronary heart disease. Serum cholesterol levels rise at the time of the menopause. There is an increase in all lipoprotein fractions with a decrease in the ratio of the high to low density fractions. There is no specific association between the menopause and hypertension.

Psychological and emotional symptoms

Many women experience severe emotional disorders at the time of the menopause with depression and anxiety states. The emotional disturbances of the menopause are often associated with feelings of inadequacy and uncertainty about the woman's role with the departure of children from the home. However, there is no doubt that in many women these symptoms are related to oestrogen deficiency and that hormone replacement therapy can return such women to a normal state. The severity of the symptoms should not be underestimated. The depression may be acute and can sometimes result in a successful suicidal attempt. There are many other symptoms ascribed to the menopause, including anorexia, excessive fatigue, nausea and vomiting and bowel disorders.

Treatment of the menopause

Many women pass through the menopause without any symptoms, and there is considerable variation in serum oestradiol levels between individuals after the menopause. Symptoms can often be treated by reassurance and explanation and occasionally by the use of tranquillisers, anti-depressants and sedatives. Flushes sometimes respond to belladonna alkaloids, but respond best to oestrogen therapy.

Hormone replacement therapy

Oestrogen therapy may be given on its own or as a combined or sequential therapy with a progestogen (Fig. 21.10). The type of therapy recommended will depend on whether the uterus has been removed and whether the therapy planned is to be short or long term.

Oral therapy. Diethylstilbestrol, ethinyl oestradiol or conjugated equine oestrogen is given continuously on a 21-day cycle with 7 days between cycles. The administration of a progestogen for the last 7 days of the oestrogen administration will result in regular withdrawal bleeding and should reduce the incidence of irregular vaginal bleeding and the development of endometrial hyperplasia or carcinoma.

Parenteral therapy. Oestrogen can also be administered by injection or by subcutaneous implants. This is best achieved with oestradiol benzoate, 100 mg, in a pellet which is inserted in the subcutaneous tissue of the anterior abdominal wall. This is often combined with testosterone, which has the advantage of a mild anabolic effect and of enhancing libido. The pellets usually last for anything up to 6 months and are particularly useful in women who have experienced a surgical menopause.

If the implants are given to a woman with an intact uterus, then it is important to give a progestogen,

Fig. 21.10   Treatment protocol for the management of menopausal symptoms with the use of hormone replacement therapy (HRT)

such as norethisterone acetate 5 mg, for the first 7 days of each month. This will provoke withdrawal bleeding as long as active oestrogen absorption occurs.

Complications. The potential complications of hormone replacement therapy include an increased incidence of carcinoma of the endometrium and possibly of the breast. Some women develop hypertension on oestrogen therapy and, therefore, periodic checks on blood pressure are important. Caution should be taken when there is a history of gall bladder disease.

The development of irregular uterine bleeding is an indication for diagnostic curettage.

Contraindications. Hormone replacement therapy is contraindicated in the presence of endometrial and breast carcinoma, acute thrombotic disease, fibrocystic disease of the breast, uterine fibroids, familial hyperlipidaemia, diabetes and gall bladder disease. However, with the exception of malignant disease of the breast and endometrium, none of the

other conditions provide an absolute contraindication, and relief of symptoms may sometimes be more important than other considerations.

Menopause

> • Onset 49–50 years
> • FSH rises, oestradiol falls
> • Menstrual irregularity with short follicular phase
> • Associated with vasomotor instability, atrophic changes in genital tract and skin, osteoporosis, cardiovascular complications
> • Hormone replacement therapy (HRT) requires additional progestogens if woman still has uterus
> • HRT contraindicated by breast/endometrial carcinoma

BIBLIOGRAPHY

Dewhurst J 1980 Practical pediatric and adolescent gynecology. Marcel Dekker, New York
Shearman R P 1985 Clinical reproductive endocrinology. Churchill Livingstone, Edinburgh

22. Disorders of the menstrual cycle

AMENORRHOEA

Primary amenorrhoea has been previously described in Chapter 20.

Secondary amenorrhoea is defined as the cessation of menses for 3 or more months.

Aetiology

There are numerous causes of amenorrhoea although the commonest are physiological. Amenorrhoea may result from any disorder of the endocrine or central nervous system or abnormalities of the target organ.

Physiological causes. These include pregnancy, the puerperium, lactation and the menopause.

Psychogenic factors. Emotional stress is a common cause of amenorrhoea. It often occurs where the environment is changed, as for example when a woman changes her occupation or leaves her home environment for institutional life. This problem usually resolves itself, but may persist for some years.

Pseudocyesis

Pseudocyesis, or false pregnancy, occurs in women who have a strong desire to have a child, but are unsuccessful in conceiving. Cessation of the periods is accompanied by abdominal distension, breast enlargement and occasional galactorrhoea. When confronted with evidence that she is not pregnant, menstruation usually returns and the abdominal distension subsides. Further supportive measures, reassurance and investigation and treatment of the underlying subfertility are also required.

Anorexia nervosa

There is a critical relationship between body weight and menstruation. Thus, if body weight falls between the 10th and 15th centile, there is a high probability that amenorrhoea will develop. This may result from vigorous dieting, but it is often a manifestation of anorexia nervosa (Fig. 22.1). This condition is characterized by an extreme neurotic aversion to food. There is usually an underlying emotional problem with conflicts over sexuality, obsession with weight loss associated with a persistent refusal to eat adequately, and self-induced vomiting or purgation.

The patient often complains of pain intolerance

Fig. 22.1 Anorexia nervosa is associated with profound weight loss and amenorrhoea

and develops a widespread growth of fine body hair. Gonadotrophin and oestrogen levels are low but, unlike panhypopituitarism, other hormone levels are normal. This is a serious condition which results in death in 10–15% of the subjects involved. Early recognition is important because it is essential to supplement dietary replacement with long-term psychiatric therapy.

Hypothalamic and pituitary disorders

Hypogonadotrophic amenorrhoea

The commonest condition encountered in this group is one of hypothalamic amenorrhoea. The patient develops amenorrhoea, but has normal prolactin levels and a normal pituitary fossa. This form of amenorrhoea often occurs in women who are underweight and who have a previous history of menstrual irregularity. Gonadotrophin, prolactin and oestradiol levels are all low.

Galactorrhoea—amenorrhoea syndromes

These are associated with hyperprolactinaemia and the presence of pituitary microadenomas. All patients with secondary amenorrhoea should have a prolactin estimation and, if the levels are abnormally raised, then an X-ray of the pituitary fossa is essential. If this film shows evidence of distortion of the sella turcica with 'double flooring' of the

Fig. 22.2 Lateral skull X-ray in the presence of 'double' flooring' of the pituitary fossa (arrow)

pituitary fossa then further tomographic views must be taken (Fig. 22.2). This condition is also known as the **Chiari–Frommel syndrome**.

Pituitary disorders

Apart from the presence of pituitary adenomas, pituitary amenorrhoea may occur where there is destruction from postpartum damage as in Sheehan's syndrome, or where there is surgically inflicted damage.

Secondary hypothalamic dysfunction

This condition can be iatrogenic and is sometimes induced by the administration of sex steroids as in the pill or by the use of psychotropic drugs such as the phenothiazines. These compounds are associated with hyperprolactinaemia. Thyroid and adrenocortical diseases or severe chronic systemic disease may also cause amenorrhoea.

Ovarian insufficiency

Surgical removal of the ovaries or destruction by radiation or infection results in secondary amenorrhoea. Ovarian neoplasms, particularly those associated with excessive production of oestrogen or testosterone, may cause amenorrhoea but constitute only a very small percentage of known causes. Auto-immune disease of the ovaries is a rare condition which sometimes presents as a premature menopause. Polycystic ovarian syndrome (Stein-Leventhal syndrome) usually causes oligomenorrhoea rather than true secondary amenorrhoea.

Failure of uterine response

Damage to the target organ may result in secondary amenorrhoea (Fig. 22.3). This includes surgical removal of the uterus or damage to the endometrium as with Asherman's syndrome. In this condition, overvigorous curettage, particularly when performed in the presence of endometritis, results in the formation of intra-uterine adhesions or synechiae. Destruction of the endometrium may also result from tuberculous infection. Cervical stenosis may cause retention of endometrial products within the uterine cavity — a condition known as **cryptomenorrhoea**.

Asherman's syndrome   Cervical stenosis

Fig. 22.3 Abnormalities of the cervix and uterine cavity resulting in secondary amenorrhoea

Investigations

A great deal of important information can be obtained from a careful history and examination. In the majority of cases nothing abnormal is found on clinical examination. In the absence of clinical evidence of thyroid or adrenal diseases it is unusual to find biochemical evidence. The differential diagnosis is established by the measurement of serum oestradiol, FSH and LH, prolactin and progesterone levels.

The administration of medroxyprogesterone acetate 10 mg daily for 5 days will produce withdrawal bleeding only in a functional uterus with an intact endometrium and a patent outflow tract.

Secondary amenorrhoea may result from stenosis of the cervix secondary to previous surgical trauma.

Management

The treatment depends on the cause. Outside of the physiological group, the vast majority of cases are hypothalamic in origin. Most of these will eventually resolve spontaneously. However, the uterus is often small and oestradiol levels are low. This also applies in the 'postpill' group and, in some cases, it is useful to administer cyclical oestrogen therapy.

Where the amenorrhoea is associated with a desire to conceive, it is appropriate to treat it by the administration of exogenous gonadotrophins, but if amenorrhoea is the only problem then it is inappropriate to stimulate ovulation.

Cryptomenorrhoea

Secondary amenorrhoea may be due to retention of menstrual products because of cervical stenosis, as a result of surgical trauma or infection. This may occur in the presence of malignant disease of the cervix.

Amenorrhoea

- No period for 3 or more months
- Most common cause physiological
- Can also be iatrogenic or associated with chronic illness or body weight < 10th centile
- Drug history, history of previous curettage/cervical surgery

DYSMENORRHOEA

Dysmenorrhoea or painful menstruation is the commonest of all gynaecological symptoms.

Primary dysmenorrhoea occurs in the absence of any significant pelvic pathology. It usually develops within the first 2 years of the menarche and is often familial, with a strong likelihood that the attitude of the mother may influence the response of the daughter. Nevertheless, it would be a mistake to underestimate the severity of dysmenorrhoea in some women. The pain is often intense and cramping and can be crippling and severely incapacitating so that it becomes a major interference in social activities. It is usually associated with the onset of menstrual blood loss but may begin on the day preceding menstruation. The pain only occurs in ovulatory cycles, is lower abdominal in nature but sometimes radiates down the anterior aspect of the thighs (Fig. 22.4). The pain often disappears or improves after the birth of the first child. Dysmenorrhoea is often associated with vomiting and diarrhoea. Pelvic examination reveals no abnormality of the pelvic organs.

Secondary or **acquired dysmenorrhoea** is caused by organic pelvic pathology and it usually has its onset many years after the menarche.

Any woman who develops secondary dysmenorrhoea should be considered to have organic pathology in the pelvis until proved otherwise.

Pelvic examination is particularly important in this situation and, if the findings are negative, laparoscopy is indicated. Common associated path-

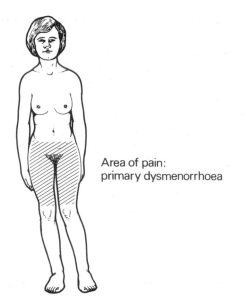

Area of pain:
primary dysmenorrhoea

Fig. 22.4   Distribution of pain experienced in dysmenorrhoea; there may also be symptoms of lumbar and sacral backache

ologies include endometriosis, adenomyosis, pelvic infections and intra-uterine lesions such as submucous fibroid polyps.

Investigations

A careful history is of great importance in this condition. Pelvic examination may not be helpful in primary dysmenorrhoea but it is advisable to perform either a vaginal or rectal examination to exclude any obvious pelvic pathology. However, in secondary dysmenorrhoea a pelvic examination is essential and, if pelvic pathology is not palpable, laparoscopy is advisable. This is only performed in cases with primary dysmenorrhoea if the condition is particularly resistant to therapy.

Management

Primary dysmenorrhoea

Discussion and reassurance are an essential part of management. Primary dysmenorrhoea tends to present some months after the menarche and is associated with ovulatory cycles, early cycles frequently being anovulatory. The intensity of pain may be aggravated by apprehension and fear,

and reassurance that the pain does not indicate any serious disorder may lessen the symptoms. It is also common for the pain to either disappear or substantially lessen after the birth of the first child.

Drug therapy

Dysmenorrhoea can be effectively treated by drugs that inhibit prostaglandin synthesis and hence uterine contractility. These drugs include aspirin, mefenamic acid, naproxen or ibuprofen. As dysmenorrhoea is often associated with vomiting, headache and dizziness, it may be advisable to start therapy either on the day before the period is expected, or as soon as the menstrual flow commences. Mefenamic acid is given in a dose of 250 mg 6-hourly. This drug also reduces menstrual flow in some women with menorrhagia.

If these drugs are inadequate, suppression of ovulation with the contraceptive pill is highly effective in reducing the severity of dysmenorrhoea. Where it is ineffective, then careful consideration should be given to the possibility of underlying pathology.

If all conservative medical therapy fails, then relief may sometimes be achieved by mechanical dilatation of the cervix or by the surgical removal of the pain fibres to the uterus in an operation known as presacral neurectomy, but these methods of treatment should be approached with considerable caution.

In cases of secondary dysmenorrhoea, the treatment is dependent on the nature of the underlying pathology. If the pathology is not amenable to medical therapy, the symptoms may only be relieved by hysterectomy.

Dysmenorrhoea

- Primary: usually normal pelvic examination and improves spontaneously
- Secondary: endometriosis, infection and intra-uterine lesions
- Management: treat any underlying cause, prostaglandin inhibitors, suppression of ovulation.

DYSFUNCTIONAL UTERINE BLEEDING

This term describes the occurrence of abnormal uterine bleeding for which an organic cause cannot

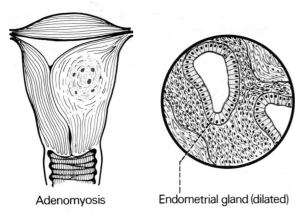

Adenomyosis   Endometrial gland (dilated)

Fig. 22.5 Adenomyosis may cause dysmenorrhoea and menorrhagia and is an important consideration in the differential diagnosis of dysfunctional uterine bleeding (left); histological features (right)

possible to exclude some types of benign organic disease.

Adenomyosis is associated with invasion of the myometrium by endometrial glands and may cause menorrhagia and dysmenorrhoea, but is not associated with any histological abnormality of the endometrium (Fig. 22.5).

The pathophysiology of dysfunctional uterine bleeding is poorly understood and therefore classification is generally unsatisfactory. Abnormalities of uterine bleeding most commonly occur at the extremes of menstrual life and particularly in the premenopausal years. These conditions are classified as ovular or anovular.

be found. The diagnosis can be made only by excluding any pathology both by examination and by diagnostic curettage. It may, however, be im-

Ovular dysfunctional uterine haemorrhage (Fig. 22.6)

The pattern of the menstrual cycle and menstrual loss may be altered by defects of the corpus

Defective degeneration of corpus luteum

Menorrhagia

Epimenorrhagia

Fig. 22.6 Disturbance of menstrual flow in dysfunctional uterine bleeding luteum or by shortening of the follicular phase of development.

Functional epimenorrhoea and epimenorrhagia

Factors which affect the pituitary–ovarian axis will alter the periodicity of the menstrual cycle. The follicular phase is shortened but the luteal phase tends to remain constant. Changes in the periodicity of the menstrual cycle and, in particular, shortening of the cycle commonly occur:

1. After pregnancy.
2. Following the menarche.
3. Preceding the menopause.

Functional menorrhagia

Abnormalities of menstrual loss may occur on a regular cyclical basis. The number of days of bleeding may remain constant and the loss become heavy or the number of days of bleeding may become prolonged, although the loss may be slight for many of these days. Two common abnormal forms of ovular dysfunctional bleeding occur:

1. Defective corpus luteum formation — irregular spotting and blood loss occurs for some days preceding the onset of menstruation. The endometrium shows only patchy progestational changes.

2. Defective degeneration of the corpus luteum — slow degeneration of the corpus luteum results in slight bleeding which persists for several days after completion of the normal period. The endometrium in such patients shows patchy progestational changes in the early proliferative phase.

Anovular dysfunctional uterine haemorrhage

Metropathia haemorrhagica

This condition most commonly occurs around the time of the menopause but may also occur in the adolescent female. The history classically involves a period of amenorrhoea followed by prolonged, heavy and irregular bleeding of such severity that it may occasionally be life threatening. The persistence of an unruptured follicular cyst in one ovary results in extended and excessive oestrogen production causing cystic or adenomatous endometrial hyperplasia. The endometrium becomes greatly thickened and when it can no longer be sustained by the continuing high levels of oestrogen it eventually breaks down in a patchy fashion. The haemorrhage commonly follows a period of 6–8 weeks amenorrhoea. Myometrial hyperplasia also occurs so that the uterus is often bulky, the endometrium being up to one centimetre thick and having the characteristic 'Swiss cheese' appearance (Fig. 22.7).

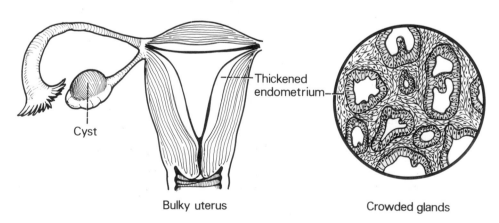

Fig. 22.7 Metropathia haemorrhagica—caused by persistent production of high levels of oestrogen (left); histological features (right)

Differential diagnosis

The diagnosis of dysfunctional uterine haemorrhage is made partly on the actual history and findings and partly by excluding other factors. It is, therefore, important to:

1. Obtain an accurate medical and menstrual history.
2. Perform a careful general examination to look for signs of endocrine disorders such as the Stein–Leventhal syndrome, hyperthyroidism or myxoedema and Cushing's disease.
3. Perform a pelvic examination to exclude any obvious local pathology.
4. Obtain a cervical smear. In practical terms this is unlikely to be productive, as most malignant lesions of the cervix that cause irregular bleeding are readily apparent on clinical examination. Nevertheless it is an essential part of the pelvic examination in a woman with irregular bleeding in the latter part of her menstrual life.

The cause of abnormal uterine haemorrhage is at least, in part, related to the age of the patient (Fig. 22.8). Around the time of puberty it most commonly results from dysfunctional uterine haemorrhage. During the reproductive years, the commonest causes of abnormal vaginal bleeding are disorders of pregnancy. Near the menopause the incidence of uterine malignancy rises sharply and abnormal bleeding most commonly results from malignancy, benign pelvic tumours and dysfunctional uterine haemorrhage.

Any of these conditions may occur in any age group, but the balance of probabilities may significantly affect the scope of clinical investigation. In the older age group, examination under anaesthesia and diagnostic curettage is essential. The presence of pelvic tumours does not exclude the possibility of uterine malignancy and diagnostic curettage may still be necessary. Uterine pathology such as endometrial polyps and submucous fibroids may be missed at curettage. The diagnosis in such cases may be established by hysterography. This involves the injection of small quantities of radio-opaque dye into the uterine cavity, which will outline space-occupying lesions. The diagnosis may also be established by hysteroscopy and clinical examination of the uterine cavity.

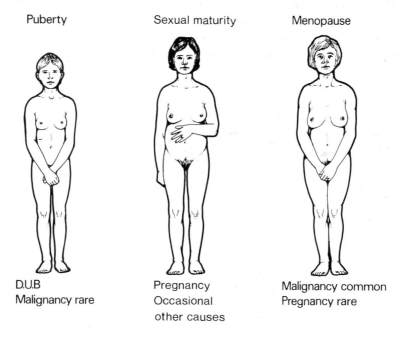

Puberty	Sexual maturity	Menopause
D.U.B Malignancy rare	Pregnancy Occasional other causes	Malignancy common Pregnancy rare

Fig. 22.8 Irregular vaginal blood loss poses a different diagnostic and management problem at different ages (DUB = dysfunctional uterine bleeding)

Treatment

The management of dysfunctional uterine haemorrhage depends in part on the age of the female.

Dysfunctional uterine haemorrhage around the menarche

Abnormal uterine haemorrhage around the time of the menarche is nearly always hormonally based as malignant disease at this age is extremely rare. It is therefore reasonable to introduce medical management without initial curettage. Initial assessment should include clinical examination and haemoglobin estimation with a complete blood picture. It is important to exclude blood dyscrasia and pregnancy. Abnormal bleeding can sometimes be controlled by the combined contraceptive pill with a high dose combination of oestrogen and progestogen. Occasionally, it may be necessary to give a loading dose of oestrogen using a compound such as Premarin® (conjugated equine oestrogen) followed by cyclical combined therapy for a period of 3 months. The problem will usually resolve itself after medical treatment but occasionally a therapeutic curettage might be necessary, as well as blood transfusion or iron therapy. Compounds such as Danol® may also be given for 3 months on a continuous basis; this compound will completely suppress menstruation.

Perimenopausal dysfunctional uterine haemorrhage

In the older age group, it is essential to perform diagnostic curettage to exclude the possibility of uterine malignancy. Once the diagnosis has been established, curettage may itself effect a cure, particularly following a single episode, and is sufficient to resolve the problem in 60% of cases. If the bleeding has been prolonged and irregular, it is sensible to suppress menstruation for 3 months with Danol® or to regulate menstrual bleeding and suppress ovulation by using a combined contraceptive pill for three cycles. The prognosis for conservative management is not good if:

1. The uterus is bulky.
2. The haemoglobin level is less than 10 g% at presentation.

3. Irregular bleeding has persisted for more than 1 year.

Under these circumstances, it may be necessary to proceed to hysterectomy.

Dysfunctional uterine bleeding

- Abnormal uterine bleeding with no apparent organic cause
- Pattern of bleeding and age of patient key features in history
- Essential to exclude pregnancy in young patients and malignancy in old
- Treatment by high dose progestogens or Danol®, curettage/hysterectomy

PREMENSTRUAL TENSION

Premenstrual tension or the premenstrual syndrome is a common episodic condition that afflicts many women and can sometimes be incapacitating in its severity. Most women experience some changes in mood during the menstrual cycle and minor symptoms of breast tenderness and weight gain. If these symptoms become severe in the premenstrual week,

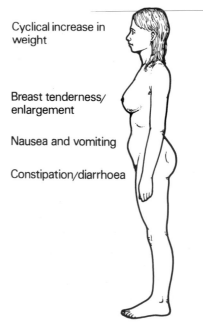

Cyclical increase in weight

Breast tenderness/enlargement

Nausea and vomiting

Constipation/diarrhoea

Fig. 22.9 Premenstrual syndrome presents with a variety of physical and psychological symptoms that tend to be worse in the week before menstruation then the condition is defined as the premenstrual syndrome (Fig. 22.9).

Symptoms and signs

The condition is commonly precipitated by stress and tension, either at home or at work, and particularly afflicts women during the third decade of life. The common symptoms include:

1. Behavioural changes — there are symptoms of depression and tension often associated with unreasonable outbursts of temper. Suicide occurs more often in the premenstrual week and minor crimes are also more frequent in the second half of the cycle.
2. Symptoms of bloatedness — many women experience these symptoms. Their clothing feels uncomfortably tight and this symptom does not subside until the onset of menstruation. Although there is a cyclical increase in weight in both symptomatic and asymptomatic women in the premenstrual week, weight gain is not usually excessive in those with premenstrual tension. The exception is the small group of women who suffer from cyclical oedema, where generalized oedema and oliguria occur in the second half of the cycle.
3. Breast symptoms — breast tenderness, enlargement of the breast and heaviness and pain are features of the syndrome in most women.
4. Gastrointestinal symptoms — nausea and vomiting and constipation or diarrhoea occur occasionally but are not major symptoms.

Pathogenesis

The mechanism of premenstrual tension remains unclear. The difficulty in studying this condition is one of definition as the symptoms are so protean. Various hypotheses have been explored, particularly in relation to the balance between oestrogen and progesterone, to the excessive production of prolactin, aldosterone or antidiuretic hormone, or to hypoglycaemia. None of these hypotheses have been substantiated.

Management

The first important aspect of management is to discuss the symptoms fully and to explore the social background particularly in relation to domestic and work tensions.

Some women lose their symptoms when they take the contraceptive pill but this is not invariably the case. Progesterone therapy administered as intramuscular injections or suppositories produces relief of symptoms. Bromocriptine is effective only in the relief of breast symptoms.

Diuretics have been widely employed and most of them produce some relief in symptoms of bloatedness. Of these compounds, the most effective is probably spironolactone given from day 12 to 26 of a 28-day cycle.

Complete suppression of the menstrual cycle will reduce the symptoms but is rarely acceptable as a method of treatment.

The simplest form of treatment is to give pyridoxine 100 mg daily. This produces a reduction in prolactin synthesis and is a safe and effective form of therapy.

Reassurance and support must be an important and continuing requirement in the treatment of premenstrual tension and it may be necessary to try a variety of therapies before a satisfactory response can be obtained.

The assessment of any form of therapy is particularly difficult because of a 70–80% placebo response. It is inadvisable to accept the validity of any form of drug therapy that has not been subjected to a placebo-controlled, double blind trial, as virtually any form of therapy will produce an improvement in symptoms in some women.

Premenstrual tension

- Key features are cyclical changes occurring in the week prior to, and ceasing within 48 hours of, the onset of menstruation
- Most common symptoms are mood changes, breast tenderness, bloating and GI changes
- Management involves establishing the diagnosis, counselling, pyridoxine and suppression of ovulation in some cases

---

BIBLIOGRAPHY

Jacobs H S 1985 Reproductive endocrinology. In: Clinics in Obstetrics and Gynaecology. W B Saunders, Eastbourne
Shearman R P 1985 Clinical reproductive endocrinology. Churchill Livingstone, Edinburgh

23. Disorders of sexual function

Disorders of sexual function may be divided into those that have a strictly organic basis and those that are predominantly functional. In most disorders, there are areas of overlap.

DISORDERS WITH AN ORGANIC BASIS

Two conditions have a predominantly organic basis:

1. Apareunia

This term defines the 'absence' of intercourse or the inability to have intercourse at all.
The common causes are:

1. Congenital absence of the vagina.
2. Imperforate hymen.
3. Impotence.

The treatment depends on the cause. Surgical treatment by vaginoplasty or by incision of the imperforate hymen is effective. The treatment of impotence will be discussed later in this chapter.

2. Dyspareunia

Dyspareunia is defined as painful intercourse. It is predominantly but not exclusively a female problem. The aetiology is divided on the basis of whether the condition is superficial or deep and it is therefore particularly important to obtain a concise history.

Superficial dyspareunia (Fig. 23.1)

Pain felt on penetration is generally associated with a local lesion of the vulva or vagina from one of the following causes:

1. Infections — local infections of the vulva and

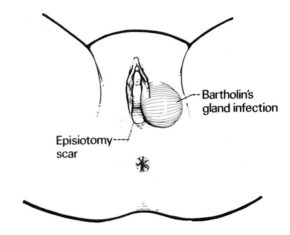

Fig. 23.1 Common causes of superficial dyspareunia

vagina. These commonly include monilial and trichomonas vulvo-vaginitis. Infections involving Bartholin's glands also cause dyspareunia.
2. Narrowing of the introitus – this may be congenital with a narrow hymenal ring or vaginal stenosis. It may sometimes be associated with a vaginal septum. The commonest cause of narrowing of the introitus is the over-vigorous suturing of an episiotomy wound or vulval laceration or following vaginal repair of a prolapse.
3. Menopausal changes — atrophic vaginitis or the narrowing of the introitus and the vagina from the effects of oestrogen deprivation may cause dyspareunia. Atrophic vulval conditions such as kraurosis vulvae can also cause pain.
4. Functional changes — lack of lubrication associated with inadequate sexual stimulation and emotional problems will result in dyspareunia. Vaginismus is a condition caused by spasm of

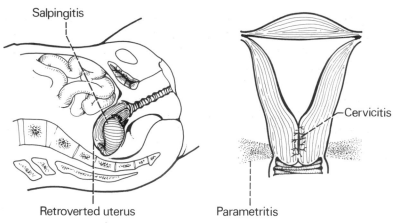

Fig. 23.2   Deep-seated dyspareunia can be caused by a variety of pelvic diseases and uterine displacement

the pelvic floor muscles and adductor muscles of the thigh, which results in pain on attempted penetration. This condition will be discussed later in this chapter.

Deep dyspareunia

Pain on deep penetration is often associated with pelvic pathology. Any woman who develops deep dyspareunia after enjoying a normal sexual life should be considered to have an organic cause for her pain until proved otherwise. The common causes of deep dyspareunia include (Figs 23.2 and 23.3):

1. Acute or chronic pelvic inflammatory disease — including cervicitis, pyosalpinx and salpingo-oophoritis. The uterus may become fixed. Ectopic pregnancy must also be considered in the differential diagnosis in this group.
2. Retroverted uterus and prolapsed ovaries — if the ovaries prolapse into the Pouch of Douglas, and become fixed in that position, intercourse is painful on deep penetration.
3. Endometriosis — both the active lesions and the chronic scarring of endometriosis may cause pain.
4. Neoplastic disease of the cervix and vagina — at least part of the pain in this situation is related to secondary infection.
5. Postoperative scarring — this may result in narrowing of the vaginal vault and loss of mobility of the uterus. The stenosis commonly occurs following vaginal repair and, less often, following

Pyosalpinx

Fig. 23.3   Chronic or acute pelvic inflammatory disease such as pyosalpinx commonly causes dyspareunia repair of a high vaginal tear. Vaginal scarring may also be caused by chemical agents such as rock salt which, in some countries, is put into the vagina in order to produce contracture.

6. Foreign bodies — occasionally, a foreign body in the vagina or uterus may cause pain in either the male or female partner. For example, the remnants of a broken needle or partial extrusion of an intra-uterine device may cause severe pain in the male partner.

Treatment

Accurate diagnosis is dependent on careful history taking and a thorough pelvic examination. The treatment will therefore be dependent on the cause.

Medical treatment includes the use of antibiotics and antifungal agents for pelvic infection and long-term Danol® or progestagen therapy for endo-metriosis. Surgical treatment includes correction of any stenosis, ventrosuspension of the retroverted uterus, excision of painful scars where appropriate, and reassurance and sexual counselling in functional disorders.

DISORDERS WITH NO ORGANIC BASIS

The most frequently occurring disorders include:

1. Premarital anxiety.
2. Frigidity.
3. Non-consummation.
4. Impotence, including premature ejaculation.

Recognition

Sexual unhappiness finds expression in many different ways. Sometimes it is accompanied by awareness of the underlying disturbance, but often, as in other emotional difficulties, the link between cause and manifestation is obscure even to the sufferer. Sexual problems may therefore appear in the guise of mental or physical illness or disturbances of behaviour and relationships and thus form a part of the working experience not only of doctors but of anyone in the 'caring' professions.

Sexual difficulties underlie many cases of vague ill health in women which defy diagnosis until repeated attempts at communication have been made. Complaints are often ill-defined but affect the life of the patient and her family. Lack of energy, backache and irritability are common problems but, understandably enough, are often treated merely by reassurance and placebos.

The patient's emphasis on a particular aspect of her difficulties is likely to determine the doctor's choice of referral. Since symptoms of anxiety and depression are often present, psychiatric advice is frequently indicated. Sexual problems may be a presenting symptom or a part of a broader symp-tomatology in mental illness but very commonly there is sexual malfunction in an otherwise sound personality.

Some patients will go to family planning clinics. This approach is likely to be chosen by those women who focus their problems upon contraception and by those who need the reassurance which is implicit in the very existence of these clinics, namely that sexual intercourse is permissible and respectable when its purpose is love and pleasure rather than procreation.

A gynaecologist will see many such cases. Some will verbalize their problems openly and directly: others will come because they have translated their emotional difficulties into physical terms. Their inability to have the 'right' feelings has found expression as something wrong with the body. In emotional and physical terms the patient is saying 'all is not well with me as a woman'.

Each one of the basic gynaecological symptoms may be wholly or partially determined by organic pathology or by psychogenic distress. When dealing with the fear of abnormality it is as important to look for the cause of the fear as for evidence of abnormality. Dread of cancer or anxiety about a non-existent vaginal discharge may be concealing the patient's real fears.

Dyspareunia means pain associated with inter-course and there may be a physical reason for it. However, particularly in early married life, it is often an expression of sexual uneasiness. Some patients are concerned about the size of the vagina, which seems too large or small. Except for the very rare cases of structural abnormality, the size of the vagina demonstrably depends, not upon its anatomy, but upon its physiology. It is determined by muscle tone or spasm, which in turn depend upon emotional factors. It is very unusual to find a hymen or a state of vaginismus which will not respond to gentle physical and psychological exploration. Resort to surgery is likely to confirm the patient's fears of abnormality and often leaves the presenting problem unchanged.

There are some unhappy women for whom all feminine functions are burdensome from menarche to menopause. They have painful periods, symptomful pregnancies, difficult labours and a suffering change of life. It would be almost out of character were they to have a joyful sexual life.

Frigidity

Definition

In medical literature the term frigidity is used to describe a variety of conditions which range from a total lack of sexual feeling and response to the infrequent event of orgasm. It seems most realistic to include here all those cases in which a woman expresses overtly, or by implication, dissatisfaction with the quality of her sexual experience. The orientation is thus based on the patient's own expectations and hopes and on her disappointment at their lack of fulfilment.

The problem of frigidity may perhaps be most readily understood in terms of the demands which active participation and pleasure in sexual intercourse make upon any woman. In fact, in feeling she has to be open and approachable, and therefore in a position in which she is undefended, vulnerable and dependent. Orgasm demands that she abandons the self-control imposed by the conventions of everyday life and allows herself to be overcome by feelings which may reach an intensity unknown in any other human activity. On the physical level, she is required to accept her genital organs as good and wholesome and as the source of pleasure and happiness. She is required to put her trust in her man and to regard him as both strong and safe and to find his body wholly acceptable. She has to accept the possibility of pregnancy or the propriety and adequacy of birth control.

This concept provides a map indicating the probable areas of tension. In each of these areas there is likely to be a conflict between the patient's needs and desires on the one hand and her defences on the other.

Secondary frigidity

It is not uncommon for a woman to declare that all was once well with her sexual life, but that later there was a gradual or sometimes sudden decline in her interest and responsiveness. Patient and doctor may well be at a loss to understand or to reverse this change. They are likely to remain so while keeping their attention focused on the presenting symptoms, although of course a careful history may be taken and appropriate examination made. Commonly it is found that other events have taken place in the life of the patient, approximately during the time under scrutiny, which have a particular meaning to this woman. One may call these 'echo situations'. It is as though she had been sensitized in childhood to certain happenings, without obvious effect on her sexual health, but that a further dose of similar trauma had tipped the balance towards loss of sexual pleasure. For example, a major quarrel with a husband may bring to the surface stormy episodes of childhood or a father's leaving home; the death or illness of a parent may re-awaken confused and conflicting feelings relating to that parent during the formative years.

Non-consummation

All that has been said about frigidity applies with equal force to those patients who not only do not enjoy intercourse but are not able to allow it to take place. Cases of impotence in the husband are not considered here, but it is noteworthy that many a man who was described as a very poor lover proves himself surprisingly virile when his wife's problems have been overcome. An element must be mentioned which is sometimes encountered in cases of frigidity but which is much more in evidence in non-consummation. This is the element of fantasy.

In contrast to the penis, which is visible, touchable and in everyday use throughout life, the vagina is mysterious and unexplored. The hymen is regarded as almost a sacred barrier guarding not simply a physical structure, but also the semimystical concept of virginity.

Reality is not readily available to confront the fantasies which flourish in the soil of sexual immaturity. The mind's eye has a picture which is undefined by structure but determined by feelings and fears scarcely affected by intellectual knowledge. The hymen may be thought of as a rigid wall which will have to be 'broken in' with much pain and bleeding. The vagina appears as tiny and fragile or as an enormous cavity communicating with everything else in the abdomen. Others have feared penetration into the urethra, the anus or the cervical os. Dread of penetration has become intelligible.

Psychopathology

Mature sexuality has a complex derivation, rooted and broadly determined in infancy but affected by events and relationships throughout childhood and adolescence. The relationship which a child forms with its mother in the first months of life provides the foundation for future emotional health and thereby of sexual health also.

The adult gender role appears to be greatly influenced by a child's capacity to find in the parent of the same sex an adequate model for its own development and to retain at the same time a sound relationship with the other parent. A boy, therefore, has to turn from his initial total involvement with his mother to finding a pattern of masculinity in his father, but nevertheless, to maintain a safe and satisfying relationship with his mother. It may be that the commoner occurrence in men of problems of sexual misdirection is partially explained by the difficulties which arise in this complex emotional change. In women, on the other hand, the common problems are those of failure of full development, rather than deviation from the accepted norm.

A study of cases of frigidity and similar sexual problems suggests that the roots of these problems are to be found in several aspects of child development.

1. The mother–infant relationships

This relationship contains on a pregenital level many elements which may later enrich a sexual relationship. It can provide the first and most deeply felt experience of warmth and tenderness and of physical closeness to another person. The child gives pleasure to its mother by being and not by doing. Its weakness and its needs are accepted without patronage. The body and that which it produces is handled lovingly and without distaste. Many fields of psychological research have provided ample evidence to confirm the damaging effect of interference with this relationship on the personality as a whole.

2. Later parent–child relationships

In several respects, childhood difficulties are mirrored in future sexual problems. Many patients demonstrate their inability to tolerate dependence upon others and scoff at any sign of weakness. They set themselves high standards of sensible behaviour and rigid self control. They are unable to accept a childish component of adult personality and attempt to put firm restrictions on all uncontrolled feeling which seems silly or noisy or messy. Often there emerges the picture of a miniature adult, an only child, or the eldest of a family, struggling hard to comply with real or imagined parental demands, tackling the sadness of unsatisfied childish needs by a denial of these needs.

Parental attitudes towards the body and its function also continue to exert their influence from childhood to adolescence, and sometimes into adult life. If these are prudish and prohibitive, it is likely that the child will learn to regard the body, and particularly the genital area, as unpleasant or even dirty. Some women find the vulva and even the breasts ugly and untouchable. Stern disapproval of masturbation will tend to endow any form of sexual excitement with guilt.

3. The mother–daughter relationship

Few patients have spoken of their mothers with easy, assured affection. Many have unhesitatingly blamed them for their sexual difficulties, while others have used excessive devotion to veil an intolerable antagonism. Criticisms have been varied and conflicting. Mothers have been accused of making sex seem a 'wife's duty' or frankly disgusting, of being too sexy or not sexy enough, of being too dominating or too submissive, of failing to tell the daughter the facts or of always talking about sex.

Like Homer's mariners who had to find their way between Scylla and Charybdis, mothers have to steer a difficult course in helping their daughters to grow towards mature womanhood by being themselves moral but not prohibitive, encouraging but not seductive, available and supporting but not intrusive. A daughter demands from her mother her blessing for her own sexuality and permission to find pleasure untainted by guilt, rivalry or envy.

4. The father–daughter relationship

A daughter seeks from her father support and affection which is a tribute to her femininity, but does not obtrude his own sexuality; she needs to see the relationship between her parents as sufficiently secure to withstand any unconscious desire of her own to have her father to herself. She will be greatly helped in establishing her own social and sexual feminine role if she can find in him an example of strength and dependability with whom she knows her mother to be safe and which will form the basis of her own attitude to men.

5. Difficulties in relationships with men

If there develops during childhood a deeply felt envy of boys, this may lead to a resentful conviction that a man always has the best of things in life and therefore engender an unwillingness to give pleasure, even though this attitude is likely to defeat her own hopes for fulfilment. Uneasiness in the feminine role is sometimes spoken of as a feeling of being 'used'.

There may be an unconscious attempt to deal with envy by the adoption of a bossy or contemptuous manner or in gentler personalities by treating men like boys or babies. The ways in which such attitudes may hinder the development of healthy sexuality can readily be imagined.

Although in some cases it seems that emotional difficulties are related to defects of personality of one or both parents, the child's contribution to family relationships must not be ignored. However irreproachable parental behaviour and personality may appear to be, it does not necessarily follow that the child will be able to accept them without prejudice or distortion.

Treatment

Congenital absence of sexual drive is unknown and therefore treatment requires to be directed towards understanding and overcoming the obstacles which prevent its free expression. It is hoped to achieve this end by the establishment of a doctor-patient relationship which has within it the potential for bringing about emotional change for the patient.

The way in which the patient enters into the relationship, her attitudes and behaviour enable the doctor to gain insight into her case. A woman's appearance and manner often provide evidence of her difficulty in accepting the feminine role. An attempt is made to understand and to help her to understand the meaning of exaggeration or denial. These patients frequently express themselves in richly symbolic language and this is freely interpreted. Some are withdrawn and hostile and need help to face their underlying conflicts. It is hoped that an atmosphere will be established in which the patient is able to express fears and feelings which had hitherto seemed quite intolerable. Although the treatment relationship which makes this possible is clearly of great importance it is usually built up with surprising rapidity. This may be because the patient enters it on the most intimate level of her personality. Against this background, vaginal examination becomes a significant experience for the patient. When indicated, she is encouraged to examine herself. Often for the first time she becomes aware of her own physical femininity and is able to confront fantasy with a reality which is not only intellectually appreciated, as it might have been through books or lectures, but which is linked by the nature of the treatment to her own feelings.

Prognosis

As a result of treatment, many patients are able to reach complete sexual fulfilment. Others find an increase of warmth and tolerance and a relief of tension, which indicate that the treatment has been worthwhile. Some remain unchanged; among these are those who are unwilling to enter into this type of treatment and do not return after one or two visits. The prognosis is best for cases of non-consummation, secondary frigidity and frigidity in the young but, commonly, good results are achieved in older women.

Impotence

Under this heading must be considered:

1. Failure to achieve erection.
2. Premature ejaculation.
3. Inability to ejaculate.
4. Lack of sexual interest.

All or any of these may be present from adolescence or have their onset at any time of life after a period of healthy sexuality.

By far the most common causes of all forms of impotence are psychological. Occasionally, a physical origin is found, probably endocrine, metabolic or neurological. It seems reasonable to suppose that where there is a capacity for masturbation, involving full erection and ejaculation, difficulties in intercourse have a psychological basis.

Depression, reactive or endogenous, is an important aetiological or concomitant condition. It appears to be a particularly common cause of loss of sexual interest in cases where this was previously lively.

A wife's contribution to the problem also requires consideration — one may not be dealing with an inability to swim but with an understandable reluctance to jump into cold water!

The effect of ageing is important and interesting. Many men who are troubled by failing sexual energy, or even by an occasional unsuccessful attempt, fear that this is due to a premature ageing process. Since many such men show no other evidence of ageing, it seems more realistic to search for signs of depression or for the kind of situation mentioned above under the heading of secondary frigidity.

Impotence can be understood, as has been suggested in the case of sexual difficulties in women, in terms of the demands which are made upon a man and his response, conscious and unconscious, to those demands. It is required that he should be able to establish a relationship with a woman in which he is willing to give himself to her, feeling confident that he will neither suffer nor inflict pain or damage, that he will be welcomed but not devoured. He requires to be sure of his own power but, at the same time, sure of his capacity to control that power.

His confidence will be based on his past experience of relationships with women and his feelings about himself as a man. A need to settle old scores or a fear that past difficulties will be repeated is likely to present obstacles. The emotional background will have a physical counterpart and he will need to see the penis as strong but not destructive and the vagina as safe.

Treatment is by psychotherapy, somewhat along the lines mentioned earlier. The prognosis is not as good as it is for women.

Dyspareunia

- Painful intercourse
- Pain felt on penetration usually associated with local lesion of vulva/vagina
- Deep dyspareunia commonly due to pelvic inflammatory disease or endometriosis
- Organic disease needs to be excluded in new deep dyspareunia
- Non-organic causes more commonly present as superficial pain

24. Genital tract infections

The female genital tract provides direct access to the peritoneal cavity. Infection may extend to any level of the tract and, once it reaches the fallopian tubes, is usually bilateral.

The genital tract has a rich anastomosis of blood and lymphatic vessels which serve to resist infection, particularly during pregnancy.

There are other natural barriers to infection which include:

1. The physical apposition of the pudental cleft and the vaginal walls.
2. Vaginal acidity — the low pH of the vagina in the sexually mature female provides a hostile environment for most bacteria. This resistance is weakened in the prepubertal and post-menopausal female.
3. Cervical mucus, which acts as a barrier in preventing the ascent of infection.
4. The regular monthly shedding of the endometrium.

VULVOVAGINITIS

The commonest infections of the genital tract are those that affect the vulva and vagina.

Symptoms

Swelling and reddening of the vulval skin is accompanied by pruritus and occasionally proctitis and dyspareunia. When the infection is predominantly one of vaginitis, the symptoms include vaginal discharge, pruritus, dyspareunia and often dysuria.

Signs

These will depend on the cause. The appearance of the vulval skin is reddened, sometimes with ulceration and excoriation. In the sexually mature female, the vaginal walls may become ulcerated with plaques of white monilial discharge adherent to the skin or, in protozoal infections, the discharge may be copious with a greenish-white frothy appearance.

Common organisms

Protozoal infections include *Trichomonas vaginalis* – a single cell, flagellated organism which may infect the cervix, urethra and vagina. In the male the organism is carried in the urethra or prostate and infection is sexually transmitted.

Candida albicans is a yeast pathogen and occurs naturally on the skin and in the bowel. The white curd-like collections are attached to the vaginal epithelium and bleeding often occurs when removed. These infections are particularly common during pregnancy, in women taking the contraceptive pill or in diabetic women. In each instance, vaginal acidity is increased above normal and bacterial growth in the vagina is inhibited in such a way as to allow free growth of yeast pathogens which thrive well in a low-pH environment.

Diagnosis

The organisms are often seen on the Papanicolaou smear even in the absence of symptoms.

A fresh wet preparation in saline of vaginal discharge will show motile trichomonads. The characteristic flagellate motion is easily recognized and the organism can be cultured.

Candida hyphae and spores can also be seen in a wet preparation (Fig. 24.1) and can be cultured.

Candida hyphae

Fig. 24.1 Candida hyphae and spores in a wet preparation

Vulvovaginitis

- Commonest infection of genital tract
- Presents as pruritus, dyspareunia or discharge
- Common causes are *Trichomonas* and *Candida*
- Predisposing factors include pregnancy, diabetes, contraceptive pill
- Can be diagnosed by examination of fresh wet preparation of vaginal discharge

Herpes genitalis

This condition has become a major cause of concern in recent years.

The condition is caused by herpes simplex virus type 2 and is a sexually transmitted disease. The local symptoms include vaginal discharge, vulval pain, dysuria and vaginal bleeding.

The lesions include skin vesicles, multiple shallow skin ulcers and inguinal lymphadenopathy (Fig. 24.2). The infection is also associated with cervical dysplasia.

Herpes genitalis

- Caused by herpes simplex type 2 virus
- Presents with pain, bleeding and vesicles or shallow ulcers on the vagina/vulva
- Associated with cervical dysplasia
- Tends to be recurrent but with decreasing severity
- Can be transmitted to the neonate during vaginal delivery if active

Infections of Bartholin's glands

Bartholin's glands are sited between the posterior part of the labia minora and the vaginal walls and these two glands secrete mucus as a lubricant during coitus. Infection of the duct and gland results in closure of the duct and formation of a Bartholin's cyst or abscess. The condition is often recurrent and causes pain and swelling of the vulva. Bartholinitis is readily recognized by the site and nature of the swelling.

Other organisms

Non-specific bacterial infections may occur in the vagina from bowel organisms and organisms from

Herpes genitalis

Multinucleate giant cells

Fig. 24.2 Herpetic lesions of the vulva (left) are associated with the presence of multinucleate giant cells in direct smears from the vesicles (right)

the respiratory tract, such as haemophilus organisms and haemolytic streptococci. These are most commonly found in vaginal infections before puberty and after the menopause.

Vaginal discharge in the child may also be associated with the presence of a foreign body and this possibility should always be excluded. Gonococcal vulvo-vaginitis is often associated with extensive pelvic infection but may also be asymptomatic or indicated merely by vaginal discharge and dysuria.

The diagnosis can be made by demonstrating the presence of Gram negative intracellular diplococci and by anaerobic culture of discharge from the cervix and urethra. The herpes virus can be recognized from scrapings and skin biopsy and culture of vesicles in appropriate culture media. Serum antibodies are raised in well-established lesions.

Syphilis

The initial lesion appears 10–90 days after contact with the spirochaete, *Treponema pallidum*.

The primary lesion or chancre is an indurated, firm papule which may become ulcerated and has a raised firm edge (Fig. 24.3). This lesion most commonly occurs on the vulva but may also occur in the vagina or cervix. The primary lesion may be accompanied by inguinal lymphadenopathy. The chancre heals spontaneously within 2–6 weeks.

Some 6 weeks after the disappearance of the chancre, the manifestations of secondary syphilis appear. A rash develops which is maculopapular and is often associated with alopecia. Papules occur, particularly in the anogenital area and in the mouth, and give the typical appearance known as **condylomata lata.**

Swabs taken from either the primary or secondary lesions are examined microscopically under dark-ground illumination and the spirochaetes can be seen (Fig. 24.3). The serological tests have been described in a previous chapter.

The disease then progresses from the secondary phase to a tertiary phase. It may mimic almost any disease process and affect every system in the body, but the common long-term lesions are cardiovascular and neurological.

Syphilis

- Spirochaete *Treponema pallidum*
- Primary infection occurs 10–90 days after contact
- Secondary symptoms 6 weeks after primary lesion
- Can be diagnosed serologically or by detection of the organism in vesicle fluid
- Responds to penicillin

Granuloma inguinale and lymphogranuloma venereum

Both of these conditions present with infected skin eruptions on the vulva. They are sexually transmitted diseases which are rare in Western Europe but are most commonly seen in tropical countries. Granuloma inguinale is caused by *Calymmatobacterium granulomatis* and is diagnosed by the recog-

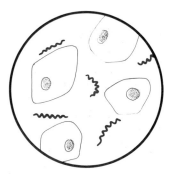

Syphilis (chancre)   Spirochaetes

Fig. 24.3 The typical lesion of primary syphilis is the chancre (left); diagnosis is established by dark-ground illumination of the spirochaetes (right) nition of Donovan bodies, bacteria encapsulated in mononuclear leucocytes. Lymphogranuloma venereum is caused by a chlamydial infection and results in a vesiculo-pustular eruption associated with a painful inguinal lymphadenitis and, in the longer term, with vulval lymphoedema which may be gross. It may also cause rectal and vaginal stenosis. The diagnosis is a positive Frei test, which involves the injection of a small volume of antigen intradermally and reading the response of the skin reaction. The histological diagnosis depends on the exhibition of a granulomatous tubercle with central fibrinoid necrosis surrounded by plasma cells.

Vulval warts (condylomata acuminata)

Vulval warts are caused by a papilloma virus. The condition is commonly, although by no means invariably, transmitted by sexual contact.

The warts have an appearance that is similar to those seen on the skin in other sites, and in the moist environment of the vulval skin are often prolific — particularly during pregnancy (Fig. 24.4). There is frequently associated pruritus and vaginal discharge. The lesions may spread to the peri-anal region, and in some cases become confluent and subject to secondary infections.

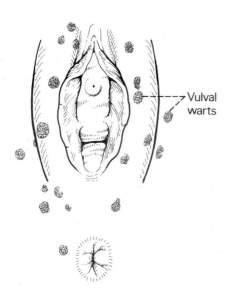

Fig. 24.4 Warts may be widespread on the vulval and peri-anal skin

Treatment of vulval and vaginal infections

When the diagnosis has been established by examination and the bacteriological tests, the appropriate treatment can be instituted.

Vulval and vaginal monilial infections are treated by topical application of nystatin, natamycin clotrimazole, miconazole nitrate, econazole nitrate of candicidin. All these compounds are inserted intravaginally as tablets, pessaries, creams or foams and should be administered over a 14-day period. Occasionally, persistent and resistant cases can be treated by painting the vagina with a 1% solution of gentian violet.

Trichomonas infections are treated with metronidazole 200 mg taken three times a day for 7 days and must be taken by both sexual partners if recurrence of the infection is to be avoided. It may be administered as a single dose of 2 g, but high dose therapy should be avoided in pregnancy. Nimorazole is also an imidazole derivative and is given as a single 2 g dose or as 1 g every 12 hours for three doses.

Chlamydial infections are treated by oral tetracycline or erythromycin in pregnancy.

Non-specific vaginal infections are common and are treated with vaginal creams including hydrargaphen, povidone–iodine, di-iodohydroxy-quinoline or sulphonamide creams.

Gonorrhoea and syphilis are treated in the first instance with penicillin and, if this fails, for example in the case of penicillin-resistant strains of the gonococcus, doxycycline hydrochloride or acrosoxacin can be used.

Infections of the vagina associated with menopausal atrophic changes are treated by the appropriate hormone replacement therapy using an oral or vaginal oestrogen preparation or lactic acid pessaries where oestrogens are contraindicated. The same therapy may be used with the local application of oestrogen creams in juvenile vulvovaginitis.

Infections of Bartholin's gland are treated with the antibiotic appropriate to the organism. If abscess formation has occurred, the abscess should be 'marsupialized' by excising an elipse of skin and sewing the skin edges to wall off the abscess cavity (Fig. 24.5). This reduces the likelihood of recurrence of the abscess.

Vulval warts are treated with either physical or

Incision   Marsupialization of cyst

Fig. 24.5 Marsupialization of a Bartholin's cyst or abscess, the incision is made over the medial aspect of the cyst (left) and the lining sutured to the skin (right)

chemical diathermy using podophyllin applied directly to the surface of the warts. Any concurrent vaginal discharge should also receive the appropriate therapy.

Herpetic infections are notoriously resistant to treatment and highly prone to recurrence. The best available treatment is acyclovir administered in tablet form 200 mg 5 times daily for 5 days or locally as a 5% cream.

INFECTIONS OF THE CERVIX

Infections that affect the vagina also produce acute and chronic cervicitis.

Acute cervicitis

Usually occurs in association with generalized infection of the genital tract and is diagnosed and treated according to the microbiology, as described in the management of vulvovaginitis.

Symptoms and signs

Acute cervicitis is associated with purulent vaginal discharge, sacral backache, lower abdominal pain, dyspareunia and dysuria. The proximity of the cervix to the bladder often results in coexistent trigonitis and urethritis, particularly in the case of gonococcal infections. The cervix appears reddened and may be ulcerated as with herpetic infections, and there is a mucopurulent discharge as the endocervix is invariably involved. The diagnosis is established by examination and taking cervical swabs for culture.

Treatment depends on the infecting organism.

Chronic cervicitis

This is an extremely common condition and is present in about 50–60% of all parous women. In many cases, the symptoms are minimal. There may be a slight mucopurulent discharge which is not sufficient to trouble the woman and may simply present as an incidental finding which does not justify active treatment.

In the more severe forms of the condition, there is profuse vaginal discharge, chronic sacral backache, dyspareunia and occasionally postcoital bleeding. The cervix is often lacerated and there is mucopurulent discharge from the cervical canal. Infection in the ducts of the endocervical glands results in obstruction of these ducts and the development of small retention cysts visible on the ectocervix. These cysts may simply contain mucus, but in more severe infections contain mucopus.

Fig. 24.6   Chronic cervicitis with infected Nabothian follicles (left); treatment is by radical cautery and needle diathermy of the follicles (right)

They are usually 2–3 mm in diameter but may be as large as 1 cm and are known as **Nabothian follicles** (Fig. 24.6). Bacteriological culture of the discharge is usually sterile. The condition may cause subfertility because of hostility of the cervical mucus to sperm invasion.

Treatment

Medical treatment is rarely effective in chronic cervicitis because it is difficult to identify an organism and antibiotics do not penetrate the chronic micro-abscesses of the cervical glands. If the cervical swab is negative, then the next most effective management is diathermy of the endocervix in order to cauterize the Nabothian follicles so that the discharge is released.

This procedure is performed under general anaesthesia as superficial chemical or physical cautery is unsatisfactory.

Following diathermy, an antibacterial cream should be placed in the vagina and the woman advised that the discharge may increase in amount for 2–3 weeks but will then diminish. She should also be advised to avoid intercourse for 3 weeks as coitus may cause secondary haemorrhage.

The two major complications of the procedure are secondary haemorrhage and postcautery stenosis. Stenosis is uncommon in the healthy parous woman but secondary haemorrhage may sometimes occur. Treatment involves packing the vaginal vault with a gauze pack soaked in an antiseptic cream such as proflavine and implementing blood

transfusion where necessary. Antibiotic cover should also be given as there will invariably be infection present.

It is occasionally necessary to suture the cervix but this is often difficult because of the oedematous state of the tissue under these circumstances.

Infections of the cervix

> - Acute (associated with generalised infection) or chronic
> - Discharge, dyspareunia, low abdominal pain or backache, urinary symptoms and postcoital bleeding
> - Can cause subfertility
> - Difficult to isolate an organism when chronic
> - Treatment includes appropriate antibiotics and cautery

Human papilloma virus (HPV)

Certain types of human papilloma virus are found in association with neoplastic changes in the cervix.

Types 6 and 11 are associated with low-grade cervical intra-epithelial neoplasia (CIN) and condylomata, whereas types 16 and 18 are associated with all grades of CIN and carcinoma of the cervix. These viruses are identified by their DNA sequences.

Factors which point towards an aetiological role for the virus in carcinoma of the cervix include:

1. Continued expression of the DNA in transferring epithelium.
2. Gene products which transform epithelial cells.
3. The particular types of HPV associated with carcinoma of the cervix will transform cells in vitro.
4. Women with the type 16 HPV have a 10-fold increased risk of developing CIN.

The immune response to this virus group appears to be relatively ineffective, and anti-HPV titres do not reflect the ability to resist further infection.

HPV DNA is present in 80–90% of cervical tumours, but it must be remembered that 30–40% of normal subjects will also be found to have HPV DNA present in cervical epithelium.

ACUTE INFECTIONS OF THE UPPER GENITAL TRACT

Acute infection of the endometrium, myometrium, Fallopian tubes and ovaries are usually the result of ascending infections from the lower genital tract (Fig. 24.7).

SITES OF INFECTION OF UPPER GENITAL TRACT

Fig. 24.7 Pelvic infections may occur by ascending from the lower genital tract or descending from the bowel or appendix

However, infection may be secondary to appendicitis or other bowel infections, which sometimes give rise to a pelvic abscess. Perforation of the appendix with pelvic sepsis remains a common cause of tubal obstruction and subfertility. Pelvic sepsis commonly occurs during the puerperium and after an abortion. Retained placental tissue and blood provide an excellent culture medium for organisms from the bowel including *E.coli*, *C. welchii* or *perfringens*, *Staphylococcus aureus* and *Streptococcus faecalis*.

The principal organism to cause acute salpingitis by sexual transmission is *Neisseria gonorrhoea*. The organism spreads across the surface of the cervix and endometrium and causes tubal infection within 1–3 days of contact. Acute infection may also be caused by *Chlamydia*.

Symptoms and signs

The symptoms of acute salpingitis include (Fig. 24.8):

1. Acute bilateral lower abdominal pain. Salpingitis is almost invariably bilateral. Where the symptoms are unilateral, an alternative diagnosis should be considered.
2. Purulent vaginal discharge.
3. A pyrexia of 38°C or more, sometimes associated with rigors.

4. Vomiting and diarrhoea.

The signs include:

1. Signs of systemic illness with pyrexia and tachycardia.
2. Signs of peritonitis with guarding or rebound tenderness.
3. On pelvic examination, acute pain on cervical excitation and thickening in the vaginal fornices which may be associated with the presence of cystic tubal swellings due to pyosalpinges or pus-filled tubes. Fullness in the Pouch of Douglas suggests the presence of a pelvic abscess.

Fig. 24.8 Acute salpingitis with reddened, oedematous Fallopian tubes and pus discharging from the fimbrial ends of the tubes

Differential diagnosis

It is often difficult to establish the diagnosis of acute pelvic infection with any degree of certainty. The differential diagnosis includes:

1. *Tubal ectopic pregnancy* — initially pain is unilateral in most cases. There are often syncopal episodes and signs of diaphragmatic irritation with shoulder tip pain. The white cell count is normal or slightly raised but the haemoglobin level is low, whereas in acute salpingitis the white cell count is raised and the haemoglobin concentration is normal.
2. *Acute appendicitis* — the most important difference in the history lies in the unilateral nature of the condition. Pelvic examination does not usually reveal as much pain and tenderness but it must be remembered that the two conditions sometimes coexist, particularly where the infected appendix lies adjacent to the right Fallopian tube.
3. *Acute urinary tract infections* — may produce similar symptoms but rarely produce signs of peritonism and are commonly associated with urinary symptoms.
4. *Torsion or rupture of an ovarian cyst.*

Investigation

When the diagnosis of acute salpingitis is suspected, the woman should be admitted to hospital. After completion of the history and general examination swabs should be taken from the cervical canal and the urethra and sent to the laboratory for culture and antibiotic sensitivity. A Gram stain of the cervical discharge should be prepared. A midstream specimen of urine should also be sent for culture.

Examination of the blood for differential white cell count, haemoglobin estimation and erythrocyte estimation rate may help to establish the diagnosis. Blood culture is indicated if there is a severe pyrexia.

Management

1. Fluid replacement by intravenous therapy. Vomiting and pain often result in dehydration.
2. Antibiotic therapy — it is sensible to treat the infection according to the organism and its sensitivity. However, the result of the cultures may not be available for 24 hours and, therefore, treatment should be started with an antibiotic such as ampicillin and metronidazole given intravenously until the acute phase of the condition begins to resolve.
3. Pain relief with opiate therapy.
4. If the uterus contains an intra-uterine device, it should be removed as soon as antibiotic therapy has been commenced.
5. Bed rest — immobilization is essential until the pain subsides.

Indications for surgical intervention

In most cases, conservative management results in complete remission. However, one episode of acute infection results in tubal obstruction in about 30% of cases and a further episode gives a 60% obstruction rate. Laparoscopy is indicated where the diagnosis is in doubt.

Laparotomy is indicated where the condition does not resolve with conservative management and where there is a pelvic mass.

In most cases, the mass will be due to a pyosalpinx or tubo-ovarian abscess. This can either be drained or a salpingectomy performed. If a pelvic abscess develops, it can be drained through the posterior fornix of the vagina by performing a posterior colpotomy.

CHRONIC PELVIC INFECTION

Acute pelvic infections may progress to a chronic state with dilatation and obstruction of the tubes forming bilateral hydrosalpinges with multiple pelvic adhesions.

Symptoms

Symptoms are varied but include:

1. Chronic pelvic pain and sacral backache.
2. Chronic purulent vaginal discharge.
3. Epimenorrhagia and dysmenorrhoea.
4. Deep-seated dyspareunia.

Chronic salpingitis is also associated with infection in the connective tissue of the pelvis known as **parametritis**.

Signs

On examination, there is a purulent discharge from the cervix. The uterus is often fixed in retroversion and there is thickening in the fornices and pain on bimanual examination.

Management

Conservative management of this condition is rarely effective and the problem is only eventually resolved by clearance of the pelvic organs.

CHRONIC TUBERCULOSIS OF THE GENITAL TRACT

Tuberculous salpingitis occurs in 5–10% of women with pulmonary tuberculosis and follows the spread of the tubercule bacillus from the primary lesion in the chest. A chronic granulomatous infection of the tubes will result in tubal obstruction and sterility.

The organism also causes chronic endometritis and the diagnosis can be established by culture and histological examination of the curettings.

Laparoscopic inspection of the tubes can also be employed to effect a diagnosis.

Management

Antibiotic therapy using drugs such as isoniazid, aminosalicylic acid, streptomycin, ethambutol and rifampicin will usually cure the condition but will not often restore fertility.

Upper genital tract infection

- Usually from ascending lower genital tract infection
- Can follow abortion or normal delivery
- Commonly due to *Neisseria gonorrhoea* or *Chlamydia* when sexually transmitted
- Presents as pain, fever, discharge and irregular periods
- Bilateral pain on cervical excitation and raised white cell count
- Differential diagnosis includes ectopic pregnancy, urinary tract infection and appendicitis
- Management includes fluid replacement, antibiotics, analgesia and rest
- Surgery is indicated to confirm diagnosis if in doubt, for drainage of pelvic mass and to clear pelvis in unresponsive chronic disease
- Major cause of infertility worldwide resulting in tubal obstruction in 60% of cases after 2 or more attacks

ACQUIRED IMMUNE DEFICIENCY SYNDROME (AIDS)

The syndrome was first recognized in 1980 with the occurrence of opportunistic infections such as *Pneumocystis carinii* in otherwise healthy young individuals, many of whom were homosexual men or drug users. There was also an increase in the incidence of Kaposi's sarcoma in young homosexual males. Various other opportunistic infections were recognized such as disseminated cytomegalovirus and toxoplasmosis infections, progressive hepatic infections and mucosal candidiasis.

AIDS occurs predominantly in homosexual males, drug users, haemophiliacs and female sexual partners of disease carriers. The disease presents with lymphadenopathy, lymphopenia and abnormal immunological markers.

Transmission of the condition is by sexual contact and by blood-borne contact. There is no evidence of direct contact transmission. There is no known treatment for the condition at the present time and there is a high mortality rate from intercurrent infections.

HIV infection

- Retrovirus infection of T helper cells and CNS
- Transmitted by sex, blood transfusion or to offspring
- Diagnosis by serology, differential lymphocyte count or opportunistic infection
- Can be asymptomatic, cause generalised malaise and lymphadenopathy or AIDS
- Incidence in heterosexuals increasing

BIBLIOGRAPHY

Spagne V A, Prior R B 1985 Sexually transmitted diseases. Marcel Dekker, New York

25. Endometriosis and adenomyosis

These terms describe the presence of endometrium in sites other than the uterine cavity. In endometriosis, the ectopic endometrium occurs in various sites outside the uterine cavity or myometrium. In adenomyosis, the endometrium exhibits aberrant growth by invading the myometrium. The glands remain in communication with the uterine cavity. Adenomyosis is sometimes known as endometriosis interna and endometriosis as endometriosis externa. Although the two conditions may coexist, they are characterized by different clinical features and do not have a common pathogenesis.

ENDOMETRIOSIS

Pathology

Aberrant endometrial deposits occur in many different sites (Fig. 25.1). Endometriosis commonly occurs in the ovaries, uterosacral ligaments and the recto-vaginal septum. It may also occur in the pelvic peritoneum covering the uterus, tubes, rectum, sigmoid colon and bladder. Remote ectopic deposits of endometrium may be found in the umbilicus, laparotomy scars, hernial scars, the appendix, vagina, vulva, cervix, lymph nodes and, on rare occasions, the pleural cavity.

Ovarian endometriosis occurs in the form of small superficial deposits on the surface of the ovary or as larger cysts known as **endometriomas**, which may grow up to 10 cm in size. These cysts have a thick whitish capsular layer and contain altered blood which has a chocolate-like appearance. For this reason, they are known as **chocolate cysts**. Endometriomas are often densely adherent both to the ovarian tissue and to other surrounding structures.

These cysts are likely to rupture and, in 8% of cases, patients with endometriosis present with symptoms of acute peritoneal irritation (Fig. 25.2).

The microscopic features of the lesions may be of endometrium that cannot be distinguished from the normal tissue lining the uterine cavity, but

Fig. 25.1 Common sites of endometriotic deposits

Fig. 25.2 Rupture of an endometriotic cyst causes acute peritonism

there is wide variation and, in many long-standing cases, desquamation and repeated menstrual bleeding may result in the loss of all characteristic features of endometrium. Underneath the lining of the cyst, there is often a broad zone containing phagocytic cells with haemosiderin. There is also a broad zone of hyalinized fibrous tissue. One of the characteristics of endometriotic lesions is the intense fibrotic reaction that surrounds them, and this may also contain muscle fibres. The intensity of this reaction often leads to great difficulty in dissection at the time of any operative procedure. The pathogenesis of endometriosis remains obscure. Sampson (1921) originally suggested that the condition was associated with retrograde spill of endometrial cells during menstruation and that some of these cells would implant under appropriate conditions in the peritoneal cavity and on the ovaries. In some cases, the spill would appear to occur from cells lining the Fallopian tubes, giving rise to a condition more appropriately known as **endosalpingiosis**.

This hypothesis does not account for endometriotic deposits outside the peritoneal cavity. An alternative theory suggests that endometrial lesions may arise from metaplastic changes in epithelium surfaces throughout the body.

Symptoms and signs

The disease most commonly presents in the third decade of life and in women of low parity. A substantial number of women are asymptomatic and present only with a history of sub-fertility. The mechanism of the association between sub-fertility and endometriosis is unknown, and cannot be explained in most instances by distention or obstruction of the tubes. An alternative explanation is that endometriosis is commonly associated with the LUF syndrome (luteinized unruptured follicles). The commonest symptom is crescendic dysmenorrhoea. Pelvic pain and swelling commence in the weeks preceding menstruation and dysmenorrhoea persists until the completion of the period. If an endometrioma ruptures, then generalized abdominal pain and peritonism may occur.

If the uterus becomes fixed or there is any adnexal mass adherent in the Pouch of Douglas, then deep-seated dyspareunia results. Menstrual disorders are not a common feature of endometriosis, but if the ovaries are extensively involved the cycle may shorten and under these circumstances menorrhagia may also occur.

The symptoms produced by lesions outside the peritoneal cavity depend on the site of the lesion. Involvement of bowel may result in melaena or, if the lesion has caused scarring and fibrosis, in bowel obstruction. Lesions of the bladder may cause haematuria. Cutaneous lesions at the umbilicus, in skin wounds and at the vulva will bleed externally on a cyclical basis. Occasional lesions in the pleural cavity cause recurrent pneumothorax.

Diagnosis

In a small number of cases, the lesion is visible on the surface, but in most patients nothing abnormal is visible or palpable on pelvic examination. In well-established disease, the uterus is often fixed in retroversion. There is thickening in the uterosacral ligaments and, if the ovaries are involved, there may be fixed cystic swellings palpable in the pelvis.

The diagnosis can be established only by direct inspection by laparoscopy or at the time of laparotomy. Cysts can be identified by ultrasound or by magnetic resonance imaging.

Management

Medical therapy

Endometriosis is a difficult condition to treat and therapy is determined by the presenting symptoms and the nature of the endometriotic lesion. It is often necessary to combine both medical and surgical treatment if the best results are to be obtained.

Endometriotic deposits respond in the same way as normal endometrium. Thus, pregnancy usually induces marked regression of the lesions. However, as the condition is commonly associated with infertility, this is rarely a practical solution to the problem. Medical therapy depends on the concept of inducing a pseudopregnancy and is most effective in the treatment of small lesions. These effects can be achieved by administration of:

1. Combined oestrogen and progestogen therapy consisting of a high dose of progestogen and a low dose of oestrogen. To prevent 'breakthrough' bleeding, it is necessary to give increasing dosages over a period of 6–9 months.

2. Progestogens-dydrogesterone 10 mg three times daily is usually sufficient to inhibit menstruation and to produce regression of small lesions. A similar effect can be achieved with oral medroxyprogesterone acetate 10 mg three times a day over a 9 month interval.

3. Androgen therapy with methyl-testosterone may produce similar effects, but has the disadvantage of its virilizing side effects and is rarely used.

An alternative approach to therapy is to induce a pseudomenopause, which is probably the most effective method of medical therapy available at the present time.

Danazol is a weak impeded androgen which causes marked gonadotrophin inhibition with minimal overt sex hormone stimulation. This produces suppression of all endogenous stimuli to the endometrium and allows regression to occur in endometriotic deposits.

Given in adequate dosage, the drug induces complete suppression of menstruation, but cessation of therapy results in the resumption of menstruation within 6 weeks. The required dosage is between 200 and 600 mg daily for 6–9 months. The drug may produce side effects which are not tolerable and may necessitate cessation of therapy. These include weight gain, oedema, fatigue, depression, increased hair growth, acne and reduced breast size. In the infertile group, success rates of 30–40% have been reported. In terms of menstrual symptoms, there is a much greater rate of relief but the symptoms often return after cessation of therapy.

Surgical treatment

Diathermy of small lesions, either at laparotomy or through the laparoscope, is the treatment of choice.

Skin lesions can be cured by excision.

Where large endometriomatous deposits occur, as with ovarian endometriomas, medical therapy is rarely effective and it is necessary to resect these lesions. Every attempt should be made to conserve ovarian tissue in these circumstances. If the uterus is fixed in retroversion and there is dyspareunia, ventrosuspension of the uterus should be performed by shortening the round ligaments and pulling the uterus anteriorly out of the Pouch of Douglas. In a limited number of situations where conservation of reproductive potential is important, pain relief can be achieved by presacral neurectomy. This procedure involves surgical transection of the presacral plexus with excision of tissue between the right ureter and superior haemorrhoidal vessels.

If all these procedures fail or there is no desire for conservation of reproductive function, then pelvic clearance is indicated with total hysterectomy and bilateral salpingo-oophorectomy. In the author's experience, hormone replacement therapy under these circumstances does not cause recurrence of the endometriotic lesions.

ADENOMYOSIS

Adenomyosis is a condition characterized by the invasion of endometrial glands and stroma into the myometrium. It is difficult to diagnose until the uterus is subjected to histological examination and, for this reason, the diagnosis is often overlooked.

Symptoms and signs

This condition, unlike endometriosis, occurs in parous women and usually arises in the fourth decade. It is associated with menorrhagia and dysmenorrhoea of increasing severity. On clinical examination, the uterus is symmetrically enlarged and tender. The condition is rare after the menopause.

Pathology

The macroscopic appearances of the uterus are those of diffuse enlargement. Adenomyosis and myomas often co-exist although the uterus is rarely enlarged to the size seen in the presence of myomas. The posterior wall of the uterus is usually thicker than the anterior wall. The cut surface of the uterus presents a characteristic whorl-like trabeculated appearance, but occasionally circumscribed nodules with dark haemorrhagic spots can be seen in the myometrium.

The microscopic diagnosis is based on the finding of islands of endometrial tissue buried deep within the myometrium. The aberrant endometrium does not respond to progesterone and the appearances are always those of proliferative endometrium. It is very rare for malignant change to occur in these lesions.

A rare variant of this condition is **stromal endometriosis**. In this condition, the stromal cells permeate into the myometrium along the lymphatic bundles and muscle fibres and, on occasions, the lesions extend through the serosa into the broad ligament. Progress of this disease is slow but it acts like a low grade malignancy and metastases are rare.

Treatment

The only satisfactory treatment of this condition is hysterectomy. The ovaries should be conserved, depending on the age of the patient. Conservative therapy with hormone preparations is rarely effective, although symptomatic relief of dysmenorrhoea with prostaglandin synthetase inhibitors is sometimes achieved.

Irradiation of the ovaries is occasionally employed to stop ovarian function, but this therapy should be reserved for women with medical problems that make surgical treatment unusually hazardous. Thus, a radiation menopause may be used in women who are excessively obese or who have a history of severe cardiac disease or thromboembolic disorders.

Endometriosis and adenomyosis

- 'Ectopic' endometrium
- Commonest sites are ovaries, uterosacral ligaments and pelvic peritoneum
- May arise from metaplastic change or implantation
- Presents as subfertility and/or crescendic dysmenorrhoea
- Management is to induce pseudopregnancy or pseudomenopause or surgical excision
- Adenomyosis is invasion of the myometrium by endometrial tissue
- Presents as menorrhagia and dysmenorrhoea

BIBLIOGRAPHY

Chalmers J A 1975 Endometriosis. Butterworths, London
Sampson A 1921 Perforating haemorrhagic (chocolate) cysts of the ovary and especially their relation to pelvic adenomas of the endometrial type. Archives of Surgery 3:245

26. Lesions of the vulva and vagina

BENIGN LESIONS OF THE VULVA

There have been numerous changes in the classification of vulvar disease, and the previous terminology of 'vulval dystrophies' has been discarded.

The following classification is now recommended:

I Non-neoplastic epithelial disorders of skin and mucosa
1. Lichen sclerosus (Lichen sclerosus et atrophicus).
2. Squamous cell hyperplasia (formerly hyperplastic dystrophy).
3. Other dermatoses.

II Classification of vulvar intra-epithelial neoplasia (VIN)
VIN I   Mild dysplasia (formally mild atypia).
VIN II   Moderate dysplasia (formally moderate atypia).
VIN III Severe dysplasia (formally severe atypia).
VIN IV   Carcinoma in situ.

This classification is based on histological appearances. The typical appearances are still described as leucoplakia and kraurosis vulvae under the general heading of squamous cell hyperplasia, and other dermatoses include psoriasis, lichen planus, lichen simplex chronicus, *Candida* infection and condyloma acuminatum. Mixed epithelial may occur and it is recommended that both descriptions should be used under these circumstances.

Where there is histological evidence of cellular atypia, the lesion should be classified as vulvar intra-epithelial neoplasia. The clinical appearances of these conditions are described under a descriptive classification which is useful only in so far as it describes the clinical appearance of these lesions.

Non-neoplastic epithelial disorders

Leucoplakia

This condition is characterized by the presence of white plaques on the vulval skin and in the perianal region and is associated with pruritus. The early stages, known as leucoplakic vulvitis, present as reddish-grey, thickened skin which later becomes white, dry and cracked.

Kraurosis vulvae

The relationship between this condition and leucoplakic vulvitis remains uncertain, but the condition consists of progressive atrophy, and shrinkage of the vulval skin (Fig. 26.1). The histological appearance is one of atrophic leucoplakic vulvitis.

Lichen sclerosus

The typical lesions of this condition, sometimes known as lichen sclerosus et atrophicus, are white papules which progress to atrophic plaques. The condition affects the perineum and peri-anal skin. However, there is considerable overlap in both the gross and histological appearances of these non-neoplastic epithelial disorders.

Aetiology

The cause of non-neoplastic epithelial disorders is unknown. These conditions are associated with a high incidence of histamine-fast achlorhydria and with pernicious anemia, hypothyroidism and hyperthyroidism. All these conditions have an auto-immune basis.

The epithelial disorders are associated with

Vaginal stenosis

Fig. 26.1 Kraurosis vulvae (left) results in stenosis of the vaginal introitus (right)

malignant change in about 5% of cases, the development of which is always preceded by atypical changes.

Treatment

It is important to biopsy the skin to establish an accurate diagnosis and classification. In addition, common infections such as trichomoniasis should be excluded. Diabetes and achlorhydria should also be excluded. The condition should be treated medically and kept under observation. Hypertrophic lesions should be treated with hydrocortisone 0.5% and occasionally topical 5-fluorouracil. In the presence of atrophic lesions, testosterone cream may sometimes be useful.

If all conservative therapy fails, it may be necessary to remove the affected skin by simple vulvectomy or by excision biopsy of visible lesions. Local treatment by laser vaporization has also been used and is appropriate where the lesions are limited and localized.

Benign tumours of the vulva

Benign cysts of the vulva include sebaceous cysts, epithelial inclusion cysts and Wolffian duct cysts, which arise from the labia minora and the periurethral region. A rare cyst may arise from a peritoneal extension along the round ligament, forming a hydrocele in the labium major. Benign

solid tumours include fibromas, lipomas and hidradenomas. Fibromas may reach an enormous size (Fig. 26.2). True squamous papillomas appear as warty growths and rarely become malignant. All of these lesions are treated by simple biopsy excision.

Vulval and vaginal trauma

Injuries to vulva and vagina may result in severe haemorrhage and haematoma formation. Vulval bruising may be particularly severe because of the rich venous plexus in the labia, and commonly results from falling astride. Lacerations of the vagina are often associated with coitus.

FIBROMA OF VULVA

Fig. 26.2 Vulval fibroids are usually pedunculated and may be very large

Vulval haematomas often subside with conservative management, but will sometimes need drainage. It is important to suture vaginal lacerations and to be certain that the injury does not penetrate into the peritoneal cavity.

Benign vulval lesions

> - Cause unknown.? auto-immune
> - Usually presents as pruritus
> - Classified by appearance or histology
> - Associated with malignant change in 5% cases
> - Need to differentiate from malignancy, infection and diabetes

MALIGNANT LESIONS OF THE VULVA

Premalignant conditions of the vulva

Carcinoma in situ of the vulva is a condition which is characterized by disorientation and loss of epithelial architecture extending through the full thickness of the epithelium. It was originally known as **Bowen's disease**. A further variant which arises from the apocrine glands is known as **Paget's disease**. The appearance of the lesions is variable but they are papular and raised and may be white, grey, dull red or various shades of brown and may be localized or widespread. These conditions are rare with an incidence of 0.53 per 100 000 and commonly occur in women over the age of 60 years.

Management

The only satisfactory treatment of this condition is local excision. It is important to establish the diagnosis by biopsy and to search for any other sites of intra-epithelial neoplasia, which are commonly found in association with the vulval lesion, particularly the cervix and vagina. Other methods of treatment include cryosurgery and the use of the CO_2 laser and, in some cases, the local application of 5-fluorouracil cream.

Carcinoma of the vulva

Carcinoma of the vulva accounts for 2–3% of female malignances. Ninety-two per cent of the lesions are squamous cell carcinomas, 5% are adenocarcinomas, 1% are basal cell carcinomas and 0.5% are malignant melanomas (Fig. 26.3). The lesions may occur at any age, but are commonest after the age of 65 years.

Chronic irritation associated with vulval dystrophies, Paget's disease of the vulva, or longstanding chronic granulomatous lesions may precede invasive carcinoma of the vulva.

Symptoms

The patient with vulval carcinoma experiences pruritis and notices a raised lesion on the vulva which may ulcerate and bleed. Malignant mela-

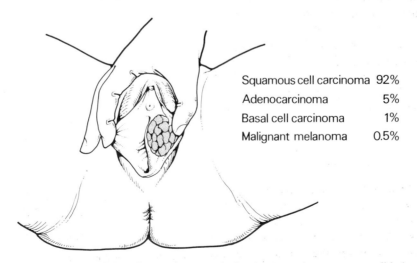

Squamous cell carcinoma 92%
Adenocarcinoma 5%
Basal cell carcinoma 1%
Malignant melanoma 0.5%

Fig. 26.3 Carcinoma of the vulva occurs at any site but is commonly a squamous cell lesion

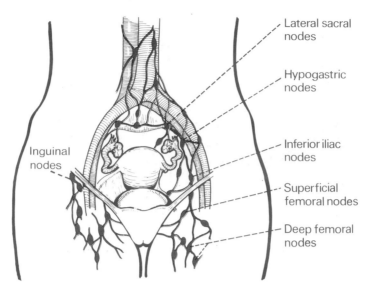

Fig. 26.4 Lymphatic drainage of the vulva

nomas are usually single, hyperpigmented and ulcerated. The tumour most frequently develops on the labia majora but may also grow on the prepuce of the clitoris, the labia minora, Bartholin's glands and in the vestibule of the vagina. Carcinoma of the vulva most commonly occurs in the sixth and seventh decades and is associated with chronic vulvitis with a high incidence of diabetes mellitus, obesity and hypertension.

Fig. 26.5 Sites of spread of vulval carcinoma

Natural history

The disease tends to progress from dysplasia through carcinoma in situ to invasion. Spread occurs both locally and through the lymphatic system (Figs 26.4, 26.5). The lymph nodes involved are the superficial and deep inguinal nodes and the femoral nodes (Fig. 26.4). Pelvic lymph nodes, except in primary lesions involving the clitoris, have usually only secondary involvement. In particular, the external iliac and obturator nodes are involved. Blood vascular spread is late and rare. The disease usually progresses slowly and the terminal stages are accompanied by extensive ulceration, infection, haemorrhage and remote metastatic disease. In some 30% of cases, lymph nodes are involved on both sides.

Classification

The most widely used classification of carcinoma of the vulva is the FIGO classification and is described as follows:

Stage I — tumour confined to the vulva — 2 cm or less in diameter. Nodes are not palpable, or are palpable in either groin, not enlarged and mobile.
Stage II — tumour confined to the vulva — more than 2 cm in diameter. Nodes are not palpable or

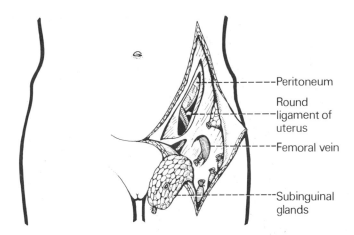

Fig. 26.6 Block dissection of the lymph nodes in surgical treatment of malignant disease of the vulva

are palpable in either groin, not enlarged and mobile.
Stage III — tumour of any size with:
1. Adjacent spread to the lower urethra and/or the vagina, the perineum and the anus, and/or:
2. Nodes palpable in either one or both groins, enlarged, firm and mobile and not fixed.

Stage IV — tumour of any size:
1. Infiltrating the bladder mucosa or the rectal mucosa, or both, including the upper part of the urethral mucosa and/or:
2. Fixed to the bone or other distant metastases. Fixed or ulcerated nodes in either one or both groins.

Therapy

Stages I to III should be treated with radical vulvectomy. This procedure involves extensive removal of the vulval and bilateral inguinal nodes and pelvic lymphadenectomy (Fig. 26.6). Radiotherapy has a limited role to play in advanced lesions in elderly patients.

Prognosis

Stages I and II have a good 5-year salvage rate with 100% survival in stage I, 80% in stage II, and 30–40% in stages III and IV.

Malignant vulval lesions

- Commonest in 6th decade
- 2–3% of female cancers
- Pre-malignant changes occur in 0.5/100 000 women
- Majority are squamous (92%) or adenocarcinomas (5%)
- Present with pruritus, bleeding lesions
- Spreads by local invasion and via inguinal and femoral nodes
- Staged according to size, lymph node involvement and spread
- Good prognosis if confined to vulva at presentation

BENIGN TUMOURS OF THE VAGINA

Vaginal cysts

Congenital

Cysts arise in the vagina from embryological remnants; the commonest varieties are those arising from Gartner's duct (Wolffian duct remnants). These are not rare and occur in the antero-lateral wall of the vagina. They are usually asymptomatic and are found on routine examination.

Histologically, the cysts are lined by cuboidal epithelium, but sometimes a flattened layer of stratified squamous epithelium is seen.

Treatment. The cysts are treated by simple surgical excision and rarely give rise to any difficulties.

Vaginal inclusion cysts

Inclusion cysts arise from inclusion of small particles or islands of vaginal epithelium under the surface. The cysts commonly arise in episiotomy scars and contain yellowish thick fluid within the cyst. They are treated by simple surgical excision.

Endometriosis

Endometriotic lesions may appear anywhere in the vagina, but occur most commonly in the posterior fornix. The lesions may appear as dark brown spots or reddened ulcerated lesions. The diagnosis is established by excision biopsy. If the lesions are multiple, then medical therapy should be instituted as for lesions in other sites.

Solid benign tumours

These lesions are rare but may represent any of the tissues that are found in the vagina. Thus polypoid tumours may include fibromyomas, myomas, fibromas, papillomas and adenomyomas. These tumours are treated by simple surgical excision.

MALIGNANT VAGINAL TUMOURS

Primary malignancies of the vagina are very rare. The lesions include squamous cell carcinomas and sarcomas and, rarely, chorio-epitheliomas.

Squamous cell carcinoma

Intra-epithelial carcinoma of the vagina is usually multicentric and tends to be multifocal and associated with similar lesions of the cervix. The condition is asymptomatic and is usually discovered because of a positive smear test or during colposcopy for abnormal cytology.

Treatment

These lesions are superficial and can be treated by surgical excision, or by cryosurgical removal, laser therapy, or partial vaginectomy if the lesion is in the vaginal vault. Radiation therapy is confined to invasive carcinoma.

Vaginal tumours

- Benign tumours are commonly, embryological remnants, inclusion cysts or endometriotic
- Primary malignancy rare, squamous carcinomas arising in upper 1/3
- Common site for spread from cervix and uterus
- Presents as pain, bleeding and fistula formation
- Spreads by local invasion and lymphatics
- Usually treated by radiotherapy
- Increased incidence in young women whose mothers were given diethylstilboestrol in pregnancy
- Premalignant changes associated with CIN

Carcinoma of the vagina

Invasive carcinoma of the vagina may be a squamous carcinoma or, occasionally, an adenocarcinoma. Primary lesions arise in the sixth and seventh decades, but are rare in the United Kingdom. In recent years, there has been an increase in adenocarcinomas in young women, which has been associated with the administration of diethylstilboestrol during the pregnancies of their mothers. These tumours are of the clear-cell or mesonephric variety.

Secondary deposits from cervical carcinoma and endometrial carcinoma are relatively common in the upper third of the vagina and can sometimes occur in the lower vagina due to lymphatic spread.

Symptoms

The symptoms include irregular vaginal bleeding and offensive vaginal discharge when the tumour becomes necrotic and infection supervenes. Infection may also cause pain, and local spread into the rectum, bladder or urethra may result in fistula formation.

The tumour may appear as an exophytic lesion or as an ulcerated, indurated mass.

Method of spread

Tumour spread, as previously stated, occurs by direct infiltration or by lymphatic extension. Lesions involving the upper half of the vagina follow a pattern of spread similar to that of carcinoma of the cervix. Tumours of the lower half of the vagina follow a similar pattern of spread to that of carcinoma of the vulva.

Clinical staging

Carcinoma of the vagina is classified as follows:

Stage 0 — intra-epithelial carcinoma.
Stage I — limited to the vaginal walls.
Stage II — involves the subvaginal tissue, but has not extended to the pelvic wall.
Stage III — the tumour has extended to the lateral pelvic wall.
Stage IV — the lesion has extended to involve adjacent organs (IVa) or has spread to distant organs (IVb).

Treatment

The diagnosis is established by biopsy of the tumour, and careful evaluation of tumour extension and staging is made before commencing treatment.

The primary method of treatment is by radiotherapy — both by external beam therapy and by interstitial gamma ray sources.

Surgical treatment includes radical vaginectomy, and anterior or posterior exenteration, but this is rarely used as the primary therapy.

Prognosis

Results of treatment depend on the initial staging and on the method of therapy. Stages I and II have a 5-year survival of around 60%, and this figure falls to 30–40% for stages III and IV. Adenocarcinoma of the vagina, which often occurs in young females, also responds well to irradiation.

Vaginal adenosis

This is the presence of columnar epithelium in the vaginal epithelium and has been found in adult females whose mothers received treatment with diethylstilboestrol during pregnancy. The condition commonly reverts to normal squamous epithelium, but in about 4% of cases the lesion progresses to carcinoma in situ. It is therefore important to follow these women carefully with serial cytology.

Sarcoma botryoides

This is a rare tumour of mixed mesodermal origin which occurs in young females of age 2–3 years. The tumour grows rapidly and may appear at the introitus as a grape-like mass. Combined treatment with radiotherapy and surgery seems to offer the best prospect for cure and may allow conservation of the bladder and rectum, although it is not possible to conserve reproductive function.

BIBLIOGRAPHY

Douglas C P 1972 Diseases of the vulva. Harper and Row
McGowan L 1978 Gynecologic oncology. Appleton-Century-Crofts, New York

27. Lesions of the cervix

EXAMINATION OF THE CERVIX

Routine examination of the cervix involves direct inspection with a good light and exposure with a bivalve or Sims' speculum. The size, shape and consistency of the cervix should be noted and the nature of any discharge recorded. The external cervical os is circular in shape and in parous women the os is a transverse slit. The nature of the epithelium should be observed, as it will vary according to the hormonal status of the woman. The normal ectocervix is covered with stratified squamous epithelium and the endocervical canal by columnar epithelium. The junction between these two epithelia is known as the **squamocolumnar junction** and it may be placed at any point across the cervix. The zone medial to the squamocolumnar junction is the transformation zone and it is in this area that most abnormal changes occur.

The term **cervical erosion** or **cervical ectopy** is used where endocervical epithelium appears to advance on to the ectocervix and gives a bright red velvety appearance (Fig. 27.1). In fact, this reflects no more than the dynamic behaviour of the transformation zone and the squamocolumnar junction. During pregnancy and adolescence, and in some women on oral contraception, the endocervical epithelium advances outwards, whereas at the menopause shrinkage occurs with diminution of the exposed area of the transformation zone. The condition is also sometimes known as **cervical erythroplakia**.

In most cases, cervical ectopy is asymptomatic, but it is sometimes associated with leucorrhoea and postcoital bleeding.

The term **cervical ectropion** describes the eversion of the cervix associated with bilateral laceration of the cervix following parturition. The

Cervical ectopy

Endocervical polyp

Fig. 27.1 Common benign lesions of the cervix include cervical ectopy or 'erosion' (top) and cervical polyps (below)

endocervical mucosa rolls out from the cervical canal and may give rise to symptoms similar to those of cervical ectopy.

MANAGEMENT

These conditions are benign and should be treated only where they produce symptoms. Treatment of cervical ectopy is by radial diathermy or cryosurgery. Squamous epithelium grows along the tracks of diathermy wounds and epithelial growth covers and replaces the endocervical epithelium. For 2 weeks after treatment, the discharge may worsen with separation of the cauterised epithelium, but within a month the symptoms will either recede or disappear.

The complications of the procedure are:

1. Secondary haemorrhage and infection.
2. Cervical stenosis.

Occasionally, it may be necessary to excise the endocervical mucosa and the laceration and thereby refashion the cervix, a procedure known as **trachelorrhaphy**.

BENIGN NEOPLASMS OF THE CERVIX

Cervical polyps

Benign polyps (Fig. 27.1) arise from the endocervix and are pedunculated with a covering of endocervical epithelium and a central fibrous tissue core. The polyps present as bright red, vascular growths which may be identified on routine examination: the presenting symptoms may include irregular vaginal blood loss or postcoital bleeding.

Less frequently, the polyps arise from the squamous epithelium when the appearance will resemble the surface of the vaginal epithelium. Malignant change may give rise to an epidermoid or adenocarcinoma, but this is rare.

Treatment

The only treatment is surgical with ligation of the pedicle and excision of the polyp.

Cervical fibroids

Cervical leiomyoma are similar to fibroids in other sites of the uterus. They are commonly pedunculated, but may be sessile and grow to a size that will fill the vagina and distort the pelvic organs.

Symptoms are similar to those caused by other cervical polyps and, in addition, the attempted extrusion of fibroid polyps may cause colicky uterine pain, particularly at the time of menstruation.

Treatment is by surgical excision. Many of these lesions have a thick peduncle which must be transfixed and ligated before excision of the polyp.

Malignant change in the form of sarcomatous degeneration is extremely rare and is no more frequent than sarcomatous change arising in the myometrium.

Benign lesions of the cervix

- Erosions are extensions of endocervical epithelium onto the ectocervix
- Ectropion is cervical eversion revealing the endocervical mucosa
- Benign polyps commonly arise from the endocervix
- Fibroids may arise from the cervix
- Benign lesions may be asymptomatic or present as vaginal bleeding or discharge

MALIGNANT LESIONS OF THE CERVIX

Screening for cervical cancer

Squamous cell carcinoma is a sexually transmitted disease and all women who have had sexual intercourse are at risk. Screening by cervical cytology should, therefore, be started with the onset of sexual activity and continued as follows:

- First smear — when sexual activity commences.
- Second smear — 1 year later (to cover 10% technical false-negative rate).
- Third and subsequent smears — at 3-year intervals to the age of 45.
- After 45 years — at 5-year intervals to the age of 60, provided there have been regular smears prior to the age of 45.
- After 60 years — regular smears *not* required.

Technique

It is essential to obtain a good view of the cervix. The speculum should be introduced with a minimum of artificial lubricant. Cells are taken from around the cervix from the whole of the transformation zone by taking a smear with a 360° sweep using an Ayre spatula. The Papanicolaou smear also includes cells from aspiration of the posterior fornix. This has the advantage of a higher detection rate for endometrial carcinoma.

Apart from assessing the cells for signs of

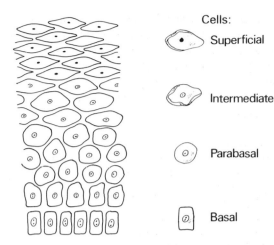

Cells:

Superficial

Intermediate

Parabasal

Basal

Fig. 27.2   Cell layers in the stratified squamous epithelium of the cervix and vagina

epithelium of the vagina and cervix is composed of four layers of cells as follows (Fig. 27.2).

1. *Basal cells* — these lie on the basement membrane and are not usually exfoliated.
2. *Parabasal cells* — these cells are oval in shape and have a centrally placed nucleus with a cytoplasm that is basophilic.
3. *Intermediate squamous cells* — these cells are polygonal in shape and have a basophilic cytoplasm, except in the presence of infection when it becomes eosinophilic. The cells lie singly or in clumps with either a flattened or a folded appearance.
4. *Superficial or mature squamous cells* — polygonal cells with a pyknotic nucleus and a cytoplasm that is eosinophilic.

Endocervical cells, which are tall and cylindrical, may also be seen as well as endometrial cells. Hormone status is assessed by counting the number of squamous cells with a pyknotic nucleus in relation to the rest of the squamous cell population, and this is known as the **Karyopyknotic index** (**KPI**). The KPI is high (50–60%) in the proliferative phase of the cycle and low (0–10%) in the secretory phase.

Characteristic appearances of malignant cells

Malignant cells show nuclear enlargement at the expense of cytoplasmic mass (Fig. 27.3.). The

malignant change, a smear from the upper third of the vagina can also be used for assessment of hormone status.

The specimen is spread immediately on to a clear glass slide in a thin, even layer. The slide is fixed with 95% ethyl alcohol alone or in combination with 3% glacial acetic acid. Fixation requires 30 minutes in solution and the preparation is then stained using the Papanicolaou technique. With this method, the nuclei stain blue, the superficial cell cytoplasm pink and the intermediate and parabasal cell cytoplasm stains blue/green. The squamous

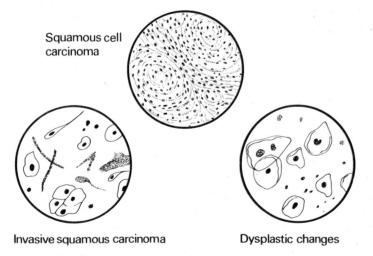

Squamous cell carcinoma

Invasive squamous carcinoma

Dysplastic changes

Fig. 27.3   Invasive carcinoma (top) is associated with 'tadpole' and 'fibre' cells in the smear (bottom left); the histology commonly shows layers of non-keratinizing squamous epithelium, although in some lesions keratinization can be seen; dysplastic appearances include nuclear changes consistent with malignancy but have normal cytoplasm (bottom right) nucleus may assume a lobulated outline. There is increased intensity of staining of the nucleus and an increase in the number of mitotic figures.

Dysplasia

Cells that lie between normal squamous and frankly malignant cells are known as dysplastic cells and exhibit degrees of nuclear changes consistent with malignancy but contain normal cytoplasm (Fig. 27.3).

The Papanicolaou grouping is described as:

Group I — normal cells only — negative.
Group II — normal variants. No suspicious cells — negative.
Group III — Unusual cells present — doubtful malignancy.
Group IV — Individual atypical cells — positive.
Group V — many atypical cells — positive.

Cervical cytology is an unreliable method for detecting endometrial carcinoma cells, but a better yield of cells can be obtained by aspiration of the posterior vaginal fornix.

Colposcopy

The presence of abnormal cytology is an indication for examination by colposcopy — a procedure that involves examination of the cervix with a binocular dissecting microscope. This enables biopsy of abnormal epithelium and local treatment unless the lesion extends into the cervical canal. Abnormal findings may include:

1. *Atypical transformation zone* — abnormal epithelium at the transformation zone.
2. *Leucoplakia* — white plaques visible without magnification.

Cervical screening

- 3–yearly from start of sexual activity
- Malignant change suggested by increased nuclear: cytoplasmic ratio, mitotic figures and intense nuclear staining
- 'Dysplasia' represents lesser degrees of abnormality
- Appearance of exfoliated cells also varies with hormonal status and infection
- Abnormal cytology requires colposcopy

---

3. *Malignant epithelium* — an increase in vascular hypertrophy; the vessels make sharp angulations. There may be a zone of red dots known as punctation and a mosaic structure of the epithelium.

Cervical cancer

The aetiology and epidemiology have been studied in considerable depth. It occurs most commonly in married women of lower socio-economic status, in women with an early age of first coitus, in women with multiple partners and in women infected with herpes virus type 2 and human papilloma virus. Cervical cancer has a direct relationship to sexual activity. It is rare in Jewish women or Moslems.

Age distribution

The peak incidence for carcinoma in situ occurs between 30 and 40 years of age, and of invasive carcinoma between 40 and 50 years of age. However, the disease may occur at any age.

Pathology

There are two types of invasive carcinoma of the cervix. The commonest variety, which accounts for 95% of these tumours, is epidermoid, and 5% are adenocarcinomas. The earliest form of these lesions is known as **cervical intra-epithelial neoplasia** (CIN). This term encompasses the spectrum of cervical dysplasia to carcinoma in situ and is described as mild, moderate and severe intra-epithelial neoplasia.

Classification

The following classification is used for carcinoma of the cervix (Fig. 27.4).

Stage 0 — carcinoma in situ or cervical intra-epithelial neoplasia (CIN).
Stage I — carcinoma confined to the cervix. This stage is subdivided into:
   Stage Ia — or microinvasion, where the tumour invades to a depth of 5 mm;
   Stage Ib — invasion extends beyond 5 mm but is confined to the cervix.

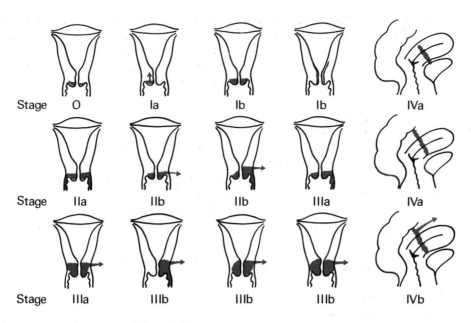

Stage	O	Ia	Ib	Ib	IVa
Stage	IIa	IIb	IIb	IIIa	IVa
Stage	IIIa	IIIb	IIIb	IIIb	IVb

Fig. 27.4 Stages of carcinoma of the cervix

Stage II — the carcinoma extends beyond the cervix but has not extended to the lateral pelvic wall. The carcinoma involves the vagina but not the lower third:

Stage IIa — no obvious parametrial involvement

Stage IIb — obvious parametrial involvement.

Stage III — the carcinoma has extended to the lateral pelvic wall and/or involves the lower third of the vagina:

Stage IIIa — no extension to the lateral pelvic wall;

Stage IIIb — extension to the pelvic wall and hydronephrosis or non-functioning kidney.

Stage IV — the carcinoma has extended beyond the true pelvis or has invaded the bladder or rectum:

Stage IVa — spread of the growth to adjacent organs;

Stage IVb — spread to distant organs.

The spread of tumour

Cervical carcinoma spreads by direct local invasion and by the lymphatics and blood vessels. Lymphatic spread occurs in approximately 40% of women with stage I and II disease and preferential spread occurs to the external iliac, internal iliac and obturator nodes. Secondary spread may also occur to inguinal, sacral and aortic nodes. Bloodborne metastases occur in the lungs, liver, bone and bowel.

Clinical features

Stage 0 and stage Ia disease are asymptomatic and are detected at the time of routine examination for cervical cytology. The common presenting symptoms from invasive carcinoma of the cervix include postcoital bleeding, foul-smelling discharge, which is thin and watery and sometimes blood stained, and irregular vaginal bleeding when the tumour becomes necrotic. Lateral invasion into the parametrium may involve the ureters, leading eventually to ureteric obstruction and renal failure. Invasion of nerves and bone produces excruciating and persistent pain, and involvement of lymphatic channels may result in lymphatic occlusion with intractable oedema of the lower limbs.

The tumour may also spread anteriorly or posteriorly to involve the bladder or rectum respectively. Involvement of the bladder produces symptoms of frequency, dysuria and haematuria; if the bowel is involved, tenesmus, diarrhoea and rectal bleeding may occur. The neoplasm may initially grow within the endocervix producing a cylindrical, barrel-shaped enlargement of the cervix with little external manifestation of the tumour.

The exophytic tumour grows over the vaginal portion of the cervix and appears as a cauliflower-like tumour. The tumour eventually sloughs and replaces the normal cervical tissue and extends on to the vaginal walls.

Death occurs from uremia following bilateral ureteric obstruction or from sepsis and haemorrhage with generalized cachexia and wasting.

Cervical cancer

- More common in lower social class, smokers, early first intercourse and multiple partners
- Associated with herpes and human papilloma virus infection
- May be asymptomatic or present with vaginal bleeding, pain, and bowel or bladder symptoms
- Spreads by local invasion and iliac/obturator nodes
- Treatment is radical hysterectomy for early stage disease, radiotherapy otherwise
- 5-year survival varies from 10–90% depending on stage
- CIN represents a premalignant stage which can be treated by local destructive therapy

Investigation

The diagnosis is established histologically by biopsy of the tumour using a punch biopsy technique under colposcopic control in stage 0 and under direct vision in all other stages. Careful evaluation and staging should be completed by vaginal and rectal examination and by cystoscopy, proctoscopy, intravenous urography, and lung and skeletal X-rays.

Treatment of cervical intra-epithelial neoplasia

If the lesion can be defined by colposcopy and can be shown to be confined to the vaginal portion of the cervix, the lesion can be treated by electro-cautery, electrocoagulation diathermy or CO_2 laser.

If the abnormal epithelium extends up the cervical canal and the upper limit is not visible, then cone biopsy should be performed (Fig. 27.5).

This procedure involves the excision of a cone of cervical tissue which includes the area of abnormal epithelium defined by the application of Lugol's

Fig. 27.5 Cone biopsy of the cervix (left); four mattress sutures are usually adequate to control bleeding from the cervical stump (right)

iodine solution and extends to the full depth of the cervical canal. Haemostasis is achieved by the use of mattress sutures to occlude the cervical branch of the uterine artery.

Complications of cone biopsy. The commonest complication is haemorrhage. This may be primary, i.e. within 12 hours of operation, or secondary, usually between the 5th and 12th postoperative day. Haemorrhage may be profuse, but can be controlled by compression with vaginal packing or by resuturing the cervix. Secondary haemorrhage is commonly associated with infection and the management therefore includes blood transfusion and antibiotic therapy.

Later complications include cervical stenosis with dysmenorrhoea and haematometra. Cone biopsy may also cause cervical incompetence and subsequent mid-trimester abortion.

Hysterectomy. Hysterectomy is indicated where:

1. Excision is not completed by cone biopsy.
2. Persistent abnormal smears follow cone biopsy.
3. Other disorders such as fibroids or prolapse are present.
4. Hysterectomy is to be used for sterilization.

Treatment of invasive carcinoma of the cervix

Treatment is by surgery or radiotherapy or a combination of both methods.

Radical hysterectomy and pelvic node dissection. Radical hysterectomy (Wertheim's hysterectomy) includes removal of the uterus, tubes and ovaries and the upper third of the vagina (Fig. 27.6). The internal and external iliac and obturator lymph

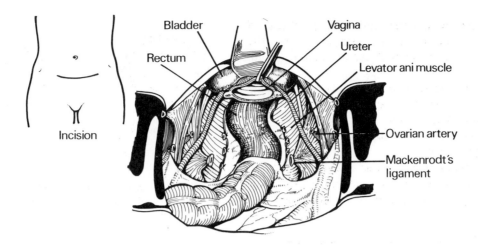

Fig. 27.6 Wertheim's hysterectomy involves block dissection of the pelvic lymph nodes and excision of the uterus, tubes, ovaries and upper third of the vagina

nodes are also removed. This method of treatment is appropriate for stage I and stage IIa cervical carcinoma.

Complications include haemorrhage, infection, pelvic haematomas and uretero-vaginal or vesico-vaginal fistulae. Where the tumour involves the bladder or rectum, but does not extend to other structures, a radical excision or exenteration is performed and includes total cystectomy or removal of the rectum.

Radiotherapy is used to treat the other stages of the disease and in some centres is used for all stages of invasive cervical carcinoma.

Radiotherapy. Radiotherapy is administered by the local insertion of a source of radium, caesium or cobalt-60 into the uterine cavity and the vaginal vault. As the radiation dose falls towards the pelvic walls, it is necessary to use external radiation to the lateral pelvic walls and lymph nodes. To prevent radiation necrosis of normal tissue, it is important to co-ordinate the intracavitary and external radiation.

Dosages are calculated at two points:

1. Point A — 2 cm cephalad from the upper vaginal fornix and 2 cm from the midline.
2. Point B — 2 cm cephalad from the upper vaginal fornix and 5 cm from the midline.

The aim is to deliver 50 Gy to the lateral pelvic wall by external radiation and 30 Gy by intracavitary radiation to point A, with a maximum dose to point B and the bowel and bladder of 25–28 Gy. These dosages may be increased with more extensive tumour growth.

Complications include the effects of excessive radiation on normal tissue and may lead to radiation cystitis and proctitis as well as fistula formation. Occasionally, there may be radiation necrosis of bone. The location of lymph nodes both pre-operatively and prior to radiotherapy can be achieved with lymphangiography.

Results of treatment

The results for 5-year survival in cancer of the cervix vary from centre to centre, but in good radiotherapy centres one can expect a figure of:

Stage I	85%
Stage II	60%
Stage III	30%
Stage IV	10%

The comparable survival figure for stage Ib using radical surgery is 90%.

A combination of limited radiation and subsequent radical surgery after 4–6 weeks has produced similar figures, with a 5-year survival in stage I disease of 77% and in stage IIa of 69%.

Recurrent cervical lesions exhibit a poor response to chemotherapy.

Vaginal and cervical clear-cell adenocarcinoma

These tumours have been described previously in relation to DES exposure and occur on both the vagina and the cervix. They are found in young females born to women who received diethylstilboestrol during the course of their pregnancy.

The tumours respond to radiation or radical surgery and there is an overall 5-year survival rate of 70%. The tumour is commonly preceded by vaginal adenosis. The condition is rare in the United Kingdom.

BIBLIOGRAPHY

Coppleson M (ed) 1991 Gynecologic oncology, fundamental principles and clinical practice, 2nd edn. Churchill Livingstone, Edinburgh.

28. Lesions of the uterus and fallopian tubes

This chapter relates to conditions of the body of the uterus and excludes lesions of the uterine cervix. Some disorders of function have been described in Chapter 22.

CONGENITAL ANOMALIES

The formation of the uterus results from the fusion of the two Müllerian ducts; this fusion gives rise to the upper two-thirds of the vagina, the cervix and the body of the uterus. Congenital anomalies arise from the failure of fusion or absence or partial development of one or both ducts. Thus, the anomalies may range from a minor indentation of the uterine fundus to a full separation of each uterine horn and cervix. These conditions are also commonly associated with vaginal septa.

Symptoms and signs

The majority of uterine anomalies are asymptomatic but are usually diagnosed in relation to complications of pregnancy. However, the presence of a vaginal septum may result in dyspareunia and postcoital bleeding.

The presence of a double uterus may also be established at routine vaginal examination when a double cervix may be seen. The separation of the uterine horns is sometimes palpable on bimanual vaginal examination, but in most cases, the uterus feels normal and there is a single cervix. The uterus may be palpable as lying obliquely in the pelvis when only one horn of the uterus is present. The abnormality of the uterine horns and one cervix is known as **uterus bicornis unicollis** (Fig. 28.1).

Partial atresia of one horn of the uterus, or a septate vagina resulting in obstruction to menstrual outflow from one horn of the uterus, may result

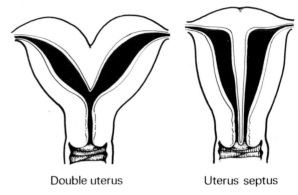

Double uterus   Uterus septus

Fig. 28.1 Common congenital abnormalities of the uterus include uterus bicornis unicollis (double uterus, one cervix) (left) and the subseptate uterus (uterus septus) (right)

in a unilateral haematocolpos and haematometra with retrograde spill of menstrual fluid. In this case, the patient may present with symptoms of dysmenorrhoea and will have a palpable mass arising from the pelvis.

The complications of pregnancy include:

1. Recurrent abortions of increasing gestational age — this problem is usually associated with the subseptate uterus and is not common in the unicornuate uterus or in uterus bicornis bicollis.
2. Premature labour.
3. Malpresentation (Fig. 28.2).
4. Retained placenta (Fig. 28.3).

Diagnosis and management

As many cases are asymptomatic, the diagnosis may arise only as a coincidental finding and requires no treatment or intervention. If there is a history of two or more consecutive abortions, then active surgical intervention is indicated.

Transverse lie

Fig. 28.2 Malpresentation and a subseptate uterus

Retained placenta

Fig. 28.3 Retention of the placenta as a feature of congenital abnormalities of the uterus

Where the diagnosis is suggested by the history, further investigation should include hysterography and hysteroscopy.

Surgical treatment

Surgical reconstruction of a double uterus should be confined to women who have experienced two or more consecutive abortions and where the abnormality is one of uterus bicornis unicollis, or there is an uterine septum.

The operation of plastic reconstruction of the uterus with unification of two uterine horns or excision of the uterine septum is known as **metroplasty** (Fig. 28.4).

An incision is made across the fundus of the uterus between the utero-tubal junctions, but taking care not to involve the intramural portion of the tube. The cavities are then reunited by suturing the surfaces together in the anteroposterior plane. If there is a septum, it is simply divided by diathermy and the cavity is then closed by suturing the transverse incision in the anteroposterior plane.

An alternative surgical management is to divide the septum by diathermy through a hysteroscope inserted through the cervix. Before undertaking a surgical procedure for the treatment of any uterine anomaly, it is essential to perform an intravenous pyelogram, as there is a high incidence of congenital urinary tract abnormalities in these cases, including ureteric reduplication and unilateral renal agenesis.

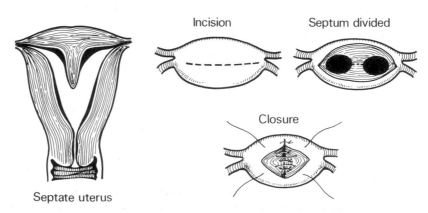

Incision   Septum divided

Closure

Septate uterus

Fig. 28.4 Metroplasty (right) for the reunification of a bicornate uterus or the division of a uterine septum (left)

Abnormalities of uterine position

The uterus normally rests in an anteverted position, but in some 10% of the female population the uterus is retroverted. In some women, this is associated with first degree descent of the cervix; in other words, it represents an early phase of uterine prolapse. If the uterus is retroverted and mobile, it is of no significance, and represents a variant of normal. However, if the uterus is fixed in retroversion, the condition is often associated with significant pelvic disease such as endometriosis or chronic pelvic inflammatory disease.

Management

Where the condition is asymptomatic, no treatment is indicated. If it is associated with deepseated dyspareunia or sacral backache, then the uterus can be fixed in anteversion by a surgical procedure known as ventro-suspension, which involves shortening the round ligaments by plication. It is advisable to test the relationship between the retroversion and the symptoms by first correcting the retroversion with a Hodge pessary before proceeding to surgical treatment. If correction of the position does not improve the symptoms, then it is unlikely that relief will be obtained from surgical procedures unless there is specific pathology which holds the uterus in fixed retroversion.

Congenital abnormalities of the uterus

- Due to failure of Müllerian ducts to fuse or develop
- Usually asymptomatic unless menstrual flow obstructed
- May cause recurrent abortion, malpresentation or retained placenta
- May be associated with abnormalities of the renal tract

BENIGN TUMOURS OF THE UTERUS

Endometrial polyps

The commonest benign tumours of the endometrium are endometrial polyps (Fig. 28.5). These occur at any age but are found most frequently in the premenopausal decade.

Polyps

Fig. 28.5 Multiple endometrial polyps may be a cause of profuse and irregular bleeding

Symptoms

Irregular bleeding and menorrhagia result from necrosis of the surface of the polyp and interference with normal endometrial shedding. Occasionally, protrusion of the polyp through the cervix may result in postcoital bleeding. Attempts by the uterus to expel the polyp may cause colicky, dysmenorrhoeic pain.

Signs

The diagnosis must be anticipated on the history, because it is unusual to be able to establish a diagnosis on the basis of the physical signs. If the polyp protrudes through the cervix, it has a bright red appearance, but is difficult to distinguish from an endocervical polyp.

Pathology

Endometrial polyps consist of a fine fibrous tissue core covered by columnar epithelium. They may be covered by functional endometrium that responds to ovarian steroids or by immature endometrium that exhibits no progesterone response even when the surrounding endometrium is in the phase of marked secretory activity. Occasionally, malignant change occurs in endometrial polyps, but there is no increase in such incidence over that seen in normal endometrium.

Treatment

These tumours are usually diagnosed at uterine curettage and are commonly cured by cervical dilatation and uterine curettage.

Benign tumours of the myometrium

It is estimated that some 20% of women over the age of 30 years have uterine myomas or 'fibroids'. These tumours are derived from smooth muscle tissue and vary enormously in size from microscopic growths to tumours that may weigh as much as 30–40 kg. They may be single or multiple and may occur in the cervix or in the body of the uterus. The site of the tumour has a considerable effect on the symptoms. Subserosal fibroids may become pedunculated, and submucous fibroids may project into the cavity of the uterus and form a fibroid polyp (Fig. 28.6). Interstitial or intramural growths may result in uniform enlargement of the uterus but can also cause irregular or nodular distention. Large subserosal tumours frequently become adherent to the omentum and eventually derive an additional blood supply. The tumour may then become separated from the uterus and form a **parasitic** or **wandering fibroid.**

The aetiology of fibroids is not known, but some 25–35% of women with myomas are sterile and the tumours occur more frequently in black than in white women. Pregnancy causes enlargement and the menopause is associated with involution.

Fig. 28.6 Uterine fibroids produce symptoms which are determined by the site of the fibroids

Histopathology

Myomas consist of whorled masses of unstriped muscle cells. There is always some admixture of connective tissue but the true nature of myomas is that of a smooth muscle benign tumour.

Pathological changes

Secondary changes may occur in fibroids. These changes include:

1. *Hyaline degeneration* — a common finding in most fibroids. Scattered islands of muscle cells are found intact in broad expanses of hyaline degeneration.
2. *Cystic degeneration* — this is an extension of hyaline degeneration with liquefaction of some areas of the fibroid and cyst formation.
3. *Calcification* — this provides evidence of degeneration and is associated with circulatory impairment. It is therefore commonly seen in fibroids after the menopause; in its most extreme form the fibroid is converted into a stony mass.
4. *Infection and abscess formation* — these are rare complications which are particularly likely to affect submucous fibroids following septic abortions or occasionally following tumours, particularly if radiotherapy is used.
5. *Necrobiosis* — impairment of blood supply is particularly likely to occur in pedunculated subserous fibroids, but there are special forms of necrosis such a red degeneration, which is seen in pregnancy. The cut surface of the tumour has a dull reddish hue and the appearance is associated with aseptic degeneration and local haemolysis.
6. *Sarcomatous change* — the incidence of malignant change in fibroids has been variably reported to be between 0.13 and 1%.

Symptoms and signs

Many myomas are asymptomatic and may be discovered during routine pelvic examination — either at the time of cervical cytology or in the management of a pregnancy.

Where symptoms do occur, they are often related to the site of the fibroids. The common presenting symptoms are:

1. *Menstrual disorders* — submucous and intramural fibroids commonly cause menorrhagia. They do not influence the length of the menstrual cycle. Submucous fibroids may cause irregular vaginal bleeding particularly if the surface of the fibroid becomes necrotic or ulcerated, or if endometrial carcinoma is also present.
2. *Pain* — colicky uterine pain may occur with pedunculated fibroids as the uterus attempts to expel them. Pain may also occur during pregnancy if red degeneration occurs or if torsion of a subserous fibroid results in necrosis of the tumour. The pain will be persistent until necrosis is complete.
3. *Pressure symptoms* — a large mass of fibroids may become apparent because of palpable enlargement of the abdomen or because of pressure on the bladder or rectum.
4. *Complications of pregnancy* — submucous fibroids interfere with nidation and therefore cause recurrent abortion.

The diagnosis may be confirmed by ultrasound scans of the pelvis or by radiological diagnosis if the fibroid is calcified.

Management

Small uterine fibroids are a common finding in asymptomatic women, but if they exceed 10 cm in size the tumour should be removed because of the difficulty of excluding the diagnosis of an ovarian tumour. There is no medical treatment of fibroids. Where the preservation of reproductive function is not important, the surgical treatment of choice is by hysterectomy. In younger women or where the preservation of reproductive function is important, the removal of the fibroids by surgical excision or myomectomy is indicated. This procedure involves incision of the pseudocapsule of the fibroid, enucleation of the bulk of the tumour and closure of the cavity by interrupted absorbable sutures. Myomectomy is associated with greater morbidity than hysterectomy because of the occurrence of haematoma formation in the cavity of the excised fibroid and also because of infection. It is also impossible to be certain that all fibroids are removed without causing excessive uterine damage; there is always a possibility that residual seedling fibroids may grow and lead to recurrence of the fibroids.

Benign uterine tumours

- Commonest are endometrial polyps and fibroids
- 20% of women over 30 have fibroids
- Symptoms depend on size and site and include menstrual disorders, pressure symptoms and complications of pregnancy
- May undergo secondary change including necrosis or malignant change (0.13–1%)
- Management depends on size and need to preserve reproductive function

---

MALIGNANT DISEASE OF THE UTERUS

Endometrial carcinoma

Adenocarcinoma of the endometrium is a common gynaecological tumour which presents after the

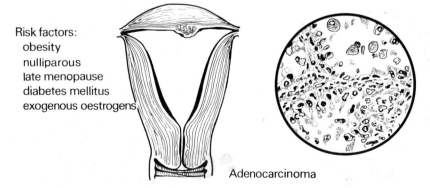

Risk factors:
  obesity
  nulliparous
  late menopause
  diabetes mellitus
  exogenous oestrogens

Adenocarcinoma

Fig. 28.7 Endometrial adenocardinoma: there are a number of risk factors associated with it (left); histological features (right)

menopause in two-thirds of all cases. Cancer of the body of the uterus is the predominant genital tract malignancy in women over the age of 50 years. The peak age of incidence occurs between 65 and 74 years of age.

There are specific risk factors associated with an increased incidence of corpus carcinoma (Fig. 28.7).

1. *Obesity* — this is a strong risk factor; approximately half of the women who develop endometrial carcinoma are grossly overweight.
2. *Parity* — the incidence of corpus carcinoma is twice as high in nulliparous women.
3. *Late menopause* — the incidence is significantly increased in women who have a menopause after the age of 50 years.
4. *Diabetes mellitus* — abnormalities of glucose tolerance are associated with a twofold increase in the incidence of endometrial carcinoma and there is also an increased incidence of hypertensive disease, although this is probably a secondary association.
5. *Exogenous oestrogens* — unopposed oestrogen action, particularly as used for hormone replacement therapy in the menopause, is associated with an increased incidence of endometrial carcinoma. The addition of a progestogen for 7 days of each month can reduce this risk.

Symptoms

The commonest symptom is postmenopausal bleeding. However, in the premenopausal woman, endometrial carcinoma is associated with irregular vaginal bleeding and menorrhagia. A serous blood-stained and offensive discharge may also accompany the history of abnormal bleeding.

Pathology

Adenocarcinoma of the endometrium may occur in a diffuse form and cover the whole surface of the endometrium, or it may be circumscribed in the form of a localized polypoid growth. The microscopic appearances include changes in the architecture with the development of closely packed polyhedral cells with dark-staining nuclei and considerable numbers of mitoses. In many tumours, the cells may retain their normal characteristics. The stromal cells almost always show marked reactive inflammatory infiltration with round cells and leucocytes. The virulence of the tumour is related to the degree of histological dedifferentiation. Endometrial cancer grows locally for a long period of time and expands the uterus. The tumour spreads by direct invasion into the myometrium and then transcervically, transtubally and by spillage of carcinomatous material. Lymphatic spread is the primary method of extrauterine extension and involves the external and internal iliac nodes and the aortic nodes. In lesions involving the fundus of the uterus, spread may occur along the lymphatics of the round ligament and metastasize to the superficial or deep inguinal nodes.

Staging

The FIGO classification of endometrial cancer takes account of the distribution of the tumour and the length of the uterine cavity (Fig. 28.8). Classification depends on the extension of the tumour and on the histological grading:

Stage 0 — carcinoma in situ.
Stage I — carcinoma confined to the corpus:

Stage   I   II   III   IV

Fig. 28.8   Staging of carcinoma of the body of the uterus

Stage Ia — uterine cavity less than 8 cm;
Stage Ib — uterine cavity larger than 8 cm.

Stage I is subgrouped with regard to histological type:

G1 — highly differentiated adenocarcinoma;
G2 — differentiated adenocarcinoma with partly solid areas;
G3 — solid or entirely undifferentiated carcinoma.

Stage II — the carcinoma involves the cervix but does not extend outside the uterus.
Stage III — the tumour has extended outside the uterus but not outside the pelvis.
Stage IV — the carcinoma extends outside the pelvis:

Stage IVa — spread of growth to adjacent organs;
Stage IVb — spread to distant organs.

Diagnosis

The diagnosis and staging of the tumour is established by diagnostic and fractional curettage and measurement of the length of the uterine cavity. Invasion of the carcinoma into the rectum or bladder can be recognized by cystoscopy and proctoscopy.

Treatment

Stage Ia G 1 and stage 0 can be treated by primary surgery alone with total hysterectomy and bilateral salpingo-oophorectomy. If the tumour is poorly differentiated, then treatment should initially include radiotherapy with hysterectomy 2–6 weeks later. Stage II and III should be treated in a similar fashion with additional postoperative irradiation. Stage IV tumours are treated with irradiation and with progestational agents such as medroxyprogesterone and megestrol acetate or, in some cases, with cytotoxic therapy.

Prognosis

Stage Ia G1 is associated with a 90% 5-year survival. In stage II, the survival falls to 55% at 5 years, and in stage III 44%. Stage IV has only a 3% 5-year survival.

Sarcoma of the uterus

Sarcoma of the uterus is a rare tumour and usually presents in women between the ages of 45 and 48 years with vaginal discharge and irregular bleeding. The overall 5-year survival rate for uterine sarcoma is approximately 20–30% following treatment by radiotherapy.

Endometrial carcinoma

- Disease of postmenopausal women
- Risk factors include obesity, nulliparity, late menopause, glucose intolerance and unopposed oestrogens
- Commonly presents as postmenopausal bleeding
- Spreads by direct invasion but tends to remain localised within the uterus initially
- Well-differentiated early stage disease can be treated by hysterectomy alone; more advanced lesions require radiotherapy +/− progestational agents
- Has 90% 5-year survival if diagnosed early

TUMOURS OF THE FALLOPIAN TUBES

Primary fallopian tube cancers are extremely rare, accounting for 0.16–1% of all gynaecological malignancies. The mean age at diagnosis is 52 years, with a range of 18–80 years. The symptoms include abnormal vaginal bleeding and a canary-yellow discharge. Tubal cancers are predominantly adenocarcinomas, which are histologically similar to epithelial ovarian tumours and are best treated by radiotherapy. In fact, most of these tumours are first diagnosed at the time of laparotomy and are therefore surgically excised with subsequent treatment with radiotherapy.

SALPINGITIS ISTHMICA NODOSA

This is a special form of chronic salpingitis, and generally represents the residue of chronic interstitial salpingitis.

The condition is characterized by the presence of one or more nodules in the isthmic portion of the tube. These nodules are usually small but may expand to a size of 2 cm.

Treatment of this rare condition is by excision of the Fallopian tubes. Once again, this diagnosis is usually established as a coincidental finding at laparotomy.

BIBLIOGRAPHY

Fox H, Buckley C H 1982 Pathology for gynaecologists.
  Edward Arnold, London
Wyann R M 1977 Biology of the uterus. Plenum, New York

29. Lesions of the ovary

Ovarian enlargement is commonly asymptomatic and the silent nature of malignant ovarian tumours is the major reason for the advanced stage of presentation. Ovarian tumours may be cystic or solid, benign or malignant. There are common factors in the presentation and complications of ovarian tumours and it is often difficult to establish the nature of a tumour without direct examination.

Symptoms

Tumours of the ovary that are less than 10 cm in diameter rarely produce symptoms. The common presenting symptoms include:

1. Abdominal enlargement. In the presence of malignant change, this may also be associated with ascites (Fig. 29.1).
2. Symptoms from pressure on surrounding structures such as the bladder and rectum.
3. Symptoms relating to complications of the tumour (Fig. 29.1). These include:
   a. **Torsion** — acute torsion of the ovarian pedicle results in necrosis of the tumour. There is acute pain and vomiting followed by remission of the pain when the tumour has become necrotic.
   b. **Rupture** — the contents of the cyst spill into the peritoneal cavity and result in generalised abdominal pain.
   c. **Haemorrhage** — haemorrhage into the tumour is an unusual complication but may result in abdominal pain and shock if the blood loss is severe.
   d. **Hormone secreting tumours** — these may present with disturbances in the menstrual cycle. In androgen-secreting tumours the patient may present with signs of virilisation.

Ascites

Torsion pedicle

Rupture haemorrhage

Fig. 29.1 Common complications of ovarian tumours which precipitate a request for medical advice

Signs

On examination, the abdomen may be visibly enlarged. Percussion over the swelling will demonstrate central dullness and resonance in the flanks. These signs may be obscured by gross ascites. Small tumours can be detected on pelvic examination and will be found by palpation in one or both fornices. However, as the tumour enlarges, it assumes a more central position and, in the case of dermoid cysts, will often be anterior to the uterus. Most ovarian tumours are not tender to palpation; if they are painful the presence of infection or torsion should be suspected. Benign ovarian tumours are palpable separately from the uterine body and are usually freely mobile.

FUNCTIONAL CYSTS OF THE OVARY

These cysts occur only during menstrual life and rarely exceed more than 6 cm in diameter.

Follicular cysts

These form the commonest functional cysts in the ovary and may be multiple and bilateral (Fig. 29.2). The cysts rarely exceed 4 cm in diameter, the walls consisting of layers of granulosa cells and the contents of clear fluid, which is rich in sex steroids. These cysts commonly occur during treatment with clomiphene or pergonal. They may produce prolonged unopposed oestrogen effects on the endometrium, resulting in cystic glandular hyperplasia of the endometrium.

Management

These cysts regress spontaneously, but if they have not involuted after 60 days then the diagnosis should be revised. The size and growth of the cysts can be monitored by ultrasound scans.

The prolonged and heavy menstrual loss caused by unopposed oestrogen action can be offset by the administration of a progestogen for 1 week followed by 'medical curettage', or through surgical intervention by cervical dilatation and uterine curettage.

Lutein cysts

There are two types of luteinized ovarian cysts (Fig. 29.3):

1. *Granulosa lutein cysts* — functional cysts of the corpus luteum may be 4–6 cm in diameter and occur in the second half of the menstrual cycle. Persistent production of progesterone may result in amenorrhoea or delayed onset of menstruation. These cysts often give rise to pain, and they therefore present a problem in terms of differential diagnosis as the history and examination findings mimic tubal ectopic pregnancy. Occasionally, haemorrhage occurs into the cyst, which may rupture and lead to a haemoperitoneum. The cysts usually regress spontaneously and require surgical intervention only when they give rise to symptoms of intra-abdominal haemorrhage.
2. *Theca lutein cysts* — these commonly arise in association with high levels of chorionic gonadotrophin and are therefore seen in cases of hyda-

Fig. 29.2 Follicular cysts are common and are generally associated with menstrual irregularity (left); histological features (right)

Fig. 29.3   Lutein cysts are a less common variant of functional ovarian cysts; regression is usually spontaneous (left); histological features (right)

tidiform mole. The cysts may be bilateral and, on occasion, will give rise to haemorrhage if they rupture. Once the cysts have been formed, they can be detected by ultrasound scans. They usually undergo spontaneous involution, but surgical intervention may be necessary if there is significant haemorrhage from the ovaries.

Polycystic ovarian disease

Polycystic ovarian disease (PCO) is associated with the **Stein–Leventhal syndrome** in which multiple cysts occur in the ovaries and are associated with hirsutism, oligomenorrhoea or amenorrhoea, subfertility and changes in body habitus with obesity (Fig. 29.4). The ovaries are clinically enlarged and are palpable vaginally.

On direct inspection, the ovaries have smooth, white surfaces. There is sometimes luteinization of the theca interna cells and focal stromal luteinization.

Biochemical investigations (Fig. 29.5) indicate abnormally raised LH levels and absence of the

LH ↑
LH surge absent
Δ^4androstenedione ↑
Dehydroepiandrosterone ↑
Normal FSH levels
Normal oestradiol levels

Fig. 29.5   Biochemical features of the Stein–Leventhal syndrome

LH surge. Oestrogen and FSH levels are normal, whilst there may be increased secretion of Δ^4-androstenedione and dehydroepiandrosterone.

Fig. 29.4   Polycystic ovaries: the capsule of the ovary is thickened and there are numerous small cysts in the ovarian cortex (left); ovarian section (right)

Treatment

Treatment depends on the underlying problem. If the problem is primarily one of subfertility, then clomiphene citrate or human menopausal gonadotrophin can be used to stimulate ovulation. Prolonged unopposed oestrogen action may result in the development of hyperplastic endometrium, which may undergo malignant change. If this occurs, the tumour will often regress following the administration of a progestational agent such as medroxy-progesterone acetate or megestrol acetate.

Functional ovarian cysts

- Usually < 6 cm size
- May arise from follicles, corpus luteum or as a result of exogenous gonadotrophins
- Can produce sex steroids and affect menstruation
- Can be monitored by ultrasound
- Usually regress spontaneously
- Require surgical intervention if the source of significant IP bleeding

---

BENIGN NEOPLASTIC LESIONS

These tumours may be cystic or solid and arise from specific cell lines in the ovary. The full WHO classification of ovarian tumours illustrates the complexity of tumours arising from the ovary; only the commoner ones will be discussed in this section.

1. Epithelial tumours

a. Serous cystadenomas

These cysts in conjunction with the mucinous cystadenomas form the commonest group of cystic ovarian tumours. The cysts may be unilocular, lined by a layer of cuboidal epithelium, or multilocular with papillary growth extending from both internal and external surfaces of the tumour (Fig. 29.6). It is often difficult to differentiate between benign and malignant appearances. The wall of the tumour sometimes contains calcified granules known as psammoma bodies.

The growths may be bilateral and may be large enough to fill the peritoneal cavity.

Treatment. The tumours often replace all normal ovarian tissue; if this is the case, the whole ovary should be removed. If the tumour is small, it may be possible to perform a local resection and to conserve ovarian tissue. If both ovaries are extensively involved or there is reason to believe that the tumours are malignant, it is better to perform bilateral oophorectomy and hysterectomy.

b. Mucinous cystadenomas

These tumours are multilocular and often reach enormous dimensions, with tumours weighing in excess of 100 kg recorded in the literature (Fig. 29.7). The fluid content consists of mucin,

Fig. 29.6 Serous cystadenomas consist of single or multiple cysts lined by cuboidal epithelium and papillary growths extending from both internal and external surfaces of the tumour (left), section through a multiple cyst (top); histological features, showing cuboidal epithelium (right)

Fig. 29.7 Mucinous cystadenomas are multilocular and often achieve enormous dimensions (left); histological features: the epithelium is columnar and stratified and the contents are mucinous (right)

and the epithelium lining the cysts presents a characteristic appearance of an epithelium of tall columnar cells with a pseudostratified appearance. This appearance is similar to the epithelium lining the endocervix. The demarcation between epithelial cells and stroma is sharply defined. There is little tendency to form papillae. These tumours are less likely to become malignant than the serous variety.

Management. The only treatment is to remove the tumour surgically. Care should be taken to avoid rupture of the cysts because mucinous epithelium may implant in the peritoneal cavity giving rise to a condition known as **pseudomyxoma peritonei**. Huge amounts of gelatinous material may accumulate in the peritoneal cavity.

c. Brenner cell tumours

Brenner cell tumours are commonly solid and occur in women after the age of 50 years (Fig. 29.8). They are only rarely malignant. The histological features of these tumours include nests of epithelial cells surrounded by fibromatous connective tissue groundwork.

The cut surface of the tumour is similar to that of an ovarian fibroma apart from a rather yellowish tinge. The tumours are occasionally bilateral and can be safely treated by local excision.

2. Sex cord stromal tumours

Hormone-secreting tumours of the ovary are a small but important group.

a. Granulosa-cell tumours

Arising from ovarian granulosa cells, these tumours produce oestrogens and are the commonest of the hormone-secreting tumours, constituting some 3% of all solid ovarian tumours. Approximately 25% exhibit the characteristics of malignancy. As granulosa cell tumours can present at any age, the

Fig. 29.8 Brenner cell tumours are solid and rarely malignant (left); histological features include nests of epithelial cells surrounded by fibrous connective tissue (right)

symptoms will depend on the age of occurrence. Tumours arising before puberty produce precocious sexual development and, in women of the reproductive age, prolonged oestrogen stimulation results in cystic glandular hyperplasia, and irregular and prolonged vaginal bleeding. Fifty per cent of cases occur after the menopause and present with postmenopausal bleeding. If the tumour is histologically benign, the surgery should be limited to ovariectomy. If there is evidence of malignancy, pelvic clearance is indicated.

Thecomas or **theca cell tumours** arise from the spindle-shaped thecal cells, but are often mixed with granulosa cells and are oestrogen secreting. The presence of a thecoma in one ovary is commonly associated with diffuse thecomatosis in the contralateral ovary.

b. Arrhenoblastomas or androblastomas

These are tumours of Sertoli–Leydig cells. They are rare androgen-secreting tumours that occur most frequently in the decade between 20 and 30 years of age. The clinical manifestations include the onset of amenorrhoea, loss of breast tissue, increasing facial and body hirsutism, deepening of the voice and enlargement of the clitoris. The diagnosis is established by the exclusion of virilizing adrenal tumours and the identification of a tumour in one ovary. The condition is treated by excision of the affected ovary. Approximately 25% of these tumours are malignant.

3. Germ cell tumours

Tumours of germ cell origin may recapitulate stages resembling the early embryo.

a. Dysgerminomas

These solid tumours may be small or large enough to fill the abdominal cavity. The cut surface of the tumour has a greyish-pink colour and the microscopic appearance is characteristic. The tumour consists of large polygonal cells arranged in alveoli or nests separated by septa of fibrous tissue. There is no doubt that these tumours are malignant. The 5-year survival is only 27%.

b. Teratomas

Solid teratomas — unlike dermoid cysts, these tumours are relatively uncommon and tend to occur in young women. Portions of any tissue or organ may be reproduced, including bone, cartilage, brain, thyroid and other structures. These tumours are commonly malignant.

Highly specialized tumours of the ovary include teratomas that consist predominantly of thyroid tissue (stroma ovarii) or carcinoid tumours. Thyroid tumours may induce a state of hyperthyroidism.

Dermoid cysts (cystic teratomas)

Benign cystic teratomas account for 12–15% of true ovarian neoplasms. They are the commonest cystic ovarian neoplasm found in young women, and contain a large number of embryonic elements such as skin, hair, adipose and muscle tissue, bone, teeth and cartilage (Fig. 29.9). Some of the components can be recognized on X-ray.

These tumours are often chance findings as they are commonly asymptomatic unless they undergo torsion or rupture when the release of sebaceous material causes an acute chemical peritonitis. Dermoid cysts tend to be anterior to the uterus.

Management. These cysts should be excised from the ovary with conservation of ovarian tissue. They are frequently bilateral and it is important to examine both ovaries before proceeding to surgical excision.

Fig. 29.9 Dermoid cysts are the commonest true ovarian neoplasms in the young female (left); histological features (right)

4. Fibromas

These solid tumours of the ovary are rare. They are associated with the presence of ascites or hydrothorax — a condition known as **Meig's syndrome**.

5. Tumour-like conditions

This group includes **endometriotic cysts**, pregnancy **luteomas** and **germinal cell cysts**. The treatment depends on the nature of the tumour and normally involves simple excision of the cyst.

Endometriotic cysts

Endometriomas contain chocolate-coloured fluid representing the accumulation of altered blood and have a thick fibrous capsule. The lining may consist of endometrial cells, but in old cysts these may disappear. Management has already been discussed in a previous chapter. The local excision of the endometrioma from the ovary should be followed by treatment with a progestagen or Danol® for 6 months postoperatively.

Benign ovarian neoplasia

- May be solid, cystic or mixed
- Commonly present as asymptomatic abdominal mass but occasionally by hormone effects or pain
- Mostly serous or mucinous epithelial tumours but germ cell tumours more common in younger patients
- Differential diagnosis includes endometriosis, functional cysts and malignant tumours

---

MALIGNANT OVARIAN TUMOURS

Ovarian cancer is the fourth commonest cause of death from malignant disease. It follows breast, large intestine and lung in frequency and makes up for approximately 5% of all cancer deaths in women. There are approximately 14 new cases of ovarian cancer every 100 000 women years. The 5-year survival figure is approximately 25–30%. The poor survival rate is attributable to late diagnosis and the resistant nature of many of these tumours.

Aetiology

The cause of ovarian cancer is not known, but there are several factors which are associated with the disease. For example, the long-term use of the contraceptive pill reduces the incidence of ovarian cancer. Denmark has the highest age-adjusted death rate for ovarian cancer in the world at 11.12 per 100 000 population, and the lowest rate occurs in Japan at 1.88 per 100 000.

Symptoms and signs

The symptoms of ovarian cancer are vague and insidious and as a result 75% of cases present at an advanced stage. There are no signs that this situation is changing, and this seems to be an instance where early diagnosis as a means of improving survival carries little prospect for the future. It is more likely that the future will depend on discovering an effective form of therapy. The common symptoms include:

1. **Abdominal pain** — this varies according to the site of involvement.
2. **Abdominal distension** — enlargement of the abdomen results from the growth of the tumour itself and the presence of associated ascites. The fluid is often blood stained and contains malignant cells shed from the tumour.
3. **Abnormal uterine haemorrhage** — some sex cord tumours produce oestrogens, but hormone production is not confined to these tumours. Cystadenocarcinomas also produce oestrogens and may cause uterine haemorrhage due to the effect of the oestrogen on the endometrium.

Pathology

Primary ovarian carcinoma

The distribution of histological type of ovarian cancers is as follows:

1. Epithelial type — such as serous and mucinous cystadenocarcinomas — make up 85% of cases; 15–20% of these cases are of borderline malignancy.
2. Sex-cord stromal tumours — granulosa cell car-

cinomas, poorly differentiated androblastomas — account for 6% of malignant tumours.

3. Germ cell tumours — dysgerminomas and embryonal carcinomas — constitute 6%.
4. Stromal soft tissue tumours make up 3%.

Secondary ovarian carcinomas

The ovaries are a common site for secondary deposits (metastases) from primary sources in the breast, genital tract, gastrointestinal system and haematopoietic system. Krukenberg's tumours are metastatic deposits from the gastrointestinal system. They are solid growths that are almost always bilateral and retain the shape of the ovary. The cut surface is variegated in appearance and, although predominantly solid, it often contains areas of cystic degeneration.

The stroma is often richly cellular and may appear to be myomatous. The epithelial elements occur as clusters of well-marked acini with cells exhibiting mucoid change. These cells are often known as **signet cells**. Secondary ovarian tumours may be much larger than the primary lesion, and tumour deposits in the liver, in particular, suggest primary malignancies in the bowel.

The mechanism by which tumour deposits occur in the ovary is not clear, but there are four possible methods that are likely:

1. Direct implantation of cancer cells on the surface of the ovary after transcoelomic spread from the primary site.
2. Lymphatic metastasis.
3. Blood-borne spread.
4. Extension of tumour by direct spread from contiguous structures.

The same principles apply to the spread of primary ovarian tumours.

Staging of primary ovarian carcinoma
(Fig. 29.10)

Staging of ovarian carcinoma is important in

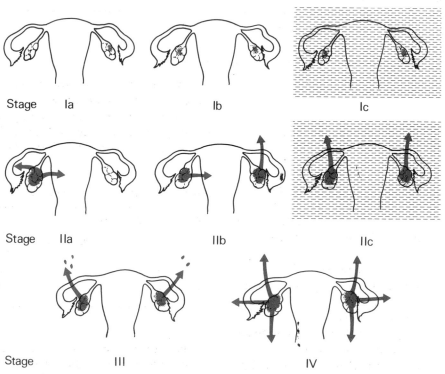

Fig. 29.10   Stages of ovarian carcinoma

determining both prognosis and the method of management.

FIGO classification

Stage I — growth limited to the ovaries:
  Stage IA — growth limited to one ovary:
  (i) no tumour on external surface: capsule intact;
  (ii) tumour present on external surface and/or capsule ruptured;
  Stage IB — growth limited to both ovaries:
  (i) no tumour on external surface: capsule intact;
  (ii) tumour on external surface: capsule ruptured;
  Stage IC — stage IA or IB with ascites or positive peritoneal fluid.
Stage II — growth involving one or both ovaries with pelvic extension:
  Stage IIA — extension and/or metastasis to uterus and tubes;
  Stage IIB — extension to other pelvic tissues;
  Stage IIC — stage IIA or IIB with ascites or positive malignant cells in the peritoneal fluid.
Stage III — growth involving one or both ovaries with intraperitoneal metastases outside the pelvis with malignant extension to small bowel and/or omentum.
Stage IV — growth involving one or both ovaries with distant metastases.

Management

Treatment is based on surgical excision or debulking of the tumour and chemotherapy.

Stage I — is treated by surgery with abdominal hysterectomy, bilateral salpingo-oophorectomy, partial omentectomy and appendicectomy. Tumours should be removed intact where possible. Stages IB and IC also merit additional treatment with cytotoxic drugs.

Stage II — treatment by surgery is the same as for stage I and this is followed by inactivation and/or the use of cytotoxic drugs.

Stages III and IV — complete removal of the tumour is usually impossible, but it is advisable to remove as much tumour tissue as possible. The main treatment of choice is chemotherapy. Alkylating agents such as cyclophosphamide produce

regression in some 40% of tumours. Similar results occur with melphalan. Single drugs are as effective as multiple therapy. *Cis*-platinum has been extensively used in recent years, but the results of all chemotherapy, whilst generally producing symptomatic relief, have had relatively little impact on 5-year survival.

It must be remembered that these drugs produce extremely unpleasant side effects with nausea, vomiting, diarrhoea, stomatitis, alopecia, cardiac toxicity and neurotoxicity. Bone marrow suppression is common and white cell counts should be checked routinely during treatment.

Malignant ovarian tumours

- Fourth commonest cause of cancer deaths in women
- Affect 1 in 75 women by age of 75
- Cause unknown.? 'super-ovulation'
- 75% cases present with advanced disease
- Most cases are epithelial in type
- Prognosis depends on stage at diagnosis and extent of residual disease after initial surgery
- 5-year survival 25–30%
- Incidence increases with age
- Shows an autosomal dominant pattern of inheritance in 4% cases

---

Prognosis

The overall 5-year survival is 25–30% and this figure has remained distressingly constant for the last 20 years. Five-year survival figures depend on the stage and on whether the tumour has or has not been completely removed (Table 29.1).

Table 29.1 Survival, stage and tumour removal

Stage	Incomplete tumour excision	Complete tumour excision
	(% 5-year survival)	
I	—	62
II	15	50
III	8	30
IV	5	—

The impact of eruption of the tumour through the capsule is seen in the difference in survival in the various grades of stage I lesions (Table 29.2).

Table 29.2   Survival rates for stage I tumours

Stage	% 5-year survivals
Stage Ia low potential malignancy	95
Stage Ia carcinomas	69
Stage Ib low potential malignancy	92
Stage Ib carcinomas	43
Stage Ic carcinomas	40

The only real prospect for survival in ovarian carcinoma is early diagnosis and complete surgical excision.

BIBLIOGRAPHY

Coppleson M 1981 Gynecologic oncology, Vol. 2. Churchill Livingstone, Edinburgh

Fox H, Buckley C H 1982 Pathology for gynaecologists. Edward Arnold, London

Lachelin G 1984 The polycystic ovary syndrome. In: Studd J (ed) Progress in obstetrics and gynaecology, Vol. 4. Churchill Livingstone, Edinburgh

30. Disorders of supports of the uterus and vagina

The position of the vagina and uterus depends on various fascial supports and ligaments derived from specific thickening of areas of the fascial support (Fig. 30.1).

The anterior vaginal wall is supported by the pubocervical fascia, which extends from the posterior surface of the pubic symphysis to the cervix and upper vagina. The posterior vaginal wall is supported by the fibrous tissue of the recto-vaginal septum and the tonus of the pelvic floor and, in particular, the integrity of the levator ani.

The uterus is supported indirectly by the supports of the vaginal walls, but directly by the cardinal or transverse cervical ligaments, which extend from the lateral pelvic wall to the upper part of the vagina and the lower part of the cervix. The uterosacral ligaments, which comprise the thickening of the pelvic floor fascia, extend from the sacrum to the lower parts of the cervix and the upper third of the vagina. The round and broad ligaments also provide weak support to the vagina and uterus. Indirect support of the vagina and uterus is provided by the integrity of the pelvic floor and the levator ani.

DEFINITIONS OF PROLAPSE

Cystocoele and urethrocoele

Prolapse of the anterior vaginal wall may affect the urethra, **urethrocoele**, and the bladder, **cystocoele** (Fig. 30.2). On examination, the urethra and bladder can be seen to descend and bulge into the anterior vaginal wall and, in severe cases, will be visible at the introitus of the vagina.

A **rectocoele** is formed by a recto-vaginal hernia, which can be seen as a visible bulge of the rectum through the posterior vaginal wall. It is often associated with deficiency and laxity of the pelvic floor.

An **enterocoele** is formed by a prolapse of the recto-uterine pouch, i.e. the Pouch of Douglas, through the upper part of the vaginal vault (Fig. 30.2). The condition may occur in isolation

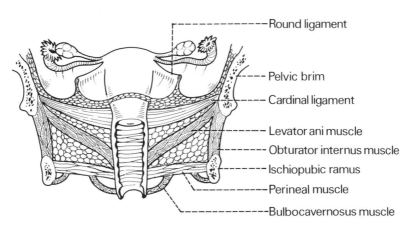

Fig 30.1 Supports of the uterus, cervix and vagina

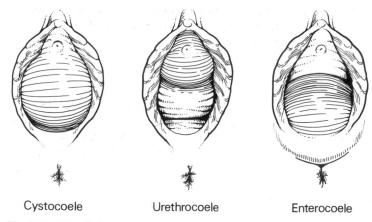

Fig. 30.2   The clinical appearance of cystocoele, urethrocoele and enterocoele

but usually in association with uterine prolapse. An enterocoele may also occur following hysterectomy when there is inadequate support of the vaginal vault.

Uterine prolapse

Descent of the uterus may occur in isolation from vaginal wall prolapse but more commonly occurs in conjunction with it. First degree prolapse of the uterus often occurs in association with retroversion of the uterus and descent of the cervix into the lower third of the vagina (Fig. 30.3).

If the cervix descends to protrude through the vaginal introitus, the prolapse is defined as second degree.

The term **procidentia** is applied to third degree prolapse where the cervix and the body of the uterus

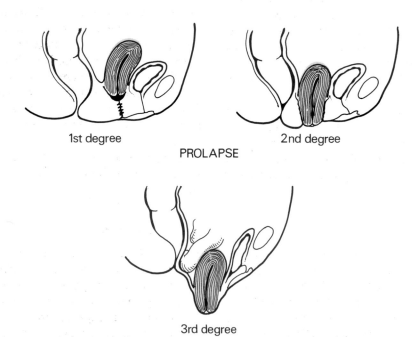

Fig. 30.3   Classification of uterine prolapse

and the vagina protrude through the introitus. The word actually means prolapse or **falling** but is generally reserved for the description of **total** or third degree prolapse.

SYMPTOMS AND SIGNS

Mild degrees of prolapse are common in parous women and may be asymptomatic. However, symptoms generally depend on the severity and site of the prolapse.

There are some symptoms which are common to all forms of prolapse and these include:

1. A sense of fullness in the vagina associated with dragging discomfort.
2. Visible protrusion of the cervix and vaginal walls.
3. Sacral backache.

Symptoms are often multiple and related to the nature of prolapse.

Urethrocoele and cystocoele

Specific symptoms relating to the urinary tract depend on the effect the prolapse has on the bladder neck. The loss of the posterior urethrovesical angle is often associated with stress incontinence, i.e. the involuntary loss of urine following raised intra-abdominal pressure. If the angle between the bladder and urethra becomes exaggerated, then there may be incomplete emptying of the bladder and this will be associated with double micturition, the desire to repeat micturition immediately after apparent completion of voiding, or recurrent urinary tract infection as a result of incomplete emptying of the bladder. The sensation of incomplete emptying or difficulty in initiating micturition can be relieved by replacing the cystocoele digitally or by the use of a vaginal pessary or tampon.

Signs

The diagnosis is established by examination with a Sims' speculum so that the vaginal wall can be seen. When the patient is asked to strain, the bulge in the anterior vaginal wall can be seen and often appears at the introitus. It is important to culture a specimen of urine to exclude the presence of infection. The differential diagnosis is limited to cysts or tumours of the anterior vaginal wall, and diverticulum of the urethra or bladder.

Rectocoele

The prolapse of the rectum through the posterior vaginal wall is commonly associated with a deficient pelvic floor, disruption of the perineal body and separation of the levator ani. It is predominantly a problem that results from overdistension of the introitus and pelvic floor during parturition.

Symptoms

The symptoms that relate in particular to rectocoele are difficulties with evacuation of faeces and the awareness of a reducible mass bulging into the vagina and through the introitus.

Signs

Examination of the vulva usually shows a deficient perineum, a lax introitus, and the rectum bulging into the posterior vaginal wall.

Enterocoele

Herniation of the Pouch of Douglas usually occurs through the vaginal vault, either through the posterior fornix or through the vaginal vault if the uterus has been removed. It is often difficult to distinguish between a high rectocoele and an enterocoele as the symptoms of vaginal pressure are identical. Occasionally, but rarely, the enterocoele occurs anterior to the vaginal vault and may mimic a cystocoele.

A large enterocoele may contain bowel and may be associated with incarceration and obstruction of the bowel.

Uterine prolapse

Descent of the uterus is initially associated with prolongation of the cervix and descent of the body of the uterus. The symptoms are those of pressure in the vagina and, ultimately, complete protrusion of the uterus through the introitus. At this stage, the prolapsed uterus may produce discomfort on sitting, and decubitus ulceration may result in haemorrhage. Cervical prolongation often leads to confusion in staging the degree of prolapse as it may appear to be in a more advanced stage than actually exists.

Urinary tract infection is common because of compression of the ureters and consequent hydronephrosis due to incomplete emptying of the bladder.

PATHOGENESIS OF UTERO-VAGINAL PROLAPSE

Prolapse may be congenital or acquired:

1. *Congenital* — uterine prolapse in young or nulliparous women is due to weakness of the supports of the uterus and vaginal vault. There is a minimal degree of vaginal wall prolapse.
2. *Acquired* — the commonest form of prolapse is acquired under the influence of multiple factors. This type of prolapse is both uterine and vaginal, but it must also be remembered that vaginal wall prolapse can also occur without any uterine descent. Predisposing factors include:
   a. *High parity* — uterovaginal prolapse is a condition of parous women. The pelvic floor provides direct and indirect support for the vaginal walls and when this support is disrupted by laceration or overdistension it predisposes to vaginal wall prolapse.
   b. *Raised intra-abdominal pressure* — tumours or ascites may result in raised intra-abdominal pressure, but a more common cause is a chronic cough.
   c. *Hormonal changes* — the symptoms of prolapse often worsen rapidly at the time of the menopause. Cessation of oestrogen production leads to thinning of the vaginal walls and the supports of the uterus. Although the prolapse is generally present before the menopause, it is at this time that the symptoms become noticeable and the degree of descent visibly worsens.

MANAGEMENT

The management of prolapse is medical or surgical.

Medical treatment

Many women have minor degrees of utero-vaginal prolapse which are asymptomatic. If the recognition of the prolapse is a coincidental finding, then the woman should be advised against any surgical treatment.

Minor degrees of prolapse are common after childbirth and should be treated by pelvic floor exercises or by the use of a pessary. Operative intervention is contraindicated for at least 6 months after delivery, as the tissues remain vascular and may undergo further spontaneous improvement.

Symptoms associated with cystocoele after the menopause are often improved by hormone replacement therapy.

Where short-term support is required or the general health of the woman makes operative treatment dangerous, then both vaginal wall and uterine prolapse can be treated by using vaginal pessaries or splinters. It is, however, necessary to have some pelvic floor support if a pessary is to be retained.

The most widely used pessaries are (Fig. 30.4).

1. *Ring pessary* — this pessary consists of a malleable plastic ring which may vary in diameter from 60 to 85 mm. The pessary is inserted in the posterior fornix and behind the pubic symphysis. Distension of the vaginal walls tends to support the vaginal wall prolapse.
2. *Hodge pessary* — a rigid, elongated curved ovoid which is inserted in a similar way to the ring pessary and is principally useful in uterine retroversion.
3. *Gelhorn pessary* — this pessary is shaped like a collar stud and is used in the treatment of severe degrees of prolapse.

The main problem with long-term use of pessaries is ulceration of the vaginal vault.

Gelhorn   Hodge   Ring

Fig. 30.4 Various types of vaginal pessaries used in the conservative management of utero-vaginal prolapse

Surgical treatment

Surgical treatment of a cystocoele is by anterior colporrhaphy (Fig. 30.5). The operation consists of a surgical excision of the excess vaginal wall and buttressing of the pubocervical fascia. In the presence of stress incontinence due to loss of the posterior urethrovesical angle, this angle is reconstructed by placing buttressing sutures under the bladder neck. These are described as **Kelly's sutures**.

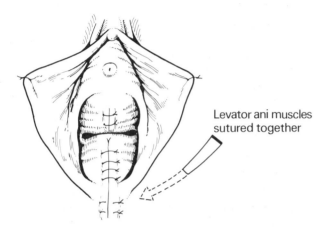

Levator ani muscles sutured together

Fig. 30.5 Anterior and posterior colporrhaphy

Rectocoele is repaired by posterior colpoperineorrhaphy with reconstruction of the pelvic floor, reapposition of the levator muscles and excision of the redundant vaginal skin.

Where there is an enterocoele, the hernial sac is opened and transfixed at its neck with excision of the redundant tissue.

The treatment of choice for uterine prolapse is vaginal hysterectomy with or without repair of the vaginal walls. If preservation of reproductive function is required, then the uterus can be conserved by simply excising the cervix and suturing the cardinal ligaments in front of the cervical stump. This procedure is known as a **Manchester** or **Fothergill repair**. The vaginal skin is then sutured into the cervical stump.

Complications

The immediate complications of vaginal hysterectomy or repair include haemorrhage, haematoma formation, infection and urinary retention. The long-term complications are those of dyspareunia and vaginal stenosis. Inadequate supportive tissue may result in recurrence of the prolapse of the vaginal vault.

Prolapse

- May involve anterior or posterior vaginal wall with varying degrees of uterine descent
- Predisposing factors include high parity, chronically raised intra-abdominal pressure and hormonal changes
- Symptoms depend on degree of prolapse and whether bowel or bladder neck involved
- May present as renal failure
- May undergo spontaneous improvement up to 6 months postpartum
- Treatment of choice is surgical repair +/− hysterectomy
- No treatment required for asymptomatic minor degrees of prolapse

BIBLIOGRAPHY

Howkins J, Hudson C N 1983 Shaw's textbook of operative gynaecology. Churchill Livingstone, Edinburgh

31. Disorders of the urinary tract

STRUCTURE AND PHYSIOLOGY OF THE LOWER URINARY TRACT

The urinary bladder is a hollow muscular organ with an outer adventitial layer, a smooth muscle layer known as the detrusor muscle and an inner layer of transitional epithelium.

The innervation of the bladder contains both sympathetic and parasympathetic components (Fig. 31.1). The sympathetic fibres arise from the lower two thoracic and upper two lumbar segments of the spinal cord and the parasympathetic fibres from the second, third and fourth sacral segments. The urethra consists of a muscle coat lined by epithelium continuous with the bladder epithelium. The muscle coat consists of a mixture of smooth muscle with an outer sleeve of striated muscle. The bladder neck does not contain a smooth muscle sphincter. The majority of muscle fibres in the bladder neck enter obliquely or longitudinally into the wall of the urethra.

During micturition, the pressure in the bladder rises to exceed the pressure within the urethral lumen and there is a fall in urethral resistance. The tonus of muscle fibres around the bladder neck is reduced by central inhibition of the motor neurones in the sacral plexus.

COMMON DISORDERS OF BLADDER FUNCTION

The common symptoms of bladder dysfunction include:

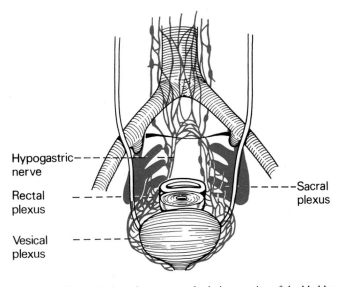

Fig. 31.1 Sympathetic and parasympathetic innervation of the bladder

Hypogastric nerve

Rectal plexus

Vesical plexus

Sacral plexus

1. Urinary incontinence.
2. Frequency of micturition.
3. Dysuria.
4. Urinary retention.

Incontinence of urine

The involuntary loss of urine may be associated with bladder or urethral dysfunction of fistula formation. The types of incontinence include:

1. **True incontinence** — this is continuous loss of urine through the vagina; it is commonly associated with fistula formation but may occasionally be a manifestation of urinary retention with overflow.
2. **Stress incontinence** — this is the involuntary loss of urine that occurs during a brief period of raised intra-abdominal pressure related to pelvic floor weakness, and in 30% of cases with detrusor instability. Examination reveals the involuntary loss of urine during coughing with descent of the anterior vaginal wall and reduction of the posterior urethrovesical angle. Digital elevation of the anterior vaginal wall leads to correction of the condition. Loss of support to the anterior vaginal wall is frequently associated with reduced pelvic floor support.
3. **Urge incontinence** — the problem of sudden detrusor contraction with uncontrolled loss of urine is known as urge incontinence. The condition may be due to idiopathic detrusor instability or associated with urinary infection, obstructive uropathy, diabetes or neurological disease. It is particularly important to exclude urinary tract infection.
4. **Mixed urge and stress incontinence** — a substantial number of women with urge incontinence also have true stress incontinence and if the latter is corrected, the detrusor instability will disappear.

Urinary frequency

The commonest cause of frequency of micturition is urinary tract infection. However, enhanced bladder contractility may occur without the presence of infection. Reduced bladder capacity may also result in frequency of micturition. The symptom may also develop because of anxiety concerning involuntary loss of urine.

Dysuria

This symptom results from infection. Local urethral infection or trauma cause burning or scalding during micturition, but bladder infection is more likely to cause pain suprapubically after micturition has been completed. It is always advisable to perform a vaginal examination on any woman who complains of scalding on micturition because urethritis is associated with vaginitis and vaginal infection.

Urinary retention and outflow obstruction

Acute urinary retention is not the common problem seen in the ageing male. It is, however, seen:

1. After vaginal delivery and episiotomy.
2. Following operative delivery.
3. After vaginal repair procedures — particularly those operations that involve posterior colpoperineorrhaphy.
4. In the menopause — spontaneous obstructive uropathy is more likely to occur in menopausal women.

DIFFERENTIAL DIAGNOSIS

The diagnosis is initially indicated by the history. Continuous loss of urine indicates a fistula, but not all fistulae leak urine continously. The fistulous communication usually occurs between the bladder and vagina, **vesico-vaginal fistula**, and the ureter and vagina, **uretero-vaginal fistula**. Fistula formation results from:

1. Surgical trauma.
2. Obstetric trauma associated with obstructed labour.
3. Malignant disease.
4. Radiotherapy.

There are other types of fistulae with communications between bowel and urinary tract and between bowel and vagina, but these are less common.

Recto-vaginal fistulae have a similar pathogenesis with the additional factor of perineal breakdown after a third degree tear.

Urinary fistulae are localised by:

1. Cystoscopy.
2. Intravenous urogram.
3. Instillation of methylene blue via catheter into the bladder; the appearance of dye in the vagina indicates a vesico-vaginal fistula.

The differential diagnosis between stress and urge incontinence is more difficult and is often unsatisfactory. Adequate pre-operative assessment is important if the correct operation is to be employed or if surgery is to be avoided.

The cystometrogram

Pressure is measured intravesically and intrarectally because intrarectal pressure represents intraabdominal pressure and is subtracted from the intravesical pressure to give a measure of detrusor pressure. The volume of fluid in the bladder at which the first desire to void occurs is usually about 150 ml. A strong desire to void occurs at 400 ml in the normal bladder. Values at a lower volume reflect an abnormally sensitive bladder associated with chronic infection. There should be no detrusor contraction during filling and any contraction that occurs under these circumstances indicates **detrusor instability**. An underactive detrusor shows no contractions on filling and indicates an abnormality of neurological control. The average bladder has a capacity of 250–550 ml but capacity is a poor index of bladder function. Thus, cystometry is a useful method for assessing detrusor muscle function or detrusor instability which may result in urge incontinence.

Pressure/flow studies (Fig. 31.2) enable a measurement to be made of the rate of flow in relation to intravesical pressure and hence indicate if there is any bladder neck obstruction. Normal flow may occur in the presence of a bladder neck obstruction if there is a powerful detrusor muscle.

Detrusor overactivity is indicated by high resting urethral pressure, good voluntary increase in urethral pressure, good ability to stop midstream, the presence of good detrusor muscle power, frequent strong bladder contractions and small volumes of urine on frequency/volume charts.

In the presence of urethral incompetence, there is low resting urethral pressure, no voluntary increase in urethral pressure, inability to stop midstream, decreased pressure transmission to the abdominal urethra and large volumes in the frequency/volume measurements. There is not always a clear-cut demarcation between the two conditions as there may be a mixture of both stress and urge incontinence. Nevertheless, it is important to differentiate between the predominant influence of bladder neck weakness and stress incontinence, and detrusor instability and urge incontinence.

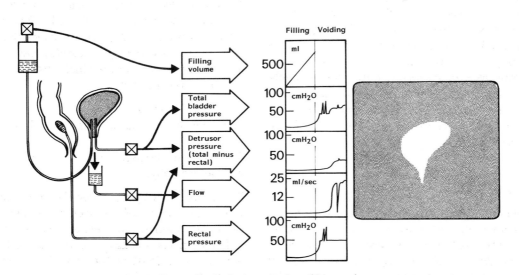

Fig. 31.2 Bladder flow studies in the investigation of lower urinary tract symptoms

Fistulae

- May present as continuous urinary or faecal incontinence
- Commonly related to surgery but may occur after radiotherapy, childbirth or in association with malignancy
- May heal with conservative treatment if small

MANAGEMENT

Urinary tract fistulae

In Western European countries, most urinary tract fistulae result from surgical trauma. The commonest fistulae are vesico-vaginal (Fig. 31.3(l)) or uretero-vaginal and result from surgical trauma at the time of hysterectomy or sometimes following Caesarean section (Fig. 31.3).

Vesico-vaginal fistula will usually become apparent in the first postoperative week. If the fistula is small, closure may be achieved spontaneously.

The patient should be treated by catheterization and continuous drainage. If closure has not occurred after 2–3 weeks, the fistula is unlikely to close spontaneously and surgical closure is recommended. The timing of further surgery is still a subject of controversy. Until recently, a delay of 6 months had been recommended but there is increasing evidence that good results can be obtained with early surgical intervention. However, the fistulous site should be free of infection.

Surgical closure may be achieved vaginally by meticulous separation of the edges of the fistula and closure in layers of the bladder and vagina (Fig. 31.3(r)). Postoperative care includes continuous catheter drainage for 1 week and antibiotic cover. An abdominal approach to the fistula can also be used and has some advantages in allowing the interposition of omentum in cases where there is a large fistula.

Uretero-vaginal fistulae are usually treated by reimplantation of the damaged ureter into the bladder.

Stress incontinence

- Presents as involuntary loss of urine on raised intra-abdominal pressure
- Commonly associated with prolapse of bladder neck outside the abdominal cavity
- Associated with detrusor instability in up to 30% of cases
- Is indicated by a low resting urethral pressure, decreased pressure transmission to abdominal urethra and inability to stop midstream during cystometry
- Treatment is surgical by elevation of the bladder neck

Once the true nature of stress incontinence has been established, then surgical correction should be attempted. A large number of operative procedures have been described and advocated. In the presence of anterior vaginal wall prolapse, **anterior repair** with the placement of buttressing sutures at the bladder neck has the virtue of simplicity. It will

Vesicovaginal fistula   Repair of fistula

Fig. 31.3 True incontinence is associated with a fistulous opening between bladder and vagina: the vesico-vaginal fistula (left); it can be closed by either the vaginal or the abdominal route (right)

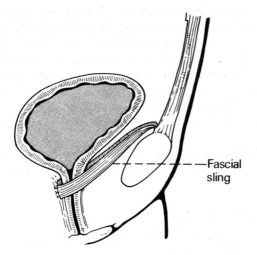

Fig. 31.4 Stress incontinence may be treated by a procedure that supports the vaginal neck such as the Aldridge sling

certainly relieve the prolapse, but the results are variable as far as the stress incontinence is concerned with relief in about 60–70% of cases.

Where there is minimal prolapse, then the following procedures are used:

1. *Marshall-Marchetti-Krantz procedure* — the bladder neck and trigone are elevated by suturing the para-urethral and paravesical tissues to the periosteum on the back of the pubic symphysis. This creates a valve-like effect at the bladder neck.
2. *Burch colposuspension* — the bladder neck is elevated by suturing the upper lateral vaginal walls to the ileo-inguinal ligaments.
3. *Sling procedures* — fascial strips from the anterior abdominal wall or inert synthetic materials attached to the anterior abdominal wall are placed in a sling under the bladder neck and cause urethral closure when the sling is stretched (Fig. 31.4).

All of these procedures have a higher success rate in curing stess incontinence but have a significant surgical complication rate and often cause detrusor instability as well as other urinary symptoms due to incomplete bladder emptying.

The unstable bladder

The features of the unstable bladder are those of frequency of micturition and nocturia, urgency and urge incontinence.

When confronted with this history, it is important to obtain some indication of the frequency as related to fluid intake and output. A chart should therefore be kept by the patient to clarify this aspect.

The assessment of predisposing factors includes urine culture, urinary flow rates and urodynamic studies.

Treatment will obviously be directed at the cause so that the presence of urinary tract infection necessitates the administration of the appropriate antibiotic therapy. Postmenopausal women with atrophic vaginal epithelium and symptoms of urgency and frequency often respond to replacement therapy with low dose oestrogens.

Detrusor instability of unknown aetiology

If the problem arises at a cerebral level, then psychotherapeutic measures are indicated. Bladder drill involves a regime of gradually increasing the voiding interval on a recorded pattern. This is effective in the short term but the relapse rate is high.

Drug treatment

The alternative approach is to use anticholinergic drugs which act at the level of the bladder wall. The most effective drugs are oxybutynin, propantheline and imipramine. The addition of tranquillisers and hypnotics may also help. Oxybutynin is prescribed in a dose of 5 mg three times daily and has a direct local anaesthetic effect on the bladder. As an anticholinergic drug, it also has side effects such as mouth dryness and blurring of vision.

Detrusor instability

- Presents as frequency, urgency, nocturia and incontinence
- Usually idiopathic but needs to be distinguished from obstructive uropathy, diabetes, neurological disorders and infection
- May occur in combination with true stress incontinence and improve when this is treated
- High resting urethral pressure and frequent strong bladder contractions at low volumes on cystometry
- Management includes bladder drill, anticholinergics and treatment of infection

Surgical treatments are not commonly used but include bladder overdistension, bladder transection and transvesical injection of 6% aqueous phenol into the trigone.

Bladder outlet obstruction

Primary bladder neck obstruction in the female probably results from the failure of the vesical neck to open during voiding and can be treated either with α-adrenergic blocking agents or by urethral dilatation. Secondary outlet obstruction is usually associated with previous surgery for incontinence and may respond to urethral dilatation but the results are not particularly good.

Conclusions

The important feature in the management of urinary tract disorders in the female is to ensure that the underlying nature of the symptoms is defined before embarking on any surgical treatment.

Simple medical measures such as bladder drill, pelvic floor exercises and anticholinergic drug therapy may give adequate relief of symptoms when administered in the appropriate situation. Surgical treatment is predominantly of value in the correction of fistulae and in the support of the bladder neck where stress incontinence is present.

BIBLIOGRAPHY

Bates C P, Taylor M C 1984 Clinical investigation of bladder function. In: Symonds E M, Zuspan F P (ed) Clinical and diagnostic procedures in obstetrics and gynecology. Marcel Dekker, New York
Raz S 1985 Gynaecological urology. In: Clinics in obstetrics and gynaecology Vol. 12, No. 2. W B Saunders, Eastbourne

Index